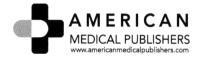

Cataloging-in-Publication Data

Ataxia : diagnosis and treatment / edited by Johnny Lopez.
    p. cm.
Includes bibliographical references and index.
ISBN 978-1-63927-571-7
1. Ataxia. 2. Ataxia--Diagnosis. 3. Ataxia--Treatment. 4. Movement disorders. I. Lopez, Johnny.
RC376.5 .A83 2023
616.83--dc23

American Medical Publishers,
41 Flatbush Avenue,
1st Floor, New York,
NY 11217, USA

ISBN 978-1-63927-571-7 (Hardback)

Contents

Preface

Ataxia is a neurological disorder that is usually caused by damage and the eventual dysfunction of those parts of the nervous system, which are responsible for coordinating movements. Cerebellar ataxia is one type of ataxia that affects brain's cerebellum. The most evident symptoms of ataxia include neurological dysfunction patterns such as gait abnormality, speech changes, deterioration of fine motor skills, and abnormalities in eye movements. Some other symptoms of ataxia include difficulty in swallowing leading to choking or coughing, tremors, shaking, or trembling in parts of the body, nystagmus, problems in maintaining balance, walking difficulties, and vision and hearing problems. Although there is no cure for ataxia, certain treatments can help relieve symptoms and ensure an improved quality of life for the patients. A patient's functionality and progress can be evaluated using certain diagnostic tools including imaging tests, blood tests, lumbar puncture and genetic testing. The book strives to provide a fair idea about the diagnosis and treatment of ataxia. It is meant for students looking for an elaborate reference text on this disease. This book will provide comprehensive knowledge to the readers.

This book has been the outcome of endless efforts put in by authors and researchers on various issues and topics within the field. The book is a comprehensive collection of significant researches that are addressed in a variety of chapters. It will surely enhance the knowledge of the field among readers across the globe.

It gives us an immense pleasure to thank our researchers and authors for their efforts to submit their piece of writing before the deadlines. Finally in the end, I would like to thank my family and colleagues who have been a great source of inspiration and support.

Editor

Redox Imbalance Associates with Clinical Worsening in Spinocerebellar Ataxia Type 2

Almaguer-Gotay Dennis [1,2] Luis E. Almaguer-Mederos [1,2] Rodríguez-Aguilera Raúl [1,2]
Rodríguez-Labrada Roberto [1] Velázquez-Pérez Luis [1,3] Cuello-Almarales Dany [1,2]
González-Zaldívar Yanetza, [1,2] Vázquez-Mojena Yaimeé [1] Estupiñán-Domínguez Annelié, [1]
Peña-Acosta Arnoy, [1] and Torres-Vega Reydenis [1]

[1] Center for the Investigation and Rehabilitation of Hereditary Ataxias (CIRAH), Holguín, Cuba
[2] University of Medical Sciences of Holguín, Cuba
[3] Cuban Academy of Sciences, Cuba

Correspondence should be addressed to Almaguer-Gotay Dennis; dennisalmaguer@gmail.com

Academic Editor: Kambiz Hassanzadeh

Background. Spinocerebellar ataxia type 2 (SCA2) is a neurodegenerative disease presenting with redox imbalance. However, the nature and implications of redox imbalance in SCA2 physiopathology have not been fully understood. *Objective.* The objective of this study is to assess the redox imbalance and its association with disease severity in SCA2 mutation carriers. *Methods.* A case-control study was conducted involving molecularly confirmed SCA2 patients, presymptomatic individuals, and healthy controls. Several antioxidant parameters were assessed, including serum thiol concentration and the superoxide dismutase, catalase, and glutathione S-transferase enzymatic activities. Also, several prooxidant parameters were evaluated, including thiobarbituric acid-reactive species and protein carbonyl concentrations. Damage, protective, and OXY scores were computed. Clinical correlates were established. *Results.* Significant differences were found between comparison groups for redox markers, including protein carbonyl concentration ($F = 3.30$; $p = 0.041$), glutathione S-transferase activity ($F = 4.88$; $p = 0.009$), and damage ($F = 3.20$; $p = 0.045$), protection ($F = 12.75$; $p < 0.001$), and OXY ($F = 7.29$; $p = 0.001$) scores. Protein carbonyl concentration was positively correlated with CAG repeat length ($r = 0.27$; $p = 0.022$), while both protein carbonyl concentration ($r = -0.27$; $p = 0.018$) and OXY score ($r = -0.25$; $p = 0.013$) were inversely correlated to the disease duration. Increasing levels of antioxidants and decreasing levels of prooxidant parameters were associated with clinical worsening. *Conclusions.* There is a disruption of redox balance in SCA2 mutation carriers which depends on the disease stage. Besides, redox changes associate with markers of disease severity, suggesting a link between disruption of redox balance and SCA2 physiopathology.

1. Introduction

Spinocerebellar ataxias (SCAs) are a heterogeneous group of neurodegenerative diseases characterized by progressive neuronal loss and shared clinical manifestations, including gait ataxia, dysmetria, dysarthria, and adiadochokinesia [1]. To date, 48 molecular variants of SCAs have been reported [2]. In particular, spinocerebellar ataxia type 2 (SCA2) is due to a CAG repeat expansion mutation in the *ATXN2* gene and

it reaches the highest worldwide prevalence in Holguín province, Cuba [3].

SCA2 is a polyglutamine disorder causing neurodegeneration at different levels, including cerebellar Purkinje cells, thalamic and cholinergic basal forebrain neurons, brainstem pontine, and olivary neurons, spinal and cortical motor neurons, as a result of mutant Ataxin-2 expression [4]. However, the primary mechanisms by which the polyQ expansion in Ataxin-2 causes SCA2 remain unknown. Nonetheless, evidence shows the occurrence of cytoplasmic aggregation of mutant Ataxin-2 [5], disturbed RNA metabolism [6, 7], dysregulation of calcium homeostasis [8, 9], altered methylation patterns in the *ATXN2* promoter [10], and oxidative stress as part of SCA2 physiopathology.

Oxidative stress was initially defined as "a disturbance in the prooxidant-antioxidant balance in favor of the former" and more recently as "a disruption of redox signaling and control" [11–14]. Enzymes like superoxide dismutase (SOD), catalase (CAT), and glutathione S-transferases (GSTs), or thiols as reduced glutathione (GSH), are part of the main antioxidant systems minimizing the damage caused by free radicals on lipids and proteins and regulate the cellular redox state [11, 12]. Oxidative stress has been linked to neurodegenerative disorders, including Alzheimer's disease (AD), Parkinson's disease (PD), amyotrophic lateral sclerosis (ALS), Huntington's disease (HD), and spinocerebellar ataxias [15–18].

Opposite to oxidative stress, the concept of "reductive stress" refers to a redox condition characterized by an abnormal increase in the levels of reducing agents in the forms of NADH, NADPH, and GSH and associated with increased mitochondrial oxidation and cytotoxicity [19]. Reductive stress has been poorly studied in the context of neurodegenerative disorders; however, evidence supporting its occurrence was gathered in young healthy individuals at risk of Alzheimer's disease [20] and in cellular and *Drosophila* models for Huntington's disease [21].

Few studies have shown the occurrence of redox imbalance in SCA2 patients. Indeed, increased levels of malondialdehyde (a product of lipids' oxidative damage), increased GST activity [22, 23], and decreased extracellular superoxide dismutase activity [24], were reported in SCA2 patients' blood serum. Besides, increased mitochondrial superoxide dismutase and decreased catalase expression were found in SCA2 patients' fibroblasts [25].

Even though evidence supporting the occurrence of redox imbalance in SCA2 was collected, its nature and implications in disease physiopathology have not been fully understood. Hence, the present study is aimed at assessing the redox imbalance and its association with disease severity in SCA2 mutation carriers by examining antioxidant and prooxidant parameters in a large sample of SCA2 patients and presymptomatic individuals.

2. Materials and Methods

2.1. Reagents. Pyrogallol (Alfa Aesar Co., Ward Hill, MA 01835, USA), hydrogen peroxide (H_2O_2) (Sigma-Aldrich, St. Louis, MO 63103, USA), 1-chloro-2,4-dinitrobenzene (Alfa Aesar, Ward Hill, MA 01835, USA), reduced glutathione (GSH) (Sigma-Aldrich, St. Louis, MO 63103, USA), 1,1,3,3-tetraethoxypropane (Sigma-Aldrich, St. Louis, MO 63103, USA), and bovine albumin (Calbiochem, San Diego, CA 92121, USA).

2.2. The Study Design. A case-control study was conducted to assess the redox status in SCA2 patients and presymptomatic individuals. Thirty-six molecularly confirmed SCA2 patients

with mild to moderate clinical presentation (M/F: 4/32; aged 25 to 65 years) were recruited at the Center for the Investigation and Rehabilitation of Hereditary Ataxias, Holguín, Cuba. SCA2 patients were matched by age and gender with 36 presymptomatic individuals (mutation carriers with no clinical presentation at the time of the study) (M/F: 4/32; aged 23 to 66 years) and an equal number of healthy control individuals (M/F: 3/33; aged 23 to 65 years). To further verify differences between patients and controls regarding redox parameters, a data set consisting of 60 molecularly confirmed SCA2 patients (M/F: 27/33; aged 22 to 68 years) and 60 control individuals (M/F: 27/33; aged 23 to 70 years) matched by age and gender were assessed. A maximal age difference of two years between patients and presymptomatic and control individuals was allowed.

To assess the relationships between redox parameters, CAG repeat length, and clinical and neurophysiological variables, the sample of SCA2 patients was enlarged to one hundred (M/F: 48/52; aged 19 to 68 years). The study was approved by the institutional ethics committee, and it was conducted according to the Declaration of Helsinki. Written informed consent was obtained from all participants after a complete description of the study.

2.3. Clinical, Neurophysiological, and Genetic Assessment. The clinical diagnosis was based on the identification of gait ataxia, dysarthria, dysmetria, and dysdiadochokinesia and the slowing of saccade eye movements. Age at onset (AO) was defined as the onset of motor impairment. Disease duration (DD) was defined as the time elapsed between the clinical debut and the time when the neurological evaluation was made. Clinical severity was estimated by using the scale for the assessment and rating of ataxia (SARA) score [26]. The progression rate was calculated as the rate between the SARA score and age. Maximal saccade velocity (MSV) (in 60°/second) and saccade latency (SL) (in milliseconds) were determined as previously reported [27]. The mean estimated age at onset of the presymptomatic group was calculated with the individuals' current age and CAG repeat length at the *ATXN2* locus, as previously reported [28]. Predicted time to onset (in years) was calculated with the formula [predicted age of onset − current age]. The CAG repeat length at the *ATXN2* locus was determined by polymerase chain reaction (PCR) followed by polyacrylamide gel electrophoresis as previously reported [29].

2.4. Blood Sample Collection. Fasting blood samples were collected from subjects by venipuncture at the time when neurological and neurophysiological evaluations were made. Serum was obtained *via* blood centrifugation at 3,000 rpm at 4°C for 10 minutes, frozen immediately, and stored at −20°C until biochemical analysis.

2.5. Assessment of Antioxidant Biomarkers in Blood Serum. SOD3 and CAT enzymatic activities were measured at 37°C, following standard methods based on the use of pyrogallol and H_2O_2 as substrates [30, 31]. GST activity was measured at 37°C, following the Habig and Jacoby method, using 1-chloro-2,4-dinitrobenzene and GSH as substrates

[32]. Reducing thiol (R-SH) total concentration was assessed at 25°C, following the Ellman protocol [33].

2.6. Assessment of Oxidative Modification on Lipids and Proteins. Thiobarbituric acid-reactive species (TBARS) and protein carbonyl (PC) concentration were assessed in blood serum following Yagi [34] and Levine [35] standard methods.

All samples were assayed in triplicate using a BioMate 3 Spectrophotometer (Thermo Spectronic Company, USA).

2.7. Redox Global Index Computation. The damage score (DS), protection score (PS), and OXY score were computed following a modified procedure to that reported by Veglia et al. [36]. The DS was computed with a base on log-transformed TBARS and PC concentrations; meanwhile, the PS was computed with a base on log-transformed SOD3, CAT, and GST enzymatic activities and R-SH concentrations. Individual redox parameters were standardized following Veglia et al. [36]. The OXY score was computed as the difference between DS and PS, reflecting the balance between oxidants and antioxidants.

2.8. Statistical Analysis. Descriptive statistics were used to assess central tendencies and dispersion of data. The Kolmogorov-Smirnov test was used to assess the normality of data distribution. The chi-square test (χ^2) was used to establish comparisons between patients, presymptomatic individuals, and controls for gender. One-way ANOVA was utilized to assess differences between comparison groups for age and redox parameters. Tukey's post-hoc test was applied to identify differences between comparison groups. Student's t-test was used to compare redox parameters between patients and controls.

Pearson's correlation test was utilized to assess the relationship between redox parameters, clinical and neurophysiological variables, and CAG repeat length. Correction for repeat length or disease duration was applied to redox and clinical variables by simple or multiple linear regression analyses. Statistical significance was defined as $p \leq 0.05$.

Type-I error in multiple comparisons was adjusted by the Benjamini-Hochberg (BH) method for controlling the false discovery rate [37]. Analyses were performed using the commercially available Statistica software package (StatSoft Inc., 2003 Statistica data analysis software system, version 6. http://www.statsoft.com).

3. Results

3.1. Redox Balance in SCA2 Mutation Carriers. To know if redox disturbances are present in SCA2 mutation carriers and to determine if these disturbances take place since the presymptomatic stage of the disease, comparisons for redox parameters were established between affected SCA2 patients and presymptomatic and control individuals. No significant differences were found between comparison groups for gender ($\chi^2 = 0.20$; $p = 0.904$) or age distributions ($F = 0.656$, $p = 0.521$). Also, no significant associations were found between age or gender and redox parameters in the comparison groups ($p > 0.05$).

There was no significant difference between SCA2 patients and presymptomatic and control individuals regarding SOD3 or CAT activities, SOD3/CAT index, R-SH, or TBARS concentrations. However, there were significant differences in GST activity, protein carbonyl concentration, damage score, and protective and OXY scores (Table 1). Nonetheless, only GST activity and protective and OXY scores remained significant after adjustment for multiple comparisons.

Post-hoc analyses showed significant decreases in GST activity and protection score and significant increases in protein carbonyl concentration and OXY score in presymptomatic individuals relative to affected patients. A significant decrease in the protection score was found in presymptomatic individuals relative to control individuals, and a significant decrease in the damage score was found in patients relative to control individuals (Figure 1). After correction for multiple comparisons, only the difference between presymptomatic individuals and affected patients relative to protein carbonyl concentration and the decrease in the damage score between patients and control individuals lost their statistical significance.

In the enlarged data consisting of 60 patients and 60 control subjects, significant decreases in the protein carbonyl concentration ($t = -3.44$; $p < 0.001$), damage score ($t = -3.15$; $p = 0.002$), and the OXY score ($t = -2.55$; $p = 0.012$) were found in patients relative to control individuals. These differences remained significant after adjustment for multiple comparisons.

3.2. Associations between Redox Parameters, CAG Repeat Length, and Clinical Biomarkers in SCA2 Mutation Carriers. Taking into account that the CAG repeat length in the *ATXN2* gene is the major determinant of clinical severity in SCA2, correlations were established between CAG repeat length and redox parameters in presymptomatic individuals and the enlarged sample of one hundred SCA2 patients. Besides, the relevance of redox parameters to clinical severity was assessed.

In presymptomatic individuals, a highly significant negative correlation between time to onset and repeat length ($r = -0.48$; $p = 0.005$) was found. However, no significant correlation was obtained between repeat length and redox parameters ($p > 0.05$). As expected, in the enlarged sample of one hundred SCA2 patients, the age at onset showed a highly significant negative correlation with the repeat length ($r = -0.73$; $p < 0.001$), and the SARA score was significantly correlated to the disease duration ($r = 0.57$; $p < 0.001$) and repeat length ($r = 0.21$; $p = 0.038$). Also, the progression rate showed significant correlations with repeat length ($r = 0.71$; $p < 0.001$) and disease duration ($r = 0.23$; $p = 0.022$). Besides, saccade velocity was significantly correlated to repeat length ($r = -0.46$; $p < 0.001$). Nonetheless, saccade latency showed no significant correlations with repeat length or disease duration.

On correlation analysis, the repeat length showed a significant association only with protein carbonyl concentration. Similarly, the disease duration showed significant negative correlations with protein carbonyl concentrations and OXY score (Figure 2).

TABLE 1: Comparison of redox parameters between SCA2 mutation carriers and control individuals.

Redox parameters	Controls ($n = 36$)		Presymptomatics ($n = 36$)		Patients ($n = 36$)		F	p
	Mean	SD	Mean	SD	Mean	SD		
SOD3 (KU/L)	2.02	0.52	1.85	0.46	1.99	0.38	1.46	0.238
CAT (KUI/L)	19.14	8.74	15.48	7.68	20.00	13.81	1.91	0.153
CAT/SOD3	9.97	5.46	9.30	6.39	10.35	6.86	0.26	0.773
GST (UI/L)	14.00	4.73	11.54	5.08	15.09	4.98	4.88	*0.009*
R-SH (μmol/L)	136.92	71.29	105.09	43.30	124.32	63.17	2.54	0.084
TBARS (μmol/L)	2.17	0.72	1.90	0.72	1.97	1.07	0.88	0.420
PC (nmol/mg)	1.65	0.43	1.74	0.41	1.48	0.43	3.30	*0.041*
DS	0.03	0.74	−0.11	0.83	−0.44	0.86	3.20	*0.045*
PS	−0.01	0.51	−0.49	0.50	0.01	0.41	12.75	*<0.001*
OXY score	0.04	0.97	0.38	0.87	−0.46	0.97	7.29	*0.001*

SOD3: superoxide dismutase activity; CAT: catalase activity; GST: glutathione S-transferase activity; R-SH: reducing thiol total concentration; TBARS: thiobarbituric acid-reactive species; PC: protein carbonyl concentration; DS: damage score; PS: protection score; SD: standard deviation.

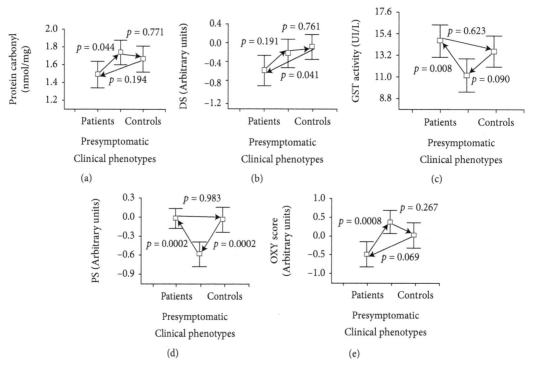

FIGURE 1: Post-hoc analyses for comparison of redox parameters between SCA2 mutation carriers and control individuals. DS: damage score; PS: protection score.

Significant effects were obtained for the repeat length ($\beta = 0.283$, SE $= 0.11$; $p = 0.012$) and disease duration ($\beta = -0.280$, SE $= 0.11$; $p = 0.014$) on protein carbonyl concentration by multiple linear regression analysis ($R = 0.387$; $p = 0.003$). Besides, significant effects were obtained for the repeat length ($\beta = 0.268$, SE $= 0.10$; $p = 0.009$) and disease duration ($\beta = -0.240$, SE $= 0.10$; $p = 0.019$) on the OXY score ($R = 0.357$; $p = 0.003$).

Regarding the associations between redox parameters and clinical biomarkers, the time to onset in presymptomatic individuals showed significant correlations with R-SH ($r = 0.41$; $p = 0.025$) and protein carbonyl concentration ($r = 0.35$; $p = 0.049$). However, after correction for repeat length, only the association with protein carbonyl concentration remained significant. Also, a correlation of marginal significance was obtained for the damage score (Table 2).

In affected patients, there was no significant correlation between the age at onset and redox parameters. Nonetheless, after correction for repeat length, the age at onset showed significant negative correlations with R-SH concentration and the protection score. Corrected age at onset also showed significant positive correlations with protein carbonyl concentration and the OXY score (Table 2).

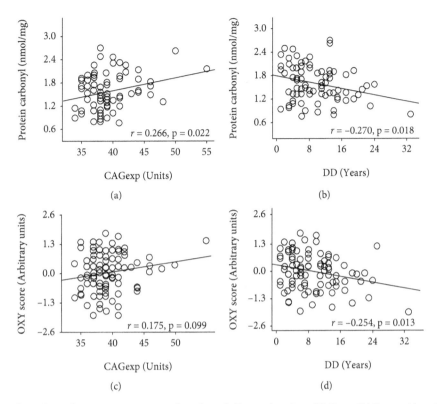

FIGURE 2: Correlation analyses for redox parameters, repeat length, and disease duration. CAGexp: CAG repeat length in ATXN2 expanded alleles; DD: disease duration.

TABLE 2: Correlation analyses for redox and clinical parameters.

Redox/clinical parameters	Correlation coefficient (p level)					
	TTO[♦]	AO[♦]	SARA score[◊]	PR[◊]	Sac. veloc.[♦]	Sac. lat.
SOD3	−0.04 (0.811)	−0.04 (0.714)	0.09 (0.428)	0.10 (0.358)	−0.031 (0.824)	0.15 (0.294)
CAT	−0.06 (0.751)	−0.07 (0.504)	0.44 (*<0.001*)	0.50 (*<0.001*)	-0.31 (*0.025*)	0.31 (*0.022*)
CAT/SOD3	0.08 (0.650)	−0.06 (0.574)	0.34 (*0.002*)	0.38 (*<0.001*)	−0.21 (0.127)	0.14 (0.303)
GST	−0.03 (0.885)	−0.09 (0.407)	0.25 (*0.017*)	0.21 (0.051)	0.17 (0.221)	−0.16 (0.249)
R-SH	0.28 (0.131)	−0.23 (*0.027*)	0.07 (0.493)	0.17 (0.112)	−0.26 (0.060)	0.21 (0.122)
TBARS	−0.18 (0.347)	0.07 (0.510)	−0.19 (0.083)	−0.16 (0.16)	−0.05 (0.742)	0.06 (0.653)
PC	−0.43 (*0.014*)	0.29 (*0.013*)	−0.20 (0.094)	−0.25 (*0.033*)	−0.04 (0.799)	0.006 (0.971)
DS	−0.34 (0.058)	0.18 (0.084)	−0.24 (*0.025*)	−0.22 (*0.036*)	−0.04 (0.782)	−0.02 (0.880)
PS	−0.05 (0.774)	−0.30 (*0.004*)	0.35 (*0.001*)	0.44 (*<0.001*)	−0.21 (0.134)	0.25 (0.072)
OXY score	−0.29 (0.111)	0.30 (*0.005*)	−0.38 (*<0.001*)	−0.41 (*<0.001*)	0.09 (0.528)	−0.15 (0.261)

SOD3: superoxide dismutase activity; CAT: catalase activity; GST: glutathione S-transferase activity; R-SH: reducing thiol total concentration; TBARS: thiobarbituric acid-reactive species; PC: protein carbonyl concentration; DS: damage score; PS: protection score; SD: standard deviation; TTO: time to onset (in presymptomatic individuals); AO: age at onset; PR: progression rate. [♦]Corrected for repeat length; [◊]corrected for disease duration and CAG repeat length.

The SARA score showed significant correlations with GST activity ($r = 0.22$; $p = 0.036$), CAT activity ($r = 0.29$; $p = 0.004$), CAT/SOD3 index score ($r = 0.29$; $p = 0.006$), protein carbonyl concentration ($r = -0.30$; $p = 0.01$), damage score ($r = -0.27$; $p = 0.008$), protection score ($r = 0.31$; $p = 0.002$), and OXY score ($r = -0.39$; $p < 0.001$). After correction for disease duration and repeat length, the SARA score showed significant positive correlations with GST and CAT activities, the CAT/SOD3 index score, and the protection score.

Likewise, corrected the SARA score showed significant negative correlations with the damage and OXY scores (Table 2). Similarly, the progression rate showed significant correlations with CAT ($r = 0.25$; $p = 0.015$) activity and the CAT/SOD3 index score ($r = 0.32$; $p = 0.002$). After correction for repeat length and disease duration, the progression rate was positively correlated to CAT activity, the CAT/SOD3 index score, and the protection score. Besides, the corrected progression rate was negatively correlated to protein carbonyl concentration and the damage and OXY scores

(Table 2). On the other hand, saccade velocity showed significant correlations with CAT activity ($r = -0.35$; $p = 0.008$) and the CAT/SOD3 index score ($r = -0.33$; $p = 0.013$). After correction for repeat length, saccade velocity showed a highly significant negative correlation with CAT activity. On the contrary, saccade latency showed a significant positive correlation with CAT activity (Table 2).

4. Discussion

In this study, taking advantage of the largest and genetically homogeneous SCA2 population worldwide, the evidence is provided for the role of oxidative stress in the presymptomatic stage of the disease, which seems to evolve into reductive stress in symptomatic stages, then contributing to clinical worsening. To our knowledge, this is the first study on redox balance in SCA2 which includes presymptomatic individuals, showing a redox shift in the transition from presymptomatic to symptomatic stages of the disease.

Presymptomatic individuals presented a significantly higher protein carbonyl concentration and OXY score, in parallel to lower GST activity than affected patients. Besides, presymptomatic individuals presented significantly lower protection scores than affected patients and healthy controls. Overall, this evidence indicates the occurrence of oxidative stress in the presymptomatic stage of the disease, which seems to be harmful as the corrected protein carbonyl concentration is negatively associated with the time to disease onset. This finding suggests that protein carbonyl concentration might be a good predictor of disease onset in mutation carriers.

As far as we know, only two studies have assessed the relevance of redox parameters in presymptomatic individuals for polyglutamine disorders. In presymptomatic individuals for Huntington's disease, higher levels of lipid peroxidation and protein carbonyl concentration and lower GSH concentration were found, suggesting the occurrence of oxidative stress before the onset of HD symptoms [38]. Also similar to our findings in SCA2, no significant associations were found for repeat length and redox parameters in HD presymptomatic individuals [38].

Contrary to our results in SCA2 presymptomatic individuals, higher SOD3 and glutathione peroxidase activities and decreased levels of reactive oxygen species were found in presymptomatic individuals with spinocerebellar ataxia type 3 (SCA3), suggesting a potential antioxidant adaptive response to an oxidative challenge taking place before disease onset. Nonetheless, these results seem to be of limited pathological significance as no correlations of redox markers with the predicted age of onset or repeat length were found [18].

Though oxidative stress has been suggested to be playing key roles in neurodegenerative disorders, this oxidative stress-centered view was challenged by evidence of little or no protection by free radical-scavenging antioxidants [39–41] and by evidences showing no association between clinical progressions and the oxidation induced by free radicals in the brain [42, 43]. In addition, findings relative to increased glucose 6-phosphate dehydrogenase (G6PDH) in AD and PD [44, 45] and increased thiore-doxin reductase (TrxR) [46], neuronal thiols, and GSH/GSSG ratio in AD [44, 47] suggest that reductive reprogramming has an important role in these disorders. Also, the occurrence of lower GSSG and P-p38 levels and higher expression of glutamylcysteinyl ligase and glutathione peroxidase in young healthy individuals at risk of Alzheimer's disease [20] and the enhancing of the neurodegenerative phenotype in cellular and Drosophila models for Huntington's disease by treatment with N-acetyl-L-cysteine and overexpression of SOD1 support a relevant role for reductive stress in these neurodegenerative disorders [21].

In this study, it was found that affected SCA2 patients show a significant decrease in the protein carbonyl concentration and damage and OXY scores relative to controls, probably as a result of increased antioxidant activity. In addition, longer CAG repeats were associated to increased protein carbonyl concentration, as a reflection of the damaging effects of mutant Ataxin-2. Unexpectedly, there was a decrease in protein carbonyl concentration and OXY score with the advance of the disease, suggesting the sustained activation of the antioxidant machinery. Indeed, increased GST activity was observed in our patients and increased concentration of GSH was found in the white matter of SCA2 patients in a previous report [48].

Similar increases in the antioxidant defenses have been traditionally interpreted as an adaptive response to counteract the damaging effects of prooxidants on the cellular major macromolecular components, with a global protective effect [15, 16, 49]. However, we found that SCA2 patients with early disease onset show higher reducing thiol total concentration and protection score, suggesting harmful effects for increased antioxidant defenses. Moreover, positive associations were found for antioxidant parameters and SARA score, progression rate, and saccade latency, as well as a negative association with saccade velocity, reinforcing the suggestion that increased antioxidant defenses have worsening effects on the clinical presentation. In particular, catalase activity seems to be of great relevance as it was associated with the SARA score, disease progression, saccade velocity, and latency. In addition, SCA2 patients with early disease onset show lower protein carbonyl concentration and there were inverse significant associations between prooxidant parameters and disease severity.

Overall, this evidence suggests the potential occurrence of reductive stress in the symptomatic stage of SCA2, which reinforces the neurodegenerative process probably by contributing to the loss of ROS physiological effects on normal neuronal development and function.

It has been shown that ROS are important in the establishment of neuronal polarity and growth cone pathfinding [50, 51] and in the regulation of synaptic transmission and plasticity [52, 53]. Indeed, superoxide is essential to induce long-term depression in the cerebellar Purkinje neurons [54] and physiological concentrations of hydrogen peroxide are necessary for structural plasticity dependent on neuronal activity and for the maintenance of evoked synaptic transmission in Drosophila [55]. On the contrary, activation of catalase inhibited the adaptive morphological changes of the neuromuscular junction in Drosophila [55]. Besides, overexpression of mitochondrial catalase, producing an astrocyte-specific decrease of endogenous mitochondrial ROS in mice, causes profound changes in brain energy and redox metabolism, eventually leading to neuronal dysfunction and cognitive impairment [56]. This evidence suggests that overactivation of the antioxidant machinery might have negative effects on the physiology of the nervous system.

It has been proved that neuronal polarization depends heavily on the activity of protein kinases including PI3K, whose signaling can be regulated by ROS-mediated inhibition of PTEN [57]. PTEN and PI3K were also involved in synaptic terminal growth by DJ-1β oxidation in *Drosophila* [58, 59]. In addition, the release of calcium from intracellular stores was involved in the mechanisms by which ROS contribute to neuronal polarity and to synaptic plasticity [54, 60, 61]. Importantly, Ataxin-2 protein was implicated in calcium signaling and PI3K/Akt/mTOR pathways [8, 9, 62]. These findings provide potential links between Ataxin-2 and redox-mediated neuronal development and function.

In conclusion, there is a disruption of redox balance in SCA2 mutation carriers which depends on the disease stage. Besides, redox changes associate with markers of disease severity, suggesting a link between disruption of redox balance and SCA2 physiopathology. Further studies are needed to confirm these findings, to clarify the molecular mechanisms involved and to assess the usefulness of redox parameters as biomarkers of disease progression and to monitor the effects of therapeutic interventions.

Acknowledgments

The authors are grateful to patients and control individuals for their cooperation with this research. We are also indebted to M.D. Patrick MacLeod and to the Cuban Ministry of Public Health for technical and financial support.

References

[1] Y. M. Sun, C. Lu, and Z. Y. Wu, "Spinocerebellar ataxia: relationship between phenotype and genotype - a review," *Clinical Genetics*, vol. 90, no. 4, pp. 305–314, 2016.

[2] D. Genis, S. Ortega-Cubero, H. S. Nicolás et al., "Heterozygous STUB1 mutation causes familial ataxia with cognitive affective syndrome (SCA48)," *Neurology*, vol. 91, no. 21, pp. e1988–e1998, 2018.

[3] L. C. Velázquez-Pérez, R. Rodríguez-Labrada, and J. Fernandez-Ruiz, "Spinocerebellar ataxia type 2: clinicogenetic aspects, mechanistic insights, and management approaches," *Frontiers in Neurology*, vol. 8, p. 472, 2017.

[4] A. Antenora, C. Rinaldi, A. Roca, C. Pane, M. Lieto, and F. Saccà, "The multiple faces of spinocerebellar ataxia type 2," *Annals of Clinical Translational Neurology*, vol. 4, no. 9, pp. 687–695, 2017.

[5] D. P. Huynh, H. T. Yang, H. Vakharia, D. Nguyen, and S. M. Pulst, "Expansion of the polyQ repeat in ataxin-2 alters its Golgi localization, disrupts the Golgi complex and causes cell death," *Human Molecular Genetics*, vol. 12, no. 13, pp. 1485–1496, 2003.

[6] E. Damrath, M. V. Heck, S. Gispert, M. Azizov, J. Nowock, and C. Seifried, "ATXN2-CAG42 sequesters PABPC1 into insolubility and induces FBXW8 in cerebellum of old ataxic knock-in mice," *PLoS Genetics*, vol. 8, no. 8, p. e1002920, 2012.

[7] S. Paul, W. Dansithong, K. P. Figueroa, D. R. Scoles, and S. M. Pulst, "Staufen1 links RNA stress granules and autophagy in a model of neurodegeneration," *Nature Communications*, vol. 9, no. 1, p. 3648, 2018.

[8] J. Liu, T. S. Tang, H. Tu, O. Nelson, E. Herndon, and D. P. Huynh, "Deranged calcium signaling and neurodegeneration in spinocerebellar ataxia type 2," *The Journal of Neuroscience*, vol. 29, no. 29, pp. 9148–9162, 2009.

[9] M. V. Halbach, S. Gispert, T. Stehning, E. Damrath, M. Walter, and G. Auburger, "Atxn2 knockout and CAG42-knock-in cerebellum shows similarly dysregulated expression in calcium homeostasis pathway," *Cerebellum*, vol. 16, no. 1, pp. 68–81, 2017.

[10] J. M. Laffita-Mesa, P. O. Bauer, V. Kourí, L. P. Serrano, J. Roskams, and D. Almaguer-Gotay, "Epigenetics DNA methylation in the core ataxin-2 gene promoter: novel physiological and pathological implications," *Human Genetics*, vol. 131, no. 4, pp. 625–638, 2012.

[11] I. Mironczuk-Chodakowska, A. M. Witkowska, and M. E. Zujko, "Endogenous non-enzymatic antioxidants in the human body," *Advances in Medical Sciences*, vol. 63, no. 1, pp. 68–78, 2018.

[12] A. E. Azab, A. A. Adwas, A. S. I. Elsayed, A. A. Adwas, A. S. I. Elsayed, and F. A. Quwaydir, "Oxidative stress and antioxidant mechanisms in human body," *Journal of Applied Biotechnology & Bioengineering*, vol. 6, no. 1, pp. 43–47, 2019.

[13] H. Sies, "Oxidative stress: introductory remarks," in *Oxidative Stress*, H. Sies, Ed., pp. 1–8, London, London, Academic Press, 1985.

[14] D. P. Jones, "Redefining oxidative stress," *Antioxidants & Redox Signaling*, vol. 8, no. 9-10, pp. 1865–1879, 2006.

[15] H. Sies, C. Berndt, and D. P. Jones, "Oxidative stress," *Annual Review of Biochemistry*, vol. 86, no. 1, pp. 715–748, 2017.

[16] J. I. Sbodio, S. H. Snyder, and B. D. Paul, "Redox mechanisms in neurodegeneration: from disease outcomes to therapeutic opportunities," *Antioxidants & Redox Signaling*, vol. 30, no. 11, pp. 1450–1499, 2019.

[17] B. D. Paul and S. H. Snyder, "Impaired redox signaling in Huntington's disease: therapeutic implications," *Frontiers in Molecular Neuroscience*, vol. 12, p. 68, 2019.

[18] M. A. de Assis, S. J. A. Morales, A. Longoni, H. C. Branco, T. V. Rocco, and B. A. Wigner, "Peripheral oxidative stress biomarkers in spinocerebellar ataxia type 3/Machado–Joseph disease," *Frontiers in Neurology*, vol. 8, p. 485, 2017.

[19] P. Korge, G. Calmettes, and J. N. Weiss, "Increased reactive oxygen species production during reductive stress: the roles

of mitochondrial glutathione and thioredoxin reductases," *Biochimica et Biophysica Acta*, vol. 1847, no. 6-7, pp. 514–525, 2015.

[20] M. C. Badía, E. Giraldo, F. Dasí et al., "Reductive stress in young healthy individuals at risk of Alzheimer disease," *Free Radical Biology & Medicine*, vol. 63, pp. 274–279, 2013.

[21] R. B. Underwood, S. Imarisio, A. Fleming, C. Rose, G. Krishna, and P. Heard, "Antioxidants can inhibit basal autophagy and enhance neurodegeneration in models of polyglutamine disease," *Human Molecular Genetics*, vol. 19, no. 17, pp. 3413–3429, 2010.

[22] F. G. Riverón, B. O. Martínez, G. R. Gutiérrez et al., "Oxidative damage and antioxidant enzymes in blood of patients with spinocerebellar ataxia type 2," *Rev. Cubana Genet. Comunit.*, vol. 4, no. 1, pp. 42–47, 2010.

[23] D. Almaguer-Gotay, L. E. Almaguer-Mederos, R. Aguilera-Rodríguez et al., "Role of glutathione S-transferases in the spinocerebellar ataxia type 2 clinical phenotype," *Journal of the Neurological Sciences*, vol. 341, no. 1-2, pp. 41–45, 2014.

[24] D. Almaguer-Gotay, L. E. Almaguer-Mederos, R. Aguilera-Rodríguez, R. Rodríguez-Labrada, D. Cuello-Almarales, and A. Estupiñán-Domínguez, "Spinocerebellar ataxia type 2 is associated with the Extracellular loss of superoxide dismutase but not catalase activity," *Frontiers in Neurology*, vol. 8, 2017.

[25] N. Cornelius, H. J. Wardman, P. I. Hargreaves, V. Neergheen, B. A. Sigaard, and Z. Tümer, "Evidence of oxidative stress and mitochondrial dysfunction in spinocerebellar ataxia type 2 (SCA2) patient fibroblasts: effect of coenzyme Q10 supplementation on these parameters," *Mitochondrion*, vol. 34, pp. 103–114, 2017.

[26] T. Schmitz-Hübsch, S. T. du Montcel, L. Baliko, J. Berciano, S. Boesch, and C. Depondt, "Scale for the assessment and rating of ataxia: development of a new clinical scale," *Neurology*, vol. 66, no. 11, pp. 1717–1720, 2006.

[27] R. Rodríguez-Labrada, L. Velázquez-Pérez, C. Seigfried, N. Canales-Ochoa, G. Auburger, and J. Medrano-Montero, "Saccadic latency is prolonged in spinocerebellar ataxia type 2 and correlates with the frontal-executive dysfunctions," *Journal of the Neurological Sciences*, vol. 306, no. 1-2, pp. 103–107, 2011.

[28] L. E. Almaguer-Mederos, N. S. Falcon, Y. R. Almira, Y. G. Zaldivar, D. C. Almarales, and E. M. Góngora, "Estimation of the age at onset in spinocerebellar ataxia type 2 Cuban patients by survival analysis," *Clinical Genetics*, vol. 78, no. 2, pp. 169–174, 2010.

[29] G. Imbert, F. Saudou, G. Yvert, D. Devys, Y. Trottier, and J. M. Garnier, "Cloning of the gene for spinocerebellar ataxia 2 reveals a locus with high sensitivity to expanded CAG/glutamine repeats," *Nature Genetics*, vol. 14, no. 3, pp. 285–291, 1996.

[30] S. Marklund and G. Marklund, "Involvement of the superoxide anion radical in the autoxidation of pyrogallol and a convenient assay for superoxide dismutase," *European Journal of Biochemistry*, vol. 47, no. 3, pp. 469–474, 1974.

[31] B. Chance, "Catalases and peroxidases, part II. Special methods," *Methods of Biochemical Analysis*, vol. 1, pp. 408–424, 1954.

[32] W. H. Habig and W. B. Jacoby, "[51] Assays for differentiation of glutathione S-transferases," *Methods in Enzymology*, vol. 77, pp. 398–405, 1981.

[33] L. G. Ellman, "Tissue sulfhydryl groups," *Archives of Biochemistry and Biophysics.*, vol. 82, no. 1, pp. 70–77, 1959.

[34] K. A. Yagi, "A simple fluorometric assay for lipoperoxide in blood plasma," *Biochemical Medicine*, vol. 15, no. 2, pp. 212–216, 1976.

[35] R. L. Levine, J. A. Williams, E. R. Stadtman, and E. Shacter, "[37] Carbonyl assays for determination of oxidatively modified proteins," *Methods in Enzymology*, vol. 233, pp. 346–357, 1994.

[36] F. Veglia, V. Cavalca, and E. Tremoli, "OXY-SCORE: a global index to improve evaluation of oxidative stress by combining pro- and antioxidant markers," *Methods in Molecular Biology*, vol. 594, pp. 197–213, 2010.

[37] Y. Benjamini and Y. Hochberg, "Controlling the false discovery rate: a practical and powerful approach to multiple testing," *Journal of the Royal Statistical Society: Series B (Methodological)*, vol. 57, pp. 289–300, 1995.

[38] N. Klepac, M. Relja, R. Klepac, S. Hećimović, T. Babić, and V. Trkulja, "Oxidative stress parameters in plasma of Huntington's disease patients, asymptomatic Huntington's disease gene carriers and healthy subjects: a cross-sectional study," *Journal of Neurology*, vol. 254, no. 12, pp. 1676–1683, 2007.

[39] A. Lloret, D. Esteve, P. Monllor, A. Cervera-Ferri, and A. Lloret, "The Effectiveness of vitamin E treatment in Alzheimer's disease," *International Journal of Molecular Sciences*, vol. 20, no. 4, 2019.

[40] R. Filograna, M. Beltramini, L. Bubacco, and M. Bisaglia, "Anti-oxidants in Parkinson's disease therapy: a critical point of view," *Current Neuropharmacology*, vol. 14, no. 3, pp. 260–271, 2016.

[41] M. M. Essa, M. Moghadas, T. Ba-Omar, M. Walid Qoronfleh, G. J. Guillemin, and T. Manivasagam, "Protective effects of antioxidants in Huntington's disease: an extensive review," *Neurotoxicity Research*, vol. 35, no. 3, pp. 739–774, 2019.

[42] A. Nunomura, G. Perry, G. Aliev, K. Hirai, A. Takeda, and E. K. Balraj, "Oxidative damage is the earliest event in Alzheimer disease," *Journal of Neuropathology and Experimental Neurology*, vol. 60, no. 8, pp. 759–767, 2001.

[43] D. R. Galasko, E. Peskind, C. M. Clark, J. F. Quinn, J. M. Ringman, and G. A. Jicha, "Antioxidants for Alzheimer disease: a randomized clinical trial with cerebrospinal fluid biomarker measures," *Archives of Neurology*, vol. 69, no. 7, pp. 836–841, 2012.

[44] R. L. Russell, S. L. Siedlak, A. K. Raina, J. M. Bautista, M. A. Smith, and G. Perry, "Increased neuronal glucose-6-phosphate dehydrogenase and sulfhydryl levels indicate reductive compensation to oxidative stress in Alzheimer disease," *Archives of Biochemistry and Biophysics*, vol. 370, no. 2, pp. 236–239, 1999.

[45] L. Dunn, G. F. Allen, A. Mamais, H. Ling, A. Li, and K. E. Duberley, "Dysregulation of glucose metabolism is an early event in sporadic Parkinson's disease," *Neurobiology of Aging*, vol. 35, no. 5, pp. 1111–1115, 2014.

[46] M. A. Lovell, C. Xie, S. P. Gabbita, and W. R. Markesbery, "Decreased thioredoxin and increased thioredoxin reductase levels in Alzheimer's disease brain," *Free Radical Biology and Medicine*, vol. 28, no. 3, pp. 418–427, 2000.

[47] J. D. Adams, L. K. Klaidman, I. N. Odunze, H. C. Shen, and C. A. Miller, "Alzheimer's and Parkinson's disease," *Molecular and Chemical Neuropathology*, vol. 14, pp. 213–226, 1991.

[48] J. M. Joers, D. K. Deelchand, T. Lyu et al., "Neurochemical abnormalities in premanifest and early spinocerebellar ataxias," *Annals of Neurology*, vol. 83, no. 4, pp. 816–829, 2018.

[49] Y. Torres-Ramos, A. Montoya-Estrada, B. Cisneros, K. Tercero-Pérez, G. León-Reyes, and N. Leyva-García, "Oxidative stress in spinocerebellar ataxia type 7 is associated with disease severity," *Cerebellum*, vol. 17, no. 5, pp. 601–609, 2018.

[50] M. Nitti, A. L. Furfaro, C. Cevasco, N. Traverso, U. M. Marinari, and M. A. Pronzato, "PKC delta and NADPH oxidase in retinoic acid-induced neuroblastoma cell differentiation," *Cellular Signalling*, vol. 22, no. 5, pp. 828–835, 2010.

[51] R. J. Hung, U. Yazdani, J. Yoon, H. Wu, T. Yang, and N. Gupta, "Mical links semaphorins to F-actin disassembly," *Nature*, vol. 463, no. 7282, pp. 823–827, 2010.

[52] S. Sanyal, D. J. Sandstrom, C. A. Hoeffer, and M. Ramaswami, "AP-1 functions upstream of CREB to control synaptic plasticity in Drosophila," *Nature*, vol. 416, no. 6883, pp. 870–874, 2002.

[53] K. Y. Lee, K. Chung, and J. M. Chung, "Involvement of reactive oxygen species in long-term potentiation in the spinal cord dorsal hor n," *Journal of Neurophysiology*, vol. 103, no. 1, pp. 382–391, 2010.

[54] H. Fujii and T. Hirano, "Calcineurin regulates induction of late phase of cerebellar long-term depression in rat cultured Purkinje neurons," *The European Journal of Neuroscience*, vol. 16, no. 9, pp. 1777–1788, 2002.

[55] C. W. M. Oswald, S. P. Brooks, F. M. Zwart, A. Mukherjee, J. H. R. West, and N. G. C. Giachello, "Reactive oxygen species regulate activity-dependent neuronal plasticity in Drosophila," *eLife*, vol. 7, article e39393, 2018.

[56] C. Vicente-Gutierrez, N. Bonora, V. Bobo-Jimenez, D. Jimenez-Blasco, I. Lopez-Fabuel, and E. Fernandez, "Astrocytic mitochondrial ROS modulate brain metabolism and mouse behavior," *Nature Metabolism*, vol. 1, no. 2, pp. 201–211, 2019.

[57] Y. C. Kim, H. Kitaura, T. Taira, S. M. M. Iguchi-Ariga, and H. Ariga, "Oxidation of DJ-1-dependent cell transformation through direct binding of DJ-1 to PTEN," *International Journal of Oncology*, vol. 35, no. 6, pp. 1331–1341, 2009.

[58] V. Kumar, M. X. Zhang, M. W. Swank, J. Kunz, and G. Y. Wu, "Regulation of dendritic morphogenesis by Ras-PI3K-Akt-mTOR and Ras-MAPK signaling pathways," *The Journal of Neuroscience*, vol. 25, no. 49, pp. 11288–11299, 2005.

[59] S. Jordán-Alvarez, W. Fouquet, S. J. Sigrist, and A. Acebes, "Presynaptic PI3K activity triggers the formation of glutamate receptors at neuromuscular terminals of Drosophila," *Journal of Cell Science*, vol. 125, no. 15, pp. 3621–3629, 2012.

[60] R. J. Gasperini, M. Pavez, A. C. Thompson, C. B. Mitchell, H. Hardy, and K. M. Young, "How does calcium interact with the cytoskeleton to regulate growth cone motility during axon pathfinding?," *Molecular and Cellular Neurosciences*, vol. 84, pp. 29–35, 2017.

[61] B. E. Herring and R. A. Nicoll, "Long-term potentiation: from CaMKII to AMPA receptor trafficking," *Annual Review of Physiology*, vol. 78, no. 1, pp. 351–365, 2016.

[62] I. Lastres-Becker, D. Nonis, F. Eich, M. Klinkenberg, M. Gorospe, and P. Kötter, "Mammalian ataxin-2 modulates translation control at the pre-initiation complex via PI3K/mTOR and is induced by starvation," *Biochimica et Biophysica Acta*, vol. 1862, no. 9, pp. 1558–1569, 2016.

2

Comparison of Selected Parameters of Redox Homeostasis in Patients with Ataxia-Telangiectasia and Nijmegen Breakage Syndrome

Barbara Pietrucha,[1] Edyta Heropolitanska-Pliszka,[1] Mateusz Maciejczyk,[2] Halina Car,[2] Jolanta Sawicka-Powierza,[3] Radosław Motkowski,[4] Joanna Karpinska,[5] Marta Hryniewicka,[5] Anna Zalewska,[6] Malgorzata Pac,[1] Beata Wolska-Kusnierz,[1] Ewa Bernatowska,[1] and Bozena Mikoluc[4]

[1]Clinical Immunology, The Children's Memorial Health Institute, Av. Dzieci Polskich 20, 04-730 Warsaw, Poland
[2]Department of Experimental Pharmacology, Medical University of Bialystok, Szpitalna 37 Str., 15-295 Bialystok, Poland
[3]Department of Family Medicine, Medical University of Bialystok, Bialystok, Poland
[4]Department of Pediatrics Rheumatology, Immunology, and Metabolic Bone Diseases, Medical University of Bialystok,
 Waszyngtona 17 Str., 15-274 Bialystok, Poland
[5]Institute of Chemistry, University of Bialystok, Bialystok, Poland
[6]Department of Conservative Dentistry, Medical University of Bialystok, Bialystok, Poland

Correspondence should be addressed to Bozena Mikoluc; bozenam@mp.pl

Academic Editor: Mohamed M. Abdel-Daim

This study compared the antioxidant status and major lipophilic antioxidants in patients with ataxia-telangiectasia (AT) and Nijmegen breakage syndrome (NBS). Total antioxidant status (TAS), total oxidant status (TOS), oxidative stress index (OSI), and concentrations of coenzyme Q10 (CoQ10) and vitamins A and E were estimated in the plasma of 22 patients with AT, 12 children with NBS, and the healthy controls. In AT patients, TAS (median 261.7 μmol/L) was statistically lower but TOS (496.8 μmol/L) was significantly elevated in comparison with the healthy group (312.7 μmol/L and 311.2 μmol/L, resp.). Tocopherol (0.8 μg/mL) and CoQ10 (0.1 μg/mL) were reduced in AT patients versus control (1.4 μg/mL and 0.3 μg/mL, resp.). NBS patients also displayed statistically lower TAS levels (290.3 μmol/L), while TOS (404.8 μmol/L) was comparable to the controls. We found that in NBS patients retinol concentration (0.1 μg/mL) was highly elevated and CoQ10 (0.1 μg/mL) was significantly lower in comparison with those in the healthy group. Our study confirms disturbances in redox homeostasis in AT and NBS patients and indicates a need for diagnosing oxidative stress in those cases as a potential disease biomarker. Decreased CoQ10 concentration found in NBS and AT indicates a need for possible supplementation.

1. Introduction

Ataxia-telangiectasia (AT; OMIM #208900) and Nijmegen breakage syndrome (NBS; OMIM #251260) belong to a group of genetically determined primary immunodeficiency disorders (PID) whose course involves defects in DNA repair processes [1]. AT is caused by null mutations in the *ATM* (*ataxia-telangiectasia mutated*) *gene* located on chromosome 11q.26 which encodes a protein of the same name. The main role of ATM protein is the coordination of cellular response to DNA double strand breaks, oxidative stress, signal transduction, and cell-cycle control. The clinical picture of the disease is characterised by cerebellar degeneration, telangiectasia, immunodeficiency, cancer susceptibility, and radiation sensitivity. Experimental studies have provided direct evidence for the presence of mitochondrial dysfunctions in AT

Comparison of Selected Parameters of Redox Homeostasis in Patients with Ataxia-Telangiectasia...

11

cells. They have demonstrated that the structural organisation of mitochondria in AT cells is abnormal compared to wild-type cells [2, 3].

NBS, similarly to AT, belongs to a group of the XCIND syndrome. The XCIND syndrome is named after Eaton et al. who found distinct hypersensitivity to ionizing (X-ray) irradiation, cancer susceptibility, immunodeficiency, neurological abnormality, and double-strand DNA breakage in these cases [4]. Mutations causative of NBS occur in the NBS1 gene, located on human chromosome 8q21. NBS1 encodes for nibrin, the key regulatory protein of the R/M/N (RAD50/MRE11/NBS1) protein complex which senses and mediates cellular response to DNA damage caused by ionizing radiation [5, 6]. The chromosome instability in AT and NBS patients results from a defective response to DNA double-strand breaks. In addition, AT and NBS patients display a few common characteristics such as growth retardation, premature aging, and neurodegeneration. It is believed that these symptoms can be caused not only by chromosomal instability and aberrant DNA damage response but also by oxidative stress and mitochondrial abnormalities [1, 2].

Recent studies indicate new, alternative sources of ROS and oxidative stress in AT and NBS cells, including NADPH oxidase 4, oxidised low-density lipoprotein (ox-LDL), or poly (ADP-ribose) polymerases (PARP-1, PARP-2, and PARP-3) [1, 7–10]. Mitochondrial dysfunction such as aberrant structural organisation of mitochondria, excess mitochondrial ROS (mROS) production and mitochondrial injury have also been reported in AT and NBS cells [1, 3, 11]. Valentin-Vega et al. [11] showed increased mROS production in AT cells, which resulted from a decline in the activity of complex I of the electron transport chain in mitochondria. Noteworthy is a study conducted by Weyemi et al. [9] who stressed that NADPH oxidase 4 (the main source of free radicals in the cell) was highly upregulated in AT cells and correlated with higher oxidative damage and apoptosis. To date, however, little is still known about the oxidant/antioxidant abnormalities in AT and NBS patients. Therefore, the purpose of our study was to measure selected parameters of redox homeostasis in patients with AT and NBS. Both disorders are characterised by symptoms typical of the XCIND syndrome, and therefore we intended to evaluate total antioxidant status (TAS), total oxidant status (TOS), and oxidative stress index (OSI) as well as concentrations of the most common lipophilic antioxidants, CoQ10, and vitamins A and E. It appears that the thorough understanding of disturbances in the body's antioxidant defense mechanisms could lead to new therapeutic strategies in AT and NBS, similarly as in other oxidative stress-related genetic disorders.

2. Materials and Methods

2.1. Patients. The study included 12 Caucasian children with NBS (5 females, 7 males) whose average age was 12 years and 1 month with a confirmed mutation in the *NBS1 gene* and 22 patients with AT (9 females, 13 males) whose average age was 13 years and 7 months with a confirmed mutation in *ATM gene*. All study participants were under the medical care of the Department of Immunology at the Children's Memorial Health Institute in Warsaw, Poland. The patients were included in the study on the basis of their medical history and physical examination, and they were found to be in good health at the time of enrollment (normal biochemical and morphological blood parameters, negative markers of inflammation). Diagnosis was based on clinical symptoms and genetic and biochemical tests according to ESID (European Society for Immunodeficiencies) criteria. None of the patients enrolled in the study were diagnosed with cancer, diabetes, hypertension, and HIV infection. The control group consisted of, respectively, 12 and 22 healthy individuals matched for age and sex. Plasma samples of the study and the control group were collected between February 2016 and January 2017.

The study was approved by the Bioethical Committee at the Medical University, Bialystok, Poland. Parents of all respondents gave informed written consent for their children's participation in the study.

2.2. Determination of Plasma Total Antioxidant Status (TAS), Total Oxidant Status (TOS), and Oxidative Stress Index (OSI). Total antioxidant status (TAS) and total oxidant status (TOS) were determined using commercial colorimetric kits (ImAnOx (TAS/TAC) Kit, Immundiagnostik, Bensheim, Germany and PerOx (TOS/TOC) Kit, Immundiagnostik, Bensheim, Germany, resp.) in accordance with the manufacturer's instructions. The determination of TAS was based on a reaction between antioxidants contained in the sample with exogenous hydrogen peroxide, while the determination of TOS was performed by the reaction of peroxidase with total lipid peroxides in the sample. The resulting coloured products were measured colorimetrically at a wavelength of 450 nm using Mindray MR-96 Microplate Reader, China. All assays were performed in duplicate samples. To assess the redox balance disorders, we have also used the oxidative stress index (OSI), which may be considered as a gold indicator of oxidative stress in biological systems. OSI was calculated according to the formula $OSI = TOS/TAS \times 100$ [12].

2.3. Determination of Plasma Vitamin A (All-Trans-Retinol), Vitamin E (L-Tocopherol), and Coenzyme Q10. Analyses were performed using high performance liquid chromatograph coupled with MS detector equipped with triple quadrupole (Shimadzu LCMS/MS-8040). Ionization was conducted using APCI (atmospheric pressure chemical ionization) mode. Data acquisition and processing were performed using Shimadzu LabSolutions LCMS Software.

The compounds were separated with a Kinetex XB-C18 100A analytical column (50 mm × 3.0 mm, 1.7 μm). The mobile phase consisted of an isocratic solvent A (methanol) 0.01-2 min and then isocratic solvent B (methanol-n-hexan, 72 : 28, *v/v*) 2.5–6 min. The flow rate was 0.4 mL/min, and the temperature of the analytical column was 400°C. The injection volumes of standard and sample solutions were 10 μL. Acquisition settings and method were optimized by the infusion of a 10 μg/mL solution of each fixed compound. The mass spectrometer was operated in the positive ion atmospheric pressure chemical ionization mode. The APCI temperature was set at 350°C and the ion current 4.5 μA.

The flow of the drying gas (N2) and the flow of the nebulizing gas were 10 L/min and 3 L/min, respectively. The desolvation line (DL) and heat block temperature was 230°C.

All analytes were detected in the MS/MS multiple reaction monitoring (MRM) with unit resolution at both Q1 and Q3. The MS conditions for generation of the positive ions are presented in Table 1. The described above chromatographic conditions were used for quantification of target analytes in plasma samples. The chromatogram of real sample is visualized in Figure 1. Plasma samples were prepared according to the procedure published previously [13].

2.4. Statistical Analysis. The examined variable distribution was assessed by means of the Kolmogoroff-Smirnow test. Due to the fact that the tested variables were inconsistent with normal distribution, the Mann–Whitney U test was used. Results are expressed as median, minimum, and maximum. The Spearman's method was applied in assessing correlations between variables. In calculations, the relevance level of $p < 0.05$ was accepted as statistically significant, authorising the rejection of individual zero hypotheses. The data were processed using the Polish version of Statistica 12.0 statistical software for PC with Windows.

3. Results

Our study demonstrated that in patients with AT plasma TAS levels were statistically lower ($p = 0.002$) and plasma TOS was statistically significantly elevated ($p = 0.001$) in comparison with the control group. Similarly to TOS, OSI was elevated in AT patients ($p = 0.001$) (Figure 2).

Tocopherol plasma concentrations were significantly reduced in AT patients as compared to the control group ($p = 0.021$). The concentrations of endogenous free radical scavenger coenzyme Q10 were statistically decreased in the plasma of AT patients versus the healthy controls ($p = 0.001$). There were no significant differences in the concentrations of plasma retinol between both groups ($p = 0.076$) (Figure 2).

Similarly to the AT group, NBS patients displayed statistically lower plasma TAS levels in comparison with the control group ($p = 0.044$). In contrast to AT, plasma TOS in NBS was not significantly different in comparison with the healthy controls ($p = 0.102$). The OSI value, similarly to AT, was higher in comparison with the controls ($p = 0.004$) (Figure 3).

We demonstrated that in patients with NBS the concentration of vitamin A precursor, beta carotene, was significantly elevated in comparison with that in the control group ($p = 0.011$). The difference in CoQ10 concentration in NBS patients and healthy controls points to a significantly lower level in NBS patients ($p = 0.001$). The concentrations of plasma vitamin E were similar in the control group and NBS patients ($p = 0.582$) (Figure 3).

It is worth noting that we did not observe statistically significant differences between the evaluated parameters in patients with AT and those with NBS (Table 2). In addition, we did not find significant correlations in the assessed

TABLE 1: The MS conditions for generation of positive ions of the analytes.

Compound	Precursor ion (m/z)	Product ions (m/z)	Collision energy [eV]
Retinol	269.10	213.20	−12
		93.10	−23
α-Tocopherol	429.30	165.10	−25
		137.05	−48
Coenzyme Q10	863.60	197.15	−45
		109.10	−47

m/z: mass-to-charge ratio.

markers of oxidative stress between the study groups and controls.

4. Discussion

This study compared the redox balance as well as major lipophilic antioxidants in patients with AT and NBS diseases. We have shown that AT and NBS are associated with impaired redox homeostasis including disturbances in lipophilic free radical scavengers such as coenzyme Q10 and alpha-tocopherol (Figure 4).

We aimed to investigate the oxidant/antioxidant status via the measurement of plasma TAS and TOS, which could provide a systemic reflection of redox homeostasis in biological systems. Concentration of TAS was significantly reduced in AT and NBS patients, which suggests the exhaustion or inefficiency of protective antioxidant systems resulting from the overproduction or enhanced activity of reactive oxygen species (ROS). It is believed that oxidative stress plays a key role in the development of many systemic complications including growth retardation, endocrine abnormalities, neurodegeneration, and premature aging as well as immunodeficiency [14–16], which are the major phenotypic hallmarks in AT and NBS diseases [1]. Our study did not directly demonstrate oxidative stress in patients with AT and NBS, since it would have been necessary to measure oxidative modification products. Nevertheless, we showed the existence of cellular redox abnormalities in the AT (↓ TAS, ↑ OSI, and ↑ TOS) and NBS groups (↓ TAS and ↑ OSI), which can constitute the basis for the development of oxidative stress leading to DNA mutations and protein oxidation as well as lipid peroxidation. We would like to emphasise that we did not find significant differences between the researched parameters of redox balance when we compared AT with NBS. A lack of correlation may indicate a similarity of redox imbalance in AT and NBS disorders, although these changes tend to be more severe in patients with AT. However, we recorded significantly elevated TOS levels only in patients with AT and therefore, TOS may be subtle distinguishing between AT and NBS diseases.

There is a consensus in the literature regarding enhanced oxidative stress in neurodegenerative disorders such as Alzheimer's or Parkinson's disease (PD) [17, 18]. Clinical studies have confirmed increased oxidant status and comparable, decreased antioxidant status in patients with PD [19–21]. It is probable that similar changes occur in the

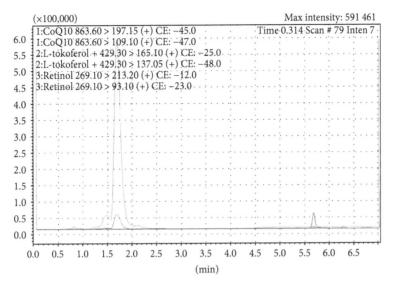

FIGURE 1: Chromatogram of a real sample (plasma).

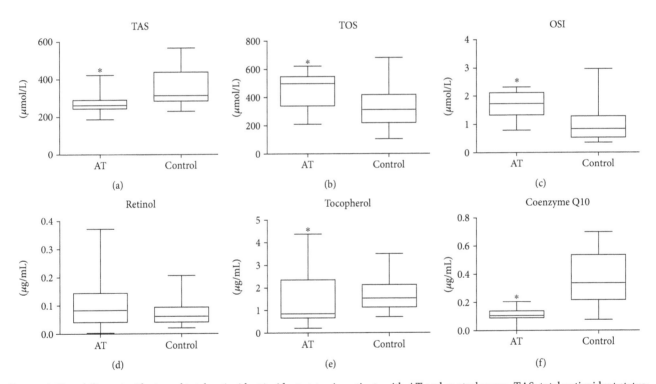

FIGURE 2: Lipophilic antioxidants and total antioxidant/oxidant status in patients with AT and control group. TAS: total antioxidant status; TOS: total oxidant status; OSI: oxidative stress index; $^*p < 0.05$.

course of AT and NBS. However, the available literature contains limited data regarding oxidative stress/redox disturbances in those cases [1]. Additionally, it should be noted that the measurement of plasma TAS and TOS provides information about antioxidant properties conditioned primarily by low molecular weight (LWMA) hydrophilic antioxidants (e.g., uric acid (UA) and ascorbic acid (AA) as well as thiol groups), but not lipophilic antioxidants [22]. Taking this into consideration, we also decided to measure levels of major lipophilic free radical scavengers (CoQ10, vitamins A and E).

Our study confirm decreased CoQ10 concentration both in AT and NBS. Coenzyme Q10 (also called ubiquinone) is a lipid soluble benzoquinone which is a key component of the mitochondrial respiratory chain for adenosine triphosphate (ATP) synthesis [23]. It has been demonstrated that most of the CoQ10 in the human body is produced endogenously; 25% of the stores are obtained from dietary intake [24]. Coenzyme Q10 deficiency results not only in abnormal respiratory chain function with inadequate cellular energy production, increased generation of free radicals, and degradation of mitochondria but also impacts on the immune

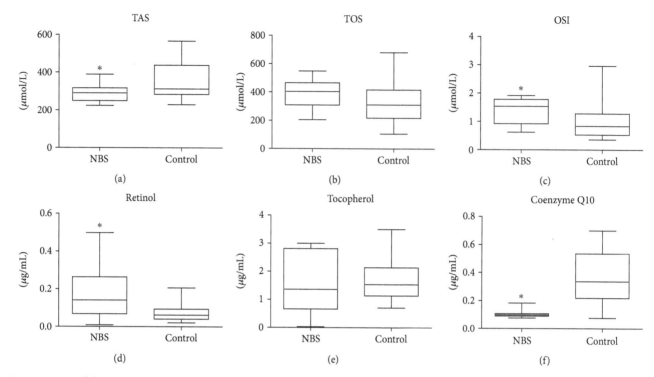

FIGURE 3: Lipophilic antioxidants and total antioxidant/oxidant status in patients with NBS and control group. TAS: total antioxidant status; TOS: total oxidant status; OSI: oxidative stress index; $^*p < 0.05$.

TABLE 2: Differences between lipophilic antioxidants and total antioxidant/oxidant status in patients with AT and NBS.

Parameters examined	AT group		NBS group		p
	Median	Min–max	Median	Min–max	
Retinol (μg/mL)	0.083	0.003–0.371	0.140	0.009–0.498	0.109
α-Tocopherol (μg/mL)	0.847	0.213–4.371	1.361	0.032–3.003	0.929
Coenzyme Q10 (μg/mL)	0.108	0.085–0.206	0.098	0.077–0.183	0.290
TAS (μmol/L)	261.745	186.852–422.515	290.288	223.966–389.895	0.327
TOS (μmol/L)	496.839	209.803–621.354	404.795	204.741–548.632	0.094
OSI	1.730	0.790–2.320	1.543	0.615–1.915	0.157

TAS: total antioxidant status; TOS: total oxidant status; OSI: oxidative stress index.

system [25]. Literature reports demonstrate that CoQ10 supplementation has improved CD4 T cell counts in patients with AIDS and outcomes in herpes and HPV infections. Furthermore, leukocyte activity is conditioned, inter alia, by proper CoQ10 activity [25]. CoQ10 deficiency may contribute to the abnormal function of mitochondria in the course of diseases such as AIDS, Alzheimer's disease, Parkinson's disease, and cancer [26, 27]. Similar disturbances have been observed in AT and NBS cells, which may suggest a potential involvement of CoQ10 in the pathogenesis of these disorders [1]. Considering the protective action of CoQ10 in neurodegenerative processes and its role in the immune system, decreased CoQ10 concentration in AT and NBS patients indicates a need for monitoring its concentration and potential supplementation. At this stage, we are unable to answer the question to what degree clinical symptoms observed in AT, such as cerebellar degeneration, immunodeficiency, cancer susceptibility, and radiation sensitivity, result from oxidative stress disturbances observed in our study. Are these

disturbances primary or secondary? However, they undeniably confirm CoQ10 involvement in the pathomechanism of the observed changes. It should be also emphasised that rare autosomal recessive disorder, CoQ10 deficiency (mutation in CABC1; COQ2; COQ9; PDSS1; PDSS2 genes), is frequently associated with seizures, cognitive decline, pyramidal track signs, myopathy, and prominent cerebellar ataxia [28, 29]. Some of these symptoms occur in both AT and NBS. Additionally, it is very likely that, in AT and NBS patients, a decrease in CoQ10 levels may be associated with impaired DNA repair mechanisms, similarly as in other bioenergetics disorders such as xeroderma pigmentosum (XP), Cockayne Syndrome (CS), Fanconi anaemia (FA), and Hutchinson-Gilford syndrome (HGS) [1].

Deficiency in lipid soluble antioxidants has been demonstrated in various conditions such as eating disorders, nicotine addiction, chronic diseases, and aging. Antioxidant vitamins and trace elements contribute to maintaining an effective immune response [30–33]. Treatments are also

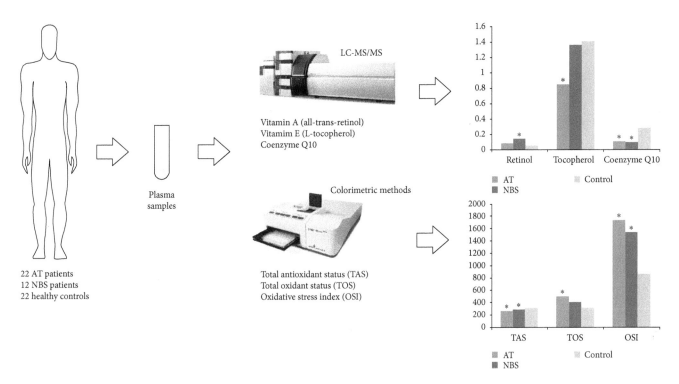

FIGURE 4: Graphical presentation of the study. $^*p < 0.05$ versus control.

available for a few autosomal recessive ataxias: vitamin E therapy for ataxia with vitamin E deficiency (AVED), chenodeoxycholic acid for cerebrotendinous xanthomatosis, CoQ10 for CoQ10 deficiency, and dietary restriction of phytanic acid for Refsum disease. Idebenone may ameliorate the cardiac and neurological manifestations of Friedreich ataxia (FRDA). No other specific treatments exist for hereditary ataxias [34]. Unfortunately, no sufficiently effective causal therapy is available for AT and NBS patients at present. Our results indicate a need for introducing CoQ10 and tocopherol into AT and NBS treatment, taking into consideration their plasma levels.

Alpha-tocopherol primarily inhibits the production of new free radicals and thus might help in preventing or delaying chronic diseases associated with reactive oxygen species molecules [35]. Decreased vitamin E concentration in AT may result in a decline in the body's antioxidant activity and anti-inflammatory as well as cell-mediated and humoral immune functions. In AT cases, we found decreased concentrations of both CoQ10 and vitamin E, which enhance disturbances in the redox balance and may increase ROS production, accumulation of damaged mitochondrial DNA (mDNA), and progressive respiratory chain dysfunction. The few experimental studies found in the available literature report that disturbances in redox processes also occur in NBS [1]. Our study of NBS cases demonstrated decreased TAS and enhanced OSI on the one hand and a reduced concentration of CoQ10 and increased concentration of vitamin A, on the other hand. Despite the fact that the interpretation of obtained results is difficult at this stage of research advancement due to a lack of comparable studies, we would like to emphasise that we did not find any differences in the tested parameters between AT and NBS.

To date, only few studies have evaluated the antioxidant defenses in AT and NBS patients [1, 36]. In one of the first reports on the subject, Reichenbach et al. showed a decrease in the levels of total antioxidant capacity, vitamin A, and vitamin E in AT patients. In contrast to our study, CoQ10 levels in AT were not significantly reduced [37]. In our study patients with AT, we found not only significantly reduced levels of CoQ10 but also of α-tocopherol. However, retinol concentration, in line with studies by Da Silva et al., was similar to the control group [38]. It is probable that the aforementioned dissimilarities result from differences in the size of study groups and research methodologies. At this point, it should be emphasized that our study is the first in which the largest group of AT and NBS patients took part.

In summary, we demonstrated a significant decrease in the level of plasma TAS in AT and NBS patients as well as an increase in the oxidative stress index. It appears that disturbances in the body's antioxidant defense mechanisms may lead to oxidative damage and altered cellular redox homeostasis and thus affect clinical manifestations of AT and NBS phenotypes. Redox imbalance in patients with AT and NBS appears to exist at a comparable level. However, a significant increase in total oxidant status (TOS) was demonstrated only in patients with AT in whom plasma TOS may be a subtle distinguishing feature of AT and NBS disorders. We are considering the theory that antioxidant supplementation with tocopherol and CoQ10 may be one of the factors enhancing treatment efficacy in AT and NBS diseases and improving patients' clinical status. Further studies regarding CoQ10 in AT and NBS are needed in order to assess its concentration not only in the blood but also in selected tissues and to evaluate the dynamics of change in relation to disease duration. The issue of a possible link between

CoQ10 deficiency and the occurrence of mutations responsible for CoQ10 deficiency remains open.

When analyzing the results of our research, one must bear in mind its limitations. We evaluated only selected parameters of redox balance in patients with AT and NBS, so determination of other markers may lead to other conclusions and clinical applications. Additionally, blood oxidative stress biomarkers cannot be mechanistically informative for some reasons. Firstly, blood and the respective tissue under study do not share common redox components and/or pathways (e.g., lack of mitochondria in erythrocytes and plasma). Secondly, both plasma and blood cells can autonomously produce significant amounts of ROS [15, 16]. However, it should be also emphasized that extremely strong point of our study is the large number of patients in the study groups compared to previously published works. Our research may also provide a new practical aspects for clinicians.

5. Conclusions

(1) Our study confirms disturbances in redox homeostasis in AT and NBS patients and indicates a need for diagnosing oxidative stress in those cases as a potential disease biomarker.

(2) The statistically significantly decreased coenzyme Q10 concentration found in NBS and AT indicates a need for possible supplementation aimed at remedying the diagnosed deficiencies in those individuals.

Abbreviations

APCI:	Atmospheric pressure chemical ionization
AT:	Ataxia-telangiectasia
ATM:	Ataxia-telangiectasia mutated
CoQ10:	Coenzyme Q10
ESID:	European Society for Immunodeficiencies
LWMA:	Low molecular weight hydrophilic antioxidants
MRM:	MS/MS multiple reaction monitoring
NBS:	Nijmegen breakage syndrome
OSI:	Oxidative stress index
PARP:	Poly (ADP-ribose) polymerase
PID:	Primary immunodeficiency disorder
ROS:	Reactive oxygen species
TAS:	Total antioxidant status
TOS:	Total oxidant status
XCIND syndrome:	Hypersensitivity to ionizing (X-ray) irradiation, cancer susceptibility, immunodeficiency, neurological abnormality, and double-strand DNA breakage.

Authors' Contributions

Barbara Pietrucha, Edyta Heropolitanska-Pliszka, and Mateusz Maciejczyk had equal participation.

Acknowledgments

The investigation was supported by Grant nos. 143-26591L and N/ST/ZB/16/001/1126 from the Medical University in Bialystok.

References

[1] M. Maciejczyk, B. Mikoluc, B. Pietrucha et al., "Oxidative stress, mitochondrial abnormalities and antioxidant defense in ataxia-telangiectasia, bloom syndrome and Nijmegen breakage syndrome," *Redox Biology*, vol. 11, pp. 375–383, 2017.

[2] F. V. Pallardó, A. Lloret, M. Lebel et al., "Mitochondrial dysfunction in some oxidative stress-related genetic diseases: ataxia-telangiectasia, down syndrome, Fanconi anaemia and Werner syndrome," *Biogerontology*, vol. 11, no. 4, pp. 401–419, 2010.

[3] M. Ambrose, J. V. Goldstine, and R. A. Gatti, "Intrinsic mitochondrial dysfunction in ATM-deficient lymphoblastoid cells," *Human Molecular Genetics*, vol. 16, no. 18, pp. 2154–2164, 2007.

[4] J. S. Eaton, Z. P. Lin, A. C. Sartorelli, N. D. Bonawitz, and G. S. Shadel, "Ataxia-telangiectasia mutated kinase regulates ribonucleotide reductase and mitochondrial homeostasis," *The Journal of Clinical Investigation*, vol. 117, no. 9, pp. 2723–2734, 2007.

[5] K. H. Chrzanowska, W. J. Kleijer, M. Krajewska-Walasek et al., "Eleven Polish patients with microcephaly, immunodeficiency, and chromosomal instability: the Nijmegen breakage syndrome," *American Journal of Medical Genetics*, vol. 57, no. 3, pp. 462–471, 1995.

[6] S. Mizutani and M. Takagi, "XCIND as a genetic disease of X-irradiation hypersensitivity and cancer susceptibility," *International Journal of Hematology*, vol. 97, no. 1, pp. 37–42, 2013.

[7] S. Squadrone, P. Brizio, C. Mancini et al., "Blood metal levels and related antioxidant enzyme activities in patients with ataxia telangiectasia," *Neurobiology of Disease*, vol. 81, pp. 162–167, 2015.

[8] M. Semlitsch, R. E. Shackelford, S. Zirkl, W. Sattler, and E. Malle, "ATM protects against oxidative stress induced by oxidized low-density lipoprotein," *DNA Repair*, vol. 10, no. 8, pp. 848–860, 2011.

[9] U. Weyemi, C. E. Redon, T. Aziz et al., "NADPH oxidase 4 is a critical mediator in ataxia telangiectasia disease," *Proceedings of the National Academy of Sciences of the United States of America*, vol. 112, no. 7, pp. 2121–2126, 2015.

[10] H. Krenzlin, I. Demuth, B. Salewsky et al., "DNA damage in Nijmegen breakage syndrome cells leads to PARP hyperactivation and increased oxidative stress," *PLoS Genetics*, vol. 8, no. 3, article e1002557, 2012.

[11] Y. A. Valentin-Vega, K. H. MacLean, J. Tait-Mulder et al., "Mitochondrial dysfunction in ataxia-telangiectasia," *Blood*, vol. 119, no. 6, pp. 1490–1500, 2012.

[12] J. Borys, M. Maciejczyk, A. J. Krętowski et al., "The redox balance in erythrocytes, plasma, and periosteum of patients

with titanium fixation of the jaw," *Frontiers in Physiology*, vol. 8, 2017.

[13] J. Karpińska, B. Mikołuć, R. Motkowski, and J. Piotrowska-Jastrzebska, "HPLC method for simultaneous determination of retinol, α-tocopherol and coenzyme Q10 in human plasma," *Journal of Pharmaceutical and Biomedical Analysis*, vol. 42, no. 2, pp. 232–236, 2006.

[14] O. I. Aruoma, "Free radicals, oxidative stress, and antioxidants in human health and disease," *Journal of the American Oil Chemists' Society*, vol. 75, no. 2, pp. 199–212, 1998.

[15] M. Valko, D. Leibfritz, J. Moncol, M. T. D. Cronin, M. Mazur, and J. Telser, "Free radicals and antioxidants in normal physiological functions and human disease," *The International Journal of Biochemistry & Cell Biology*, vol. 39, no. 1, pp. 44–84, 2007.

[16] B. Uttara, A. V. Singh, P. Zamboni, and R. T. Mahajan, "Oxidative stress and neurodegenerative diseases: a review of upstream and downstream antioxidant therapeutic options," *Current Neuropharmacology*, vol. 7, no. 1, pp. 65–74, 2009.

[17] A. Arikanoglu, E. Akil, S. Varol et al., "Relationship of cognitive performance with prolidase and oxidative stress in Alzheimer disease," *Neurological Sciences*, vol. 34, no. 12, pp. 2117–2121, 2013.

[18] A. Kirbas, S. Kirbas, M. C. Cure, and A. Tufekci, "Paraoxonase and arylesterase activity and total oxidative/anti-oxidative status in patients with idiopathic Parkinson's disease," *Journal of Clinical Neuroscience*, vol. 21, no. 3, pp. 451–455, 2014.

[19] M. Y. Sherman and A. L. Goldberg, "Cellular defenses against unfolded proteins: a cell biologist thinks about neurodegenerative diseases," *Neuron*, vol. 29, no. 1, pp. 15–32, 2001.

[20] T. B. Shea, Y. L. Zheng, D. Ortiz, and H. C. Pant, "Cyclin-dependent kinase 5 increases perikaryal neurofilament phosphorylation and inhibits neurofilament axonal transport in response to oxidative stress," *Journal of Neuroscience Research*, vol. 76, no. 6, pp. 795–800, 2004.

[21] A. K. Verma, J. Raj, V. Sharma, T. B. Singh, S. Srivastava, and R. Srivastava, "Plasma Prolidase activity and oxidative stress in patients with Parkinson's disease," *Parkinson's Disease*, vol. 2015, Article ID 598028, 6 pages, 2015.

[22] C. Rice-Evans and N. J. Miller, "Total antioxidant status in plasma and body fluids," *Methods in Enzymology*, vol. 234, pp. 279–293, 1994.

[23] L. Ernster and G. Dallner, "Biochemical, physiological and medical aspects of ubiquinone function," *Biochimica et Biophysica Acta (BBA) - Molecular Basis of Disease*, vol. 1271, no. 1, pp. 195–204, 1995.

[24] H. N. Bhagavan and R. K. Chopra, "Coenzyme Q10: absorption, tissue uptake, metabolism and pharmacokinetics," *Free Radical Research*, vol. 40, no. 5, pp. 445–453, 2006.

[25] S. Farough, A. Karaa, M. A. Walker et al., "Coenzyme Q10 and immunity: a case report and new implications for treatment of recurrent infections in metabolic diseases," *Clinical Immunology*, vol. 155, no. 2, pp. 209–212, 2014.

[26] J. Garrido-Maraver, M. D. Cordero, M. Oropesa-Ávila et al., "Coenzyme Q10 therapy," *Molecular Syndromology*, vol. 5, no. 3-4, pp. 187–197, 2014.

[27] I. P. Hargreaves, "Coenzyme Q10 as a therapy for mitochondrial disease," *The International Journal of Biochemistry & Cell Biology*, vol. 49, pp. 105–111, 2014.

[28] C. Lamperti, M. H. a Naini, D. C. De Vivo et al., "Cerebellar ataxia and coenzyme Q10 deficiency," *Neurology*, vol. 60, no. 7, pp. 1206–1208, 2003.

[29] R. Montero, M. Pineda, A. Aracil et al., "Clinical, biochemical and molecular aspects of cerebellar ataxia and coenzyme Q10 deficiency," *Cerebellum*, vol. 6, no. 2, pp. 118–122, 2007.

[30] J. A. Drisko, "The use of antioxidants in transmissible spongiform encephalopathies: a case report," *Journal of the American College of Nutrition*, vol. 21, no. 1, pp. 22–25, 2002.

[31] D. Q. Pham and R. Plakogiannis, "Vitamin E supplementation in Alzheimer's disease, Parkinson's disease, tardive dyskinesia, and cataract: part 2," *The Annals of Pharmacotherapy*, vol. 39, no. 12, pp. 2065–2072, 2005.

[32] C. Ramassamy, "Emerging role of polyphenolic compounds in the treatment of neurodegenerative diseases: a review of their intracellular targets," *European Journal of Pharmacology*, vol. 545, no. 1, pp. 51–64, 2006.

[33] D. Brambilla, C. Mancuso, M. R. Scuderi et al., "The role of antioxidant supplement in immune system, neoplastic, and neurodegenerative disorders: a point of view for an assessment of the risk/benefit profile," *Nutrition Journal*, vol. 7, no. 1, p. 29, 2008.

[34] S. Jayadev and T. D. Bird, "Hereditary ataxias: overview," *Genetics in Medicine*, vol. 15, no. 9, pp. 673–683, 2013.

[35] S. Rizvi, S. T. Raza, F. Ahmed, A. Ahmad, S. Abbas, and F. Mahdi, "The role of vitamin E in human health and some diseases," *Sultan Qaboos University Medical Journal*, vol. 14, no. 2, pp. 157–165, 2014.

[36] A. Lloret, R. Calzone, C. Dunster et al., "Different patterns of in vivo pro-oxidant states in a set of cancer- or aging-related genetic diseases," *Free Radical Biology & Medicine*, vol. 44, no. 4, pp. 495–503, 2008.

[37] J. Reichenbach, R. Schubert, C. Schwan, K. Müller, H. J. Böhles, and S. Zielen, "Anti-oxidative capacity in patients with ataxia telangiectasia," *Clinical and Experimental Immunology*, vol. 117, no. 3, pp. 535–539, 1999.

[38] R. da Silva, E. C. dos Santos-Valente, F. Burim Scomparini, R. O. Saccardo Sarni, and B. T. Costa-Carvalho, "The relationship between nutritional status, vitamin a and zinc levels and oxidative stress in patients with ataxia-telangiectasia," *Allergologia et Immunopathologia*, vol. 42, no. 4, pp. 329–335, 2014.

3

Friedreich's Ataxia: Clinical Presentation of a Compound Heterozygote Child with a Rare Nonsense Mutation and Comparison with Previously Published Cases

Vamshi K. Rao ⓘ,[1,2] Christine J. DiDonato,[2,3] and Paul D. Larsen[4]

[1]*Division of Neurology, Ann & Robert H. Lurie Children's Hospital of Chicago, Chicago, IL 60611, USA*
[2]*Department of Pediatrics, Feinberg School of Medicine, Northwestern University, Chicago, IL 60611, USA*
[3]*Human Molecular Genetics Program, Ann & Robert H. Lurie Children's Hospital, Stanley Manne Research Institute, Chicago, IL 60611, USA*
[4]*Division of Neurology, Department of Pediatrics, University of Nebraska Medical Center and Children's Hospital and Medical Center, Omaha, NE, USA*

Correspondence should be addressed to Vamshi K. Rao; vrao@luriechildrens.org

Academic Editor: Dominic B. Fee

Friedreich's ataxia is a neurodegenerative disorder associated with a GAA trinucleotide repeat expansion in intron 1 of the frataxin (FXN) gene. It is the most common autosomal recessive cerebellar ataxia, with a mean age of onset at 16 years. Nearly 95-98% of patients are homozygous for a 90-1300 GAA repeat expansion with only 2-5% demonstrating compound heterozygosity. Compound heterozygous individuals have a repeat expansion in one allele and a point mutation/deletion/insertion in the other. Compound heterozygosity and point mutations are very rare causes of Friedreich's ataxia and nonsense mutations are a further rarity among point mutations. We report a rare compound heterozygous Friedrich's ataxia patient who was found to have one expanded GAA FXN allele and a nonsense point mutation in the other. We summarize the four previously published cases of nonsense mutations and compare the phenotype to that of our patient. We compared clinical information from our patient with other nonsense FXN mutations reported in the literature. This nonsense mutation, to our knowledge, has only been described once previously; interestingly the individual was also of Cuban ancestry. A comparison with previously published cases of nonsense mutations demonstrates some common clinical characteristics.

1. Introduction

Friedrich's ataxia is the most common inherited ataxia with an estimated prevalence of 1 in 30,000-50,000 and a carrier frequency of 1 in 90-110 in the Caucasian population [1, 2]. It is characterized typically by progressive gait and limb ataxia, loss of deep tendon reflexes, and dysarthria. Additional features can include hypertrophic cardiomyopathy [3], diabetes [4], scoliosis, distal wasting, optic atrophy, and sensorineural deafness [5, 6].

The mutation causing Friedrich's ataxia was mapped to chromosome 9 by Chamberlain et al. in 1988 [7]. Subsequently in 1995 Montermini et al. [8] isolated the critical region on 9q13 and in 1996 Campuzano et al. [9] demonstrated the intronic GAA triplet repeat expansion that is associated with the disease.

The identification of the gene led to a phenotypic characterization of the disease. The classic phenotype (95-98%) associated with a homozygous GAA triplet repeat expansion (in the first intron) on both alleles has an age of onset before 25 years, wheelchair dependence within a decade, and death typically due to cardiac compromise by the fourth decade. Repeat expansion size was inversely correlated with the age at onset, duration to wheelchair, and development of cardiomyopathy [10]. Variability in clinical presentations included either late or very late presentations, retained tendon reflexes, or Acadian type (original French people living in North America, intermediate repeats, milder course, and lower incidence of cardiomyopathy) and was usually associated with lower GAA repeat expansion sizes or genetic modifiers.

Compound heterozygous (2-5%) individuals possess a GAA trinucleotide repeat expansion on one allele and a point mutation on the other allele. Diseases causing alterations include frameshift, missense, splice site, in/dels, and nonsense mutations. The two largest case series of Friedrich's ataxia patients with point mutations have been described by Cossee et al. [11] (25 patients) and Gellera et al. [12] (12 patients). Recently Galea et al. [13] compared clinical information from 131 individuals with homozygous expansions and 111 compound heterozygotes. Structural modeling and stability analyses were used to predict protein stability and protein interaction disruption of the various missense mutations. Within the 111 compound heterozygotes (81 were from previous literature review) 50 were predicted to be null alleles representing 38 different types of mutations. These consisted mostly of splice site or in/del mutations that resulted in truncating mutations. Very few were nonsense point mutations as they are rare among the point mutations that have been detected to date. It has been observed that null mutations have earlier onset and higher incidence of diabetes compared to homozygous GAA expansions. On the other hand, there is a higher rate of cardiomyopathy in homozygous GAA expansion than any type of compound heterozygous mutation.

Here we report the case of a child with Friedrich's ataxia found to harbor a W155X nonsense mutation that has to our knowledge, only been described once before [14]. We discuss the clinical phenotype while drawing comparisons with point mutations in general and the previously published cases of nonsense point mutations.

2. Case Description

A 7.5-year-old boy presented with progressive gait disturbance and falls. History included a full-term birth with no pregnancy or delivery complications. Developmental milestones including sitting up without support, walking, and speech were all within the normal range. Family history was remarkable for tremors in grandfather. He was first seen by the pediatric neurologist for unsteady gait and toe walking at the age of 3.5 years with the gait unsteadiness commencing around the age of 2.5 years with frequent falls. Tremors in the hands were noted sometime previous to the clinic visit. Examination was notable for a well-developed child with a normal funduscopic exam, no cardiac murmur, and normal mental status including speech, normal cranial nerves, and strength. He had 1+ deep tendon reflexes (DTRs) in both upper and lower extremities with down going toes. Gait was wide based and unsteady. He had a tremor in both hands.

By the age of 6.5 years he had progressed to more falls and worsening handwriting. Examination revealed pes cavus, mild scoliosis, and absence of cardiac murmur. Neurological exam was notable for trace to absent DTRs, loss of position

sense, positive Romberg, downgoing toes, slowed rapid alternating movements, tremor on finger to nose exam, and wide based unsteady gait.

By the age of 7 years he had more frequent falls and worsening handwriting. Examination showed progression with respect to ataxia in upper and lower limbs with wider based gait. DTRs were absent and a positive Babinski was noted.

At last exam around the age of 7.5 years he was falling more, and exam showed evidence of increased tone in lower extremities with foot drop and steppage gait in addition to decreased proprioception in the lower extremities and inconsistent responses in the upper extremities.

Magnetic resonance imaging of the brain was normal. Laboratory testing including quantitative immunoglobulins, alpha fetoprotein, thyroid profile, serum lactate, vitamin E levels, creatine kinase, serum amino acids, and serum acylcarnitine profile were all normal. Echocardiogram showed global hypertrophy of both ventricles. Ophthalmological examination did not show any evidence of optic atrophy.

Mutation analysis showed one allele with a GAA trinucleotide repeat expansion of approximately 1000. Since the index of suspicion was high, frataxin sequencing was done which demonstrated another allele harboring a c.464G>A nucleotide change. The nucleotide change predicted an amino acid substitution of tryptophan to a premature stop codon at residue 155 (W155X).

3. Discussion

The classic Friedreich's ataxia phenotype (95-98%) is due to a homozygous GAA triplet repeat expansion in intron 1 of the FXN gene (Figure 1(a)), which results in low frataxin protein levels, whereas compound heterozygous (2-5%) individuals possess GAA trinucleotide repeat expansion on one allele and point mutation on the other allele, as seen in our patient (Figure 1(b)).

Including our patient there are four other reported nonsense mutations. Campuzano et al. [9] published the case of a French family with 2 affected siblings with a T to G transversion in exon 3 that changed a leucine to a stop codon (L106X). De Castro et al. [14] reported a Cuban patient from Florida, USA, with a G to A nucleotide change in exon 4 that resulted in substitution of tryptophan to a stop codon, similar to our patient (W155X). Gellera et al. [12] reported an Italian patient with a C to G transversion leading to a substitution of tyrosine to a stop codon (Y118X) in exon 3 (Figure 1(c)).

Clinical features of the known nonsense Friedrich's ataxia patients are listed in Table 1. All patients were males. Age at onset of symptoms was before 15. All patients presented with gait ataxia, upper motor neuron signs, dysarthria, decreased vibration, and scoliosis. Upper and lower limb areflexia and cardiomyopathy were present in all except sibling 2 from the French family. Diabetes was not found in any patients. Hearing loss was not present in most of the patients and presence or absence of hearing was not mentioned in the siblings from France.

From the collective works of Cossee et al. [11] and Gellera et al. [12], some patterns have emerged with respect

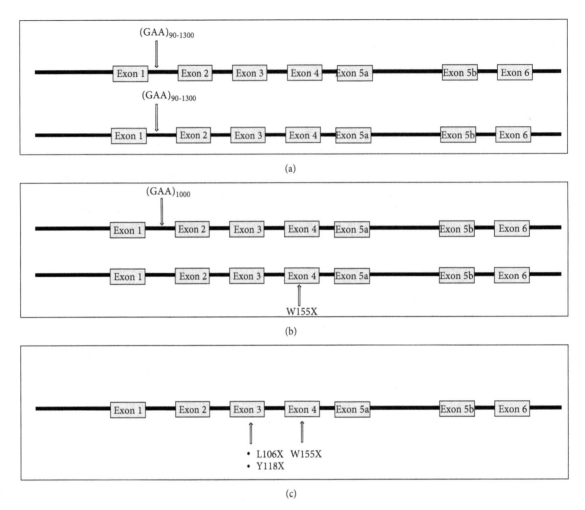

FIGURE 1: (a) Homozygous GAA triplet repeat expansion. (b) Compound heterozygosity with a point mutation in the second allele resulting in a stop codon, as in our patient. (c) Other known compound heterozygous cases resulting in a nonsense mutation from review of literature.

to disease onset and clinical features when homozygous trinucleotide repeat expansion is compared to those with compound heterozygosity. As discussed in those papers, the onset of symptoms is significantly earlier in the compound heterozygous patients (before 25 years of age). The offered explanation is that the repeat expansion in the homozygous patients is significantly smaller and becomes the determinant of the age of onset. This seems to suggest that the residual expression of frataxin protein determines the clinical phenotype. Therefore, in compound heterozygotes the frataxin protein is very low in quantity with a larger repeat expansion on one allele and no protein is expressed with the point mutation on the other allele. Other clinical features that have been noted from the work of Cossee and Gellera et al. is the lower incidence of dysarthria and higher incidence of optic atrophy (especially where expansions were greater than 700 repeats).

Interestingly enough, all the patients with the known nonsense mutations were male. The nonsense mutation hot spots seem to center in exons 3 and 4 of the frataxin gene. Some features were consistent with what is known about compound heterozygotes with an early onset, upper motor signs, gait ataxia, decreased vibratory sensation, and cardiomyopathy. Age at onset was directly proportional to the number of trinucleotide repeat expansion sizes in the nonsense mutations too. Our patient demonstrated the earliest onset which correlated with approximately 1000 repeats, higher than the other patients. Our patient's ancestry on the paternal side was Cuban which was similar to the W155X nonsense mutation described by De Castro et al. [14].

The sample size for phenotypic generalization of children presenting with nonsense mutations is small and our patient is only 8 years of age. As such clinical pattern recognition with respect to absence of diabetes, hearing loss and optic atrophy in our patient cannot be thought of as unique. Furthermore, genetic and clinical heterogeneity has emerged within compound heterozygous mutations. Although lower levels of frataxin are seen in compound heterozygotes compared to homozygous GAA repeat expansions, levels of frataxin can be significantly different in tissues among different mutations, leading to variabilities in clinical phenotype [15]. There is evidence that certain mutations such as G130V or I154F, although compound heterozygote, have milder clinical phenotypes [16].

TABLE 1: Clinical features of Friedrich's ataxia patients with nonsense mutations.

Mutation	L106X (Sibling 1)	L106X (Sibling 2)	W155X	Y118X	W155X Our patient
Geographical origin	France	France	USA (Cuban origin)	Italy	USA (Father Cuban)
GAA repeat size	733	700	850	640	1000
Gender	Male	Male	Male	Male	Male
Age at onset (years)	9	13	4	14	2.5
Age at last exam (years)	35	32	Unknown	27	8
Gait ataxia	+	+	+	+	+
Nystagmus	+	+	-	+	-
Deep Tendon Reflexes	-	+, upper limbs	-	-	-
Babinski sign	+, unilateral	+	+	+	+
Vibration sense	↓	↓	↓	↓	↓
Foot deformity	+	+	+	-	+
Cardiomyopathy	+	-	+	+	+
Scoliosis	+	+	+	+	+
Optic disks	Pallor	Pallor	No atrophy	No atrophy	No atrophy
Dysarthria	+	+	+	+	+
Diabetes	-	-	-	-	-
Hearing loss	Not reported	Not reported	-	-	-

In conclusion, if the index of suspicion is high for Friedrich's ataxia then frataxin sequencing should be performed if there is a repeat expansion detected only on one allele. Secondly, for the most part, compound heterozygous patients have an earlier age of onset that directly correlates with the trinucleotide expansion size. Finally, whether there is a unique phenotype to the nonsense mutations requires further study before counseling families regarding natural history of disease.

References

[1] A. H. Koeppen, "Friedreich's ataxia: Pathology, pathogenesis, and molecular genetics," *Journal of the Neurological Sciences* vol. 303, no. 1-2, pp. 1–12, 2011.

[2] F. Taroni and S. DiDonato, "Pathways to motor incoordination: The inherited ataxias," *Nature Reviews Neuroscience*, vol. 5, no. 8, pp. 641–655, 2004.

[3] P. Salazar, R. Indorkar, M. Dietrich, and A. Farzaneh-Far, "Cardiomyopathy in Friedreich's ataxia," *European Heart Journal* vol. 39, no. 7, p. 631, 2018.

[4] A. Pappa, M. G. Häusler, A. Veigel et al., "Diabetes mellitus in Friedreich Ataxia: A case series of 19 patients from the German-Austrian diabetes mellitus registry," *Diabetes Research and Clinical Practice*, vol. 141, pp. 229–236, 2018.

[5] A. E. Harding, "Friedreich's ataxia: a clinical and genetic study of 90 families with an analysis of early diagnostic criteria and intrafamilial clustering of clinical features," *Brain*, vol. 104, no. 3, pp. 589–620, 1981.

[6] M. B. Delatycki and L. A. Corben, "Clinical features of Friedreich ataxia," *Journal of Child Neurology*, vol. 27, no. 9, pp. 1133–1137, 2012.

[7] S. Chamberlain, J. Shaw, A. Rowland et al., "Mapping of mutation causing Friedreich's ataxia to human chromosome 9," *Nature*, vol. 334, no. 6179, pp. 248–250, 1988.

[8] L. Montermini, F. Rodius, L. Pianese et al., "The Friedreich ataxia critical region spans a 150-kb interval on chromosome 9q13," *American Journal of Human Genetics*, vol. 57, no. 5, pp. 1061–1067, 1995.

[9] V. Campuzano, L. Montermini, M. D. Moltò et al., "Friedreich's ataxia: autosomal recessive disease caused by an intronic GAA triplet repeat expansion," *Science*, vol. 271, no. 5254, pp. 1423–1427, 1996.

[10] A. Filla, G. De Michele, F. Cavalcanti et al., "The relationship between trinucleotide (GAA) repeat length and clinical features in Friedreich ataxia," *American Journal of Human Genetics*, vol. 59, no. 3, pp. 554–560, 1996.

[11] M. Cossée, A. Dürr, M. Schmitt et al., "Friedreich's ataxia: Point mutations and clinical presentation of compound heterozygotes," *Annals of Neurology*, vol. 45, no. 2, pp. 200–206, 1999.

[12] C. Gellera, B. Castellotti, C. Mariotti et al., "Frataxin gene point mutations in Italian Friedreich ataxia patients," *neurogenetics*, vol. 8, no. 4, pp. 289–299, 2007.

[13] C. A. Galea, A. Huq, P. J. Lockhart et al., "Compound heterozygous FXN mutations and clinical outcome in friedreich ataxia," *Annals of Neurology*, vol. 79, no. 3, pp. 485–495, 2016.

[14] M. De Castro, J. García-Planells, E. Monrós et al., "Genotype and phenotype analysis of Friedreich's ataxia compound heterozygous patients," *Human Genetics*, vol. 106, no. 1, pp. 86–92, 2000.

[15] M. Lazaropoulos, Y. Dong, E. Clark et al., "Frataxin levels in peripheral tissue in Friedreich ataxia," *Annals of Clinical and Translational Neurology*, vol. 2, no. 8, pp. 831–842, 2015.

[16] E. Clark, J. S. Butler, C. J. Isaacs, M. Napierala, and D. R. Lynch, "Selected missense mutations impair frataxin processing in Friedreich ataxia," *Annals of Clinical and Translational Neurology*, vol. 4, no. 8, pp. 575–584, 2017.

4

New Insights into the Hepcidin-Ferroportin Axis and Iron Homeostasis in iPSC-Derived Cardiomyocytes from Friedreich's Ataxia Patient

Alessandra Bolotta ⓘ,[1,2] Provvidenza Maria Abruzzo ⓘ,[1,2] Vito Antonio Baldassarro ⓘ,[3] Alessandro Ghezzo ⓘ,[1] Katia Scotlandi,[4] Marina Marini ⓘ,[1,2] and Cinzia Zucchini ⓘ[1]

[1]*Department of Experimental, Diagnostic and Specialty Medicine, Bologna University, 40126 Bologna, Italy*
[2]*IRCCS Fondazione Don Carlo Gnocchi, 20148 Milan, Italy*
[3]*Interdepartmental Centre for Industrial Research in Health Sciences and Technologies (ICIR-HST), University of Bologna, 40064 Ozzano, Bologna, Italy*
[4]*CRS Development of Biomolecular Therapies, Experimental Oncology Laboratory, Orthopedic Rizzoli Institute, 40136 Bologna, Italy*

Correspondence should be addressed to Provvidenza Maria Abruzzo; provvidenza.abruzzo2@unibo.it

Guest Editor: Giorgos Sakkas

Iron homeostasis in the cardiac tissue as well as the involvement of the hepcidin-ferroportin (HAMP-FPN) axis in this process and in cardiac functionality are not fully understood. Imbalance of iron homeostasis occurs in several cardiac diseases, including iron-overload cardiomyopathies such as Friedreich's ataxia (FRDA, OMIM no. 229300), a hereditary neurodegenerative disorder. Exploiting the induced pluripotent stem cells (iPSCs) technology and the iPSC capacity to differentiate into specific cell types, we derived cardiomyocytes of a FRDA patient and of a healthy control subject in order to study the cardiac iron homeostasis and the HAMP-FPN axis. Both CTR and FRDA iPSCs-derived cardiomyocytes express cardiac differentiation markers; in addition, FRDA cardiomyocytes maintain the FRDA-like phenotype. We found that FRDA cardiomyocytes show an increase in the protein expression of HAMP and FPN. Moreover, immunofluorescence analysis revealed for the first time an unexpected nuclear localization of FPN in both CTR and FRDA cardiomyocytes. However, the amount of the nuclear FPN was less in FRDA cardiomyocytes than in controls. These and other data suggest that iron handling and the HAMP-FPN axis regulation in FRDA cardiac cells are hampered and that FPN may have new, still not fully understood, functions. These findings underline the complexity of the cardiac iron homeostasis.

1. Introduction

Iron is a trace metal essential for numerous biological processes. Its homeostasis is finely regulated, since both iron excess and deficiency are potential detrimental. In fact, iron excess favors the formation of oxygen radicals, while iron deficiency impairs enzyme functionality affecting oxygen metabolism. It has been demonstrated that the dysregulation of iron homeostasis is involved in different pathological conditions, including cancer, anemia, neurodegenerative disorders, and cardiac diseases [1]. Iron deficiency was found to occur in heart failure patients, independently of normal systemic iron concentration, causing morphological and functional mitochondrial alterations and consequently ATP depletion [2]. These dysfunctions, in turn, impair cardiac contractility and relaxation. Ironically, cardiomyopathy can be induced also by systemic iron overload, as in hereditary hemochromatosis (HH) and β-thalassemia, and by iron misdistribution in the cellular organelles, as in Friedreich's ataxia (FRDA) [3]. Iron excess causes an alteration of systolic and diastolic functions through the decrease of L-type channel activity, essential for the heart contraction. In addition, at the cellular level, iron misdistribution in cellular organelles, such as the mitochondria, can damage the cells through oxygen radical production. Cardiomyocytes, being endowed of poor antioxidant defenses, are more susceptible to reactive species of oxygen (ROS) damage via Fenton and Heiber-Weiss-typereactions [3, 4]. Iron homeostasis is regulated by several proteins involved in the iron uptake, transport, storage, and export. These proteins cooperate with ferrireductases, ferroxidases, and chaperones to regulate the cellular iron trafficking and to limit the unbound labile iron pool (LIP), potential source of ROS. Iron exists within heme molecules such as hemoglobin and cytochromes or in iron-sulfur cluster- (ISC-) containing proteins such as succinate dehydrogenase; moreover, nonheme/non-ISC iron-containing proteins are present in the cells [5]. Nonheme iron is transported into the cells by iron-binding proteins, such as transferrin. Cellular uptake of iron from transferrin is initiated by the binding of transferrin to transferrin receptor 1 (TFRC). TFRC is a transmembrane protein that assists iron uptake through receptor-mediated endocytosis of iron-loaded transferrin [5]. In addition, iron chaperones such as frataxin, a nuclear-encoded protein localized into the mitochondrial matrix, act as iron sensor and storage proteins as well as iron chaperons during cellular Fe-S cluster biosynthesis [6].

In iron homeostasis, a central regulatory mechanism is the binding of the hormone hepcidin (HAMP) to the iron exporter ferroportin (FPN). FPN is the only iron-exporting protein localized in the cell membrane; it was independently discovered by three different groups [7–9]. The FPN structure has not been completely defined; it is characterized by 9-12 transmembrane domains (TMs), organized into two six-helix halves, which are connected by a large cytoplasmic loop between the 6th and the 7th domain [10, 11]. Furthermore, whether the functional form of FPN is monomeric or dimeric remains an open question. Genetic and biochemical evidences support the dimeric form [12]. However, different groups reported that FPN is a monomer, and that, in this form, it is able to bind HAMP [13, 14]. Regulation of FPN occurs at multiple levels, transcriptional, posttranscriptional, and posttranslational. FPN expression is regulated at the transcriptional level by hypoxia inducible factor-2alpha (HIF2α) in response to hypoxia and inflammation; moreover, it is induced by iron heme and other metals. Posttranscriptionally, FPN synthesis is regulated by iron regulatory proteins (IRPs), which bind to an iron responsive element (IRE) located in its $5'$UTR. In addition, posttranslational regulation of FPN is mediated by HAMP. HAMP binds FPN and triggers its internalization, ubiquitination, and subsequent lysosomal degradation [10, 11].

At systemic level, circulating HAMP is synthesized by the liver, where it is induced in iron overloading conditions and is inhibited by iron deficiency due to anemia, hypoxia, ineffective erythropoiesis, and inflammation [10, 11]. HAMP is also expressed in the heart, brain, kidney, and placenta [15]; in these tissues, its role is less defined, but it is likely involved in iron handling. HAMP expression is regulated by different members of the TGF-β superfamily, including BMP (bone morphogenetic protein) receptors, associated BMP ligands, and the cytoplasmic SMAD transcription factor [16]. Moreover, it is been shown that Atoh8 (atonal bHLH transcription factor 8) contributes to hepcidin regulation in response to iron levels by interacting with Id1 proteins [17]. Cardiac expression of HAMP is induced in response to hypoxia and inflammation [18]. Upregulation of HAMP occurs in heart ischemia [19], while its downregulation was described in a mouse model of dilated cardiomyopathy [20]. Moreover, Hsieh et al. [21] showed that apoptosis was induced by the knockdown of HAMP by siRNA in human cardiomyocytes treated with ferrous iron. Anomalies of HAMP-FPN axis affect the heart functionality. Mouse cardiac FPN knockouts show dilated cardiomyopathy and iron deposits in cardiomyocytes [22]. In addition, it has been shown that HAMP knockout at the cardiac level leads to an increase in cardiac FPN; moreover, HAMP loss or HAMP unresponsiveness is associated to cardiac hypertrophy and apoptosis [23]. In addition, heart autoptic tissue of FRDA patients revealed macrophagic inflammatory infiltrate with high levels of HAMP and iron deposits [24]. To the mechanisms of iron uptake, transport, storage, and export mentioned above, one should add those that regulate the utilization of iron and its correct subcellular distribution. Noteworthy, a still underestimated subcellular compartment involved in iron trafficking is the nucleus, where iron-sulfur clusters associated with DNA repair enzymes [25] and transcription factors have been described [26]. Iron transporters and storage proteins, such as the divalent metal transporter 1 (DMT1), lactoferrin, and ferritin, are associated to the nucleus [27].

The deregulation of iron compartmentalization is very often associated with neurodegenerative pathologies such as Friedrich's ataxia, a progressive neurodegenerative disorder characterized by degeneration of central and peripheral nervous systems and associated with hypertrophic cardiomyopathy and iron deposits [28]. Cardiomyopathy and subsequent cardiac failure is the most common cause of death in FRDA patients [29], where expanded GAA repeats in intron 1 of the frataxin gene (FXN) cause its partial deficit [30]. Physiological functions of frataxin involve iron binding and storage, biogenesis of heme and iron-sulfur clusters, and iron sensing; data suggest that further—still undetermined—functions are present. Frataxin depletion results in mitochondrial dysfunction, mitochondrial iron accumulation, and ROS production [5, 31]. In this context, the complex relationship between the mitochondrial aberrations, iron imbalance and frataxin dysfunction, has contributed to the difficulty of deciphering the molecular mechanisms underlying the iron homeostasis imbalance and consequently of identifying effective therapeutic molecules to mitigate the cardiac hypertrophy. Moreover, the lack of a model that can recapitulate the phenotypic and genotypic characteristics of FRDA contributes to the poor knowledge of the underlying mechanisms of this disease.

Aim of the present study is to generate and characterize iPSC-derived cardiomyocytes as a cellular model to explore the HAMP-FPN axis and investigate the iron homeostasis in FRDA cardiac phenotype. Differentiation of iPSC-derived cardiomyocytes was monitored by cardiac gene analysis with real-time PCR and evaluation of cardiac proteins by cytofluorimetric and immunofluorescence methods.

2. Material and Methods

2.1. Human-Induced Pluripotent Stem Cells (hiPSCs). Human iPSCs derived from a healthy subject and from a FRDA patient were obtained from the NIGMS Human Genetic Cell Repository at the Coriell Institute for Medical Research: (GM 23280∗A and GM23404∗B, respectively) and generated through fibroblast reprogramming according to the Yamanaka method [32]. Table S1 reports genotypic and phenotypic features of the subjects.

2.2. Cardiomyocyte Derivation from hiPSCs. Differentiation of hiPSCs in cardiomyocytes was performed according to the GiWi method by Lian et al. [33]. The detailed protocol and the timeline of cardiac differentiation are reported in Figure S1.

2.3. Flow Cytometric Analysis. For cytometric analysis, wells were washed with PBS 1x and cardiomyocytes were dissociated with trypsin-EDTA 0.25% and then fixed in 1% paraformaldehyde for 20 min at room temperature and 90% cold methanol for 15 min. Cells (0.5×10^6) were centrifuged and the pellet incubated with primary anti-troponin T (TNNT2) antibody (Thermo Fisher Scientific, Waltham, MD) overnight at 4°C in a buffer containing 5% BSA and 1% Triton X-100 in PBS. Secondary antibody (Alexa Fluor 488 Goat anti-mouse IgG1) was added, and the samples were incubated for 30 min at room temperature, after which the nuclei were stained with DAPI. Samples were acquired using a FACSCalibur instrument and analyzed with the CellQuest software (Becton Dickinson, Italy). The primary and secondary antibody and the dilutions used are listed in Table S2.

2.4. Immunostaining Analysis. Cardiomyocytes were washed with PBS 1x and were dissociated with trypsin-EDTA 0.25% and then seeded on 0.1% gelatin-coated coversplis at 1×10^5 cells/mL. After two days, the cells were fixed in 4% paraformaldehyde for 15 min at room temperature. The primary and secondary antibody and the dilutions used are listed in Table S2. Cardiomyocytes were incubated overnight at 4°C with the primary antibody in a buffer containing 5% nonfat dry milk and 0.4% Triton X-100 in PBS. Cells were washed three times for 5 min in PBS 1x. Subsequently, the cardiomyocytes were incubated with the secondary antibody for 20 min at room temperature, followed by nuclear staining with mounting medium containing DAPI (Santa Cruz Biotechnology, DBA, Italy). Images of cardiomyocytes were obtained using a fluorescence microscope (Leica DMLB Fluo MS15062).

2.5. RNA Isolation and cDNA Synthesis. Total RNA was extracted with TRIzol™ reagent (Invitrogen, Milan, Italy) following the manufacturer's instructions. RNA quality was measured by evaluation of 28S and 18S rRNA band sharpness after denaturing electrophoresis. RNA purity and concentration were assessed by spectrophotometer evaluation (Ultrospec 3000, Pharmacia Biotech, Cambridge, UK) at 230, 260, and 280 nm. Reverse transcription (800 ng of RNA template) was performed in a final volume of $20\,\mu L$ using the iScript cDNA Synthesis Kit (Bio-Rad, Hercules, CA) following

the manufacturer's instructions. The cDNA thus obtained was stored at -20°C and used for qRT-PCR analysis.

2.6. Quantitative RT-PCR Analysis. Quantitative RT-PCR was performed according to Abruzzo et al. [34] in a Bio-Rad CFX96 real-time thermal cycler using the SsoAdvanced™ SYBR® Green Supermix (Bio-Rad Laboratories, Hercules, CA). The primer sequences for target and housekeeping genes (β-actin, GAPDH) are listed in Table S3. Primers were designed with *PRIMER3* and *AMPLIFY* software and, whenever possible, were designed as to span an exon-exon junction. All primers were purchased from Sigma-Aldrich (St. Louis, MO). Data were analyzed with the software CFX Manager software (Bio-Rad Laboratories, Hercules, CA), by using the $2^{-\Delta\Delta CT}$ method [35]; data were normalized with the housekeeping genes β-actin and GAPDH; primer efficiency in the real-time PCR reaction was between 95% and 105% [36].

2.7. Bioinformatic Analysis of Ferroportin Protein Sequence. In order to evaluate whether a nuclear localization signal (NLS) is present in FPN, its protein sequence was analyzed by cNLS Mapper, a freely available software (http://nls-mapper.iab.keio.ac.jp/cgi-bin/NLS_Mapper_form.cgi). cNLS is a bioinformatic tool useful to predict the NLS specific for the $\alpha\beta$ importin pathway; it yields the NLS scores (levels of NLS activities). Four NLS profiles are calculated: class 1/2, class 3, class 4, and bipartite NLSs. cNLS Mapper extracts putative NLS sequences with a score equal to or more than the selected cutoff score. Each amino acid residue at each position within an NLS class yields a score that sums up in order to characterize the entire NLS activity. Higher scores (8, 9, or 10) indicate the exclusive localization in the nucleus; scores 7 or 8 indicate a partial localization in the nucleus; scores 3, 4, or 5 suggest that the protein is localized both in the nucleus and in the cytoplasm. Scores 1 or 2 define the exclusive localization in the cytoplasm [37].

2.8. Confocal Analysis of Ferroportin. Confocal microscopy was used to study the presence of the FPN in the nuclei of iPSC-derived cardiomyocytes. Sections were scanned with a Nikon Ti-E fluorescence microscope coupled to an A1R confocal system and the NIS-Elements AR 3.2 software. A diode laser system with 405 wavelength output, air-cooled argon-ion laser system with 488 wavelength output, and yellow diode-pumped solid-state laser system with 561 wavelength output were used. Images were acquired with oil immersion 60x with an optical resolution of 0.18 micron, 2x scanner zoom, and 1024×1024 pixel resolution. All the z stacks were collected in compliance with optical section separation (z interval) values suggested by the NIS-Elements AR 3.2 software. Three random fields per sample were acquired, containing at least 10 cells per sample. Stacks were $0.850\,\mu m$ for a total of 14 images. 3D images were analyzed by the Imaris software (Bitplane, Concord, MA). The algorithm of the software is able to detect the nuclei, marked by DAPI, and create an isosurface on the blue fluorescence. Then, the green fluorescence, corresponding to the total FPN signal, was quantified only inside the nuclei isosurfaces. In addition, the volume of each nucleus was measured and analyzed.

2.9. Western Blot Analysis. Cardiomyocytes were lysed in 50 mM Tris-HCl (pH 8.0), 150 mM NaCl, NP-40 1%, and protease inhibitor mix (Roche, Sigma-Aldrich, Saint Louis, MO). Protein concentration was determined using Bradford protein assay (Bio-Rad Laboratories, Hercules, CA). 45 μg of protein samples was solubilized in Laemmli buffer 4x (200 mM Tris-HCl, pH 6.8, 5% SDS, 25% glycerol, 0.04% bromophenol blue, and 5% beta-mercaptoethanol) for 1 h in ice bath. Precast gradient gels (Mini-PROTEAN TGX stain-free protein gel, 4-15% polyacrylamide) (Bio-Rad Laboratories, Hercules, CA) were used. Mini-PROTEAN TGX gels contain trihalo compounds, which, in the presence of UV light, react with tryptophan residues producing fluorescence, proportional to the total protein amount of the sample. Gels were electroblotted onto nitrocellulose membranes (pore sizes: 0.45 μm). Membranes were exposed to UV light in order to visualize the protein band integrity and the efficiency of transfer. After blocking in Tris-buffered saline (TBS 1x) containing 0.1% Tween-20 (TBS-T), nonfat milk 5%, and 1% BSA for 1 h at room temperature, membranes were probed overnight at 4°C with the primary antibodies and then washed three times with TBS-T and incubated with rabbit-IgG HRP-conjugated secondary antibody, dissolved in blocking buffer for 1 hour at room temperature. Details about primary and secondary antibodies used are listed in Table S2. Finally, membranes were incubated with ECL chemiluminescent reagent (Western Bright ECL HRP substrate, Advansta, CA, USA) and exposed to an X-ray film (Aurogene s.r.l., Rome, Italy). Densitometric analysis was performed by means of Bio-Rad Gel Doc 2000. Density of specific protein bands was normalized to the β-actin band.

2.10. Statistical Analysis. For quantitative RT-PCR, statistical analysis was performed by the CFX Manager software (Bio-Rad Laboratories, Hercules, CA) and qbase plus (http://www.biogazelle.com/). For Western blot, the statistical analysis was performed by Student's *t*-test. A value of $p < 0.05$ was considered statistically significant.

3. Results

3.1. Cardiomyocyte Differentiation from hiPSCs. The differentiation of cardiomyocytes (CMs) from iPSCs was successfully repeated four times. Movies SM1 and SM2, reported in the Supplementary Materials, show beating CMs from both control and FRDA cultures. Notably, some of the beating areas found in cardiomyocyte cultures derived from FRDA iPSCs were unsynchronized, in contrast with the remarkable synchronization of control cardiomyocyte cultures.

3.2. Cardiomyocyte Characterization. The characterization of cardiomyocyte differentiation was obtained by evaluating the synthesis of four heart-specific genes: GATA4, a transcription factor specific for the cardiac lineage; SIRPA, a nonreceptorial tyrosine protein-phosphatase, exclusively expressed on the surface of hiPSC-derived cardiomyocytes [38]; and TNNT2 and actinin 2, two cardiac structural

proteins. Messenger RNAs from control and FRDA CMs and iPSCs were compared by qRT-PCR and results are shown in Figure 1(a) as the average of four independent differentiation procedures. Cardiac-specific genes were significantly upregulated in CMs with respect to iPSCs in both control and FRDA samples.

Moreover, TNNT2 protein was evaluated by FACS analysis in CMs (Figure 1(b)). FACS analysis showed that the efficiency of CM differentiation from iPSCs was 80-90%.

Finally, the immunofluorescence analysis demonstrated that TNNT2 costained with the heavy myosin chain (MF20) proteins (Figure 1(c)) in both control and FRDA CMs. TNNT2 fluorescence suggests that both control and FRDA CMs display the typical sarcomeric organization.

3.3. Maintenance of the FRDA-Like Phenotype in iPSCs and CMs. To determine whether FRDA iPSCs and CMs maintained the FRDA-like phenotype, the gene expression of FXN was analyzed. As expected, the expression of FXN gene in FRDA iPSCs was about 30% of control iPSCs (Figure 2). Moreover, cardiac differentiation did not alter the pathological phenotype; the expression of FXN in FRDA CMs was about 55% with respect to control. An average of four independent experiments is shown.

3.4. TFRC Gene Expression Is Upregulated in FRDA CMs. The mRNA abundance of the key iron homeostasis-related genes was assessed in control and FRDA CMs by qRT-PCR. Data are shown in Figure 3 as the average of four independent differentiation procedures. The expression of transferrin receptor (TFRC) was significantly increased in iPSC-CMs FRDA. Moreover, also the mRNA levels of HAMP, FPN, and ATOH8, a transcription factor involved in HAMP regulation, showed a trend to increase. No relevant difference was evidenced in the expression of FTH1 gene.

3.5. Protein Expression of HAMP and FPN Is Increased in FRDA CMs. To validate gene expression data, the protein amount of HAMP and FPN by Western blot was evaluated in whole lysates of both CTR and FRDA CMs. A representative image and the densitometric analysis of the bands are shown in Figures 4(a) and 4(b); the average of three independent differentiation experiments is reported. A significant increase of HAMP and FPN (about 2.5 and 2.0 times, respectively) was found in FRDA CMs compared to controls. It should be noted that FPN antibody detects two bands, at about 72 kDa and 62 kDa, respectively, both of which were more intense in FRDA CMs with respect to controls. Ross et al. [39] described two FPN bands, at ~65 and ≈55 kDa, respectively, in T-REx™/FPN-V5 cells and demonstrated that the heavier isoform was glycosylated.

3.6. FPN Nuclear Localization in iPSC-Derived CMs. FPN protein localization and expression was assessed by immunostaining using confocal microscopy. Figure 5(a) clearly demonstrates a nuclear localization of FPN in both CTR and FRDA CMs. Moreover, the analysis of FITC fluorescence intensity (Figure 5(b)) showed that (i) the amount of FPN was significantly lower in the nuclei from FRDA CMs compared to controls and (ii) decrease was stronger when

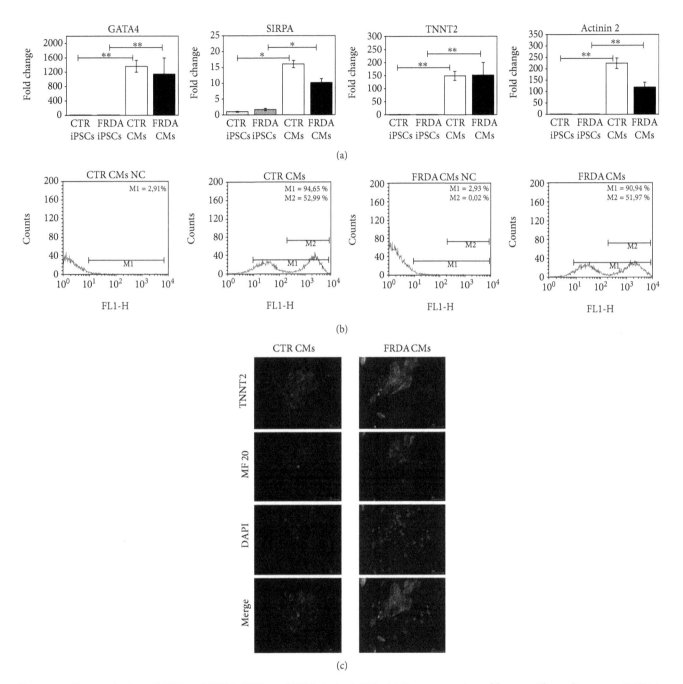

FIGURE 1: Characterization of CTR and FRDA iPSCs and iPSC-derived CMs. (a) Gene expression of four specific cardiac genes, GATA4, SIRPA, TNNT2, and actinin 2 characterized by qRT-PCR. Data were normalized with two housekeeping genes, β-actin and GAPDH; for each gene, the normalized expression value of CTR iPSCs was set to 1, and all other gene expression data were reported to that sample. PCR was run in triplicate; data are from four independent differentiation experiments and are expressed as mean ± SEM. $^*p < 0.05$; $^{**}p < 0.01$. (b) A representative flow cytometer analysis of CTR and FRDA CMs stained with TNNT2. NC negative control was stained with secondary antibody only; M1: percentage of TNNT2-positive CMs; M2: percentage of CMs highly positive to TNNT2. (c) A representative immunofluorescence image of CTR and FRDA CMs. TNNT2 is stained in green; heavy myosin chain (MF 20) is stained in red; the nuclei are stained with DAPI (blue). Scale bar 50 μm.

normalized to the volume of the nucleus, which (iii) is greater in FRDA CMs than in control. Since the nuclear localization of FPN had not been previously described, we used the cNLS Mapper software to identify, if present, nuclear localization signals (NLS) in the FPN protein sequence (NP_055400). This analysis revealed three predicted bipartite nuclear localization sequences: a sequence of 29 aa in 223 position (LWKVYQKTPALAVKAGLKEEETELKQLNL) with 3.3 score, a sequence of 32 aa (WLRRKCGLVRTGLISGLAQLSCLILCVISVF) in 362 position with 3.1 score, and finally a sequence of 29 aa (KAGLKEEETELKQLNLHKDTEPKPLEGTH) in 236 position with 3.8 score (Figure 5(c)). The NLS score analysis suggests that FPN can be localized in both the nucleus and cytoplasm.

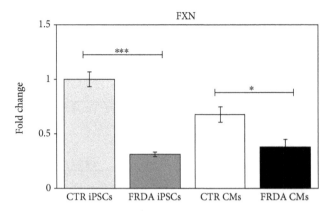

FIGURE 2: Evaluation of the FRDA-like phenotype in iPSCs and CMs. qRT-PCR of FXN gene expression in both CTR and FRDA iPSCs and CMs. Data were normalized with two housekeeping genes, β-actin and GAPDH; the normalized FXN expression value of CTR iPSCs was set to 1, and all other gene expression data were reported to that sample. Data are from four independent differentiation experiments and are expressed as mean $\pm$ SEM. $^*p < 0.05$; $^{***}p < 0.001$.

4. Discussion

In the present study, we describe some relevant features of iron homeostasis in iPSC-derived cardiomyocytes from one healthy control and one FRDA-affected patient. Cardiomyocytes were shown to fully express cardiac differentiation markers. Both FRDA iPSCs and CMs maintained the pathological phenotype, characterized by low levels of frataxin mRNA; however, frataxin expression in FRDA CMs was not as reduced as in iPSCs relative to control CMs. A similar result was reported by Hick et al. [40], who ascribed such difference to the reduced number of GAA repeats in the CM beating areas with respect to iPSCs of the same subject. Spontaneously beating areas were observed at 9-12 days from the start of the induction procedure, but FRDA beating areas were desynchronized, in agreement with similar results reported by Hick et al. [40].

Several studies pointed out the importance of iron homeostasis in the cardiac tissue; however, to date, the local regulation of iron in cardiomyocytes has not been fully characterized. In particular, the HAMP-FPN axis seems to be crucial for heart function [15, 22, 23]. Cardiac iron dysregulation was described in several disorders including FRDA, which is characterized by iron maldistribution within subcellular compartments, leading to mitochondrial iron accumulation and cytosolic iron depletion [5, 28, 41]. In the present study, cardiomyocytes were derived from CTR and FRDA human iPSCs in order to study some features of iron homeostasis, focusing the attention to the HAMP-FPN axis. This cellular model was already exploited by Lee et al. [42] to study the gene and protein expression of a group of iron-handling proteins in FRDA. To our knowledge, iron distribution within the cell compartments has not yet been evaluated in the iPSC-derived CM cellular model. The lack of such evaluation is a limitation of the present study, but this issue will be addressed in future research.

In the present study, a number of iron homeostasis-related genes and proteins were found to be dysregulated in FRDA CMs. Elevated HAMP expression has been already described in FRDA autoptic heart tissues [24], but the authors attributed HAMP overexpression to macrophagic inflammatory infiltrate. On the contrary, our results suggest that the increase in HAMP content is due to its overexpression in FRDA CMs.

In turn, HAMP downregulates the cellular amount of FPN, causing its lysosomal degradation [10, 11]. At variance with the expected decrease of FPN levels, HAMP upregulation in FRDA CMs was not accompanied by a decrease in FPN, rather a significant increase of FPN (protein) was observed.

In a different context, both FPN and HAMP were found to be significantly decreased in brain tissue of Alzheimer's disease patients, where oxidative stress is known to occur [43].

Our data show that the upregulation of HAMP and FPN in FRDA CMs is accompanied by the upregulation of TFRC. Huang et al. [44] found a decrease of FPN and an increase of TFRC in the heart of a conditional frataxin knockout (mutant) mice. It is difficult to compare our in vitro data with this study, which makes use of an animal model, where a complex interplay between local and systemic iron homeostasis takes place, and where frataxin expression is almost completely abolished. It is our opinion that our observations may reflect a dysregulation of these iron-handling proteins in FRDA CMs. Since it is known that oxidative stress affects FRDA neuronal and cardiac cells [45], it is possible that FPN loses its responsiveness to HAMP downregulation owing to the oxidation of key cysteine residues located in the HAMP- and FPN-interacting sites [46–48]. It can be envisioned that these cysteine residues are not oxidized in a "normal" low iron context, where oxidative stress is not present and HAMP downregulates FPN in order to avoid a further iron depletion. However, in the cytoplasm of FRDA cardiomyocytes, an unusual concurrence of low iron concentration AND oxidative stress is present, which would favor the inability of HAMP to downregulate FPN and to avoid iron leakage. Obviously, this is only one out of several other hypotheses, and further investigations need to be carried out for its validation or disproval.

The presence of FPN in the nuclei of CTR and FRDA CMs was demonstrated in this study for the first time. This finding suggests that FPN, traditionally considered as a transmembrane protein, could play a role in the maintenance of nuclear iron homeostasis. Henle et al. [49] described specific iron-binding sites on DNA. Moreover, other proteins involved in iron cellular trafficking, such as the divalent metal transporter 1 (DMT1), lactoferrin, and ferritin [27], have been found in the nuclear compartment. It is possible that the nuclear localization of FPN underscores a protective role from excess free iron in the nuclear compartment. Surprisingly, we found a lesser amount of nuclear FPN in FRDA cardiomyocytes with respect to controls, a result that seems to support the finding of DNA oxidative stress markers (8-OXO-dg) in FRDA patients [50]. On the other hand, the fact that FPN is less abundant in the nuclei of FRDA CMs than in controls is not necessarily in contradiction with the increase in both mRNA and protein FPN in FRDA

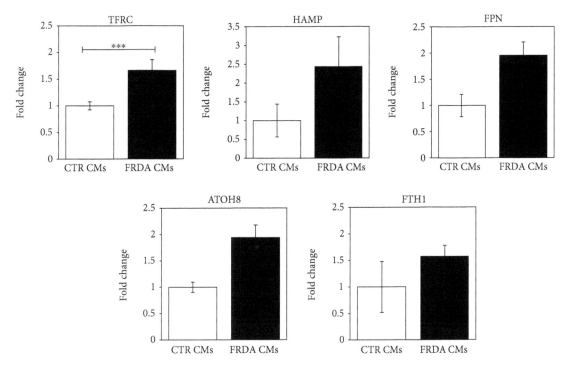

FIGURE 3: Gene expression of proteins involved in iron homeostasis in CTR and FRDA CMs. Expression levels of TFRC, HAMP, FPN, ATOH8, and FTH1 genes in CTR and FRDA CMs evaluated by qRT-PCR. Data were normalized with two housekeeping genes, β-actin and GAPDH; for each gene, the normalized expression value of CTR CMs was set to 1, and all other gene expression data were reported to that sample. Data are from four independent differentiation experiments and are expressed as mean $\pm$ SEM. ***$p < 0.001$.

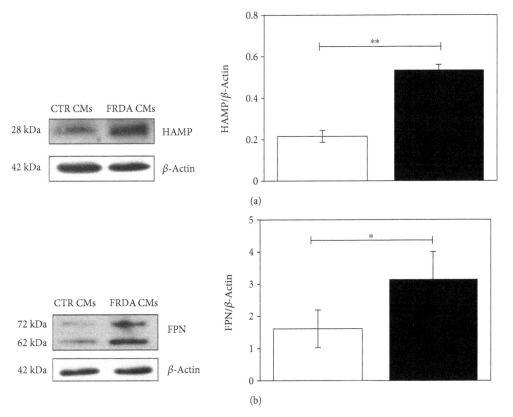

FIGURE 4: Protein expression of HAMP and FPN. (a) A representative Western blot image of HAMP expression. The band densities were analyzed by densitometry and normalized to β-actin. Histogram showing means $\pm$ Std Dev of HAMP/β-actin. (b) A representative Western blot image of FPN expression. The band densities were analyzed by densitometry and normalized to β-actin. Histogram showing means $\pm$ Std Dev of FPN/β-actin. Data are from three independent differentiation experiments. *$p < 0.05$; **$p < 0.01$.

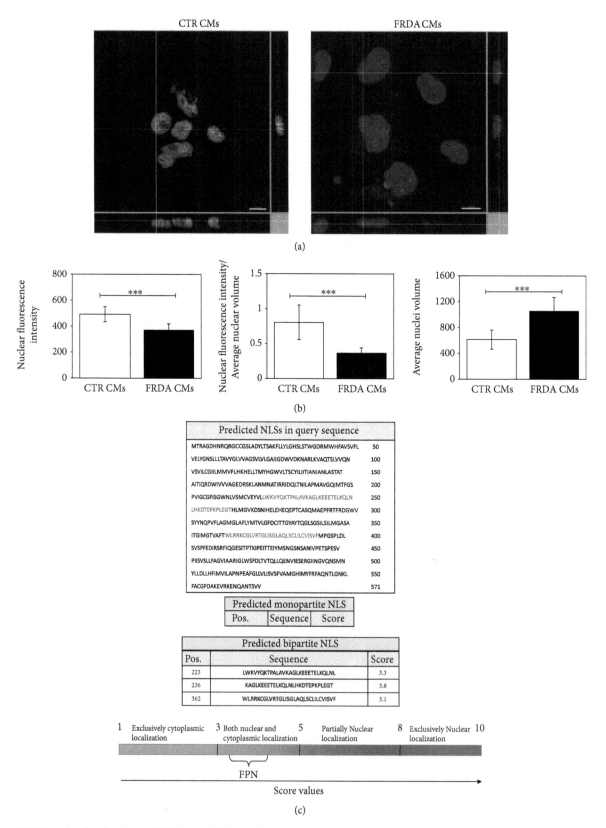

FIGURE 5: FPN nuclear localization in iPSC-derived CMs. (a) A representative confocal microscopy 3D image projection of FITC-stained FPN (green) protein expression in both CTR and FRDA CMs; the nuclei are counterstained with DAPI (blue). Scale bar equal 10 μm. (b) (i) Quantitative analysis of nuclear FITC fluorescence intensity in both CTR and FRDA CMs, (ii) quantitative analysis of nuclear FITC fluorescence intensity normalized to the average nuclear volume in both CTR and FRDA CMs, and (iii) average nuclear volume in both CTR and FRDA CMs; ***p < 0.001. (c) Bioinformatic analysis of FPN (NP_055400), using cNLS Mapper, predicted three bipartite NLS with a score value >3 indicating that the protein localizes both in the nucleus and in the cytoplasm.

cardiomyocytes, since Western blots were carried out in whole cell lysates, which include cytoplasmic FPN. A limitation of the present study is the lack of quantification of cytoplasmic FPN, either by confocal microscopy (which would require the delimitation of cell boundary by a specific staining) or by subcellular fractioning. This will be addressed by future studies.

The regulation of FPN distribution among the different subcellular compartments is a relevant issue, not yet afforded by researchers; in fact, the presence of 9-12 transmembrane domains supports its localization in the plasma membrane and its role of iron exporter and makes less likely a cytoplasmic and a nuclear localization. Thus, the nuclear localization of FPN we document here needs to be discussed not only in terms of novel FPN function(s), but also within the context of membrane and organelle trafficking and of final destination of proteins characterized by hydrophobic domains calling for a plasma membrane localization.

Finally, the presence of the enlarged nuclei, which was described here to occur in FRDA cardiomyocytes, has been reported in other cardiac pathologies, such as in hypertrophic and in dilated cardiomyopathy [51]. These morphological data need to be further investigated.

5. Conclusions

Cardiomyocytes derived from iPSCs retained the FRDA-like phenotype. Important alterations in the expression of HAMP and FPN, two proteins that play pivotal roles in cardiac iron homeostasis, are described here. Moreover, a novel nuclear localization of FPN in cardiomyocytes is reported, which suggests a potential new physiological function of this protein. These findings may have important implications in the understanding of cardiac iron homeostasis in both physiological and pathological conditions, such as FRDA. In particular, FRDA cardiomyocytes appear to be unable to exploit HAMP-operated regulation of FPN, which might be one of the reasons why iron distribution within the cell is impaired, thus leading to increase in the free iron pool. This, together with the defective assembly of mitochondrial proteins, would lead to chronic oxidative stress in FRDA cardiac cells. As pointed out by many authors [52–54], oxidative stress does not only lead to cell damage and apoptosis but also plays a role in adverse remodeling and contractile dysfunctions, as seen in FRDA patients.

Abbreviations

ATOH8:	Atonal BHLH transcription factor 8
BMPs:	Bone morphogenetic proteins
CMs:	Cardiomyocytes
DMT1:	Divalent metal transporter 1
FACS:	Flow cytometry
FPN:	Ferroportin
FRDA:	Friedreich's ataxia
FTH1:	Ferritin heavy chain 1
FXN:	Frataxin gene
GAPDH:	Glyceraldehyde-3-phosphate dehydrogenase
HAMP:	Hepcidin
HH:	Hereditary hemochromatosis
hiPSCs:	Human-induced pluripotent stem cells
IF:	Immunofluorescence
IREs:	Iron regulatory elements
IRPs:	Iron regulatory proteins
ISC:	Iron-sulfur cluster
LIP:	Labile iron pool
MF 20:	Myosin heavy chain
NLS:	Nuclear localization signal
ROS:	Reactive oxygen species
TFRC:	Transferrin receptor 1
TNNT2:	Cardiac troponin T
TMs:	Transmembrane domains.

Disclosure

The funding organizations had no role in the study design, data collection and analysis, decision to publish, or preparation of the manuscript.

Authors' Contributions

Marina Marini and Cinzia Zucchini share coseniorship.

Acknowledgments

This work has been supported by a grant from the AISA (Italian Association of Patients with Ataxic Syndrome) and by a grant from the "Fondazione Luisa Fanti Melloni," University of Bologna, Italy. The authors would like to thank Dr. Filippo Fortuna for believing in this research and for supporting it in any possible way and Dr. Martina Rossi for her help.

References

[1] R. Gozzelino and P. Arosio, "Iron homeostasis in health and disease," *International Journal of Molecular Sciences*, vol. 17, no. 1, 2016.

[2] M. F. Hoes, N. Grote Beverborg, J. D. Kijlstra et al., "Iron deficiency impairs contractility of human cardiomyocytes through decreased mitochondrial function," *European Journal of Heart Failure*, vol. 20, no. 5, pp. 910–919, 2018.

[3] S. Dev and J. L. Babitt, "Overview of iron metabolism in health and disease," *Hemodialysis International*, vol. 21, Supplement 1, pp. S6–S20, 2017.

[4] E. Gammella, S. Recalcati, I. Rybinska, P. Buratti, and G. Cairo, "Iron-induced damage in cardiomyopathy: oxidative-dependent and independent mechanisms," *Oxidative Medicine and Cellular Longevity*, vol. 2015, Article ID 230182, 10 pages, 2015.

[5] D. J. R. Lane, A. M. Merlot, M. L.-H. Huang et al., "Cellular iron uptake, trafficking and metabolism: key molecules and mechanisms and their roles in disease," *Biochimica et Biophysica Acta (BBA) - Molecular Cell Research*, vol. 1853, no. 5, pp. 1130–1144, 2015.

[6] K. C. Kondapalli, N. M. Kok, A. Dancis, and T. L. Stemmler, "Drosophila frataxin: an iron chaperone during cellular Fe-S cluster bioassembly," *Biochemistry*, vol. 47, no. 26, pp. 6917–6927, 2008.

[7] S. Abboud and D. J. Haile, "A novel mammalian iron-regulated protein involved in intracellular iron metabolism," *Journal of Biological Chemistry*, vol. 275, no. 26, pp. 19906–19912, 2000.

[8] A. Donovan, A. Brownlie, Y. Zhou et al., "Positional cloning of zebrafish ferroportin1 identifies a conserved vertebrate iron exporter," *Nature*, vol. 403, no. 6771, pp. 776–781, 2000.

[9] A. T. McKie, P. Marciani, A. Rolfs et al., "A novel duodenal iron-regulated transporter, IREG1, implicated in the basolateral transfer of iron to the circulation," *Molecular Cell*, vol. 5, no. 2, pp. 299–309, 2000.

[10] H. Drakesmith, E. Nemeth, and T. Ganz, "Ironing out ferroportin," *Cell Metabolism*, vol. 22, no. 5, pp. 777–787, 2015.

[11] D. M. Ward and J. Kaplan, "Ferroportin-mediated iron transport: expression and regulation," *Biochimica et Biophysica Acta*, vol. 1823, no. 9, pp. 1426–1433, 2012.

[12] I. De Domenico, D. M. Ward, G. Musci, and J. Kaplan, "Evidence for the multimeric structure of ferroportin," *Blood*, vol. 109, no. 5, pp. 2205–2209, 2007.

[13] E. Pignatti, L. Mascheroni, M. Sabelli, S. Barelli, S. Biffo, and A. Pietrangelo, "Ferroportin is a monomer in vivo in mice," *Blood Cells, Molecules, and Diseases*, vol. 36, no. 1, pp. 26–32, 2006.

[14] A. E. Rice, M. J. Mendez, C. A. Hokanson, D. C. Rees, and P. J. Bjorkman, "Investigation of the biophysical and cell biological properties of ferroportin, a multipass integral membrane protein iron exporter," *Journal of Molecular Biology*, vol. 386, no. 3, pp. 717–732, 2009.

[15] D. Vela, "Balance of cardiac and systemic hepcidin and its role in heart physiology and pathology," *Laboratory Investigation*, vol. 98, no. 3, pp. 315–326, 2018.

[16] P. J. Schmidt, "Regulation of iron metabolism by hepcidin under conditions of inflammation," *Journal of Biological Chemistry*, vol. 290, no. 31, pp. 18975–18983, 2015.

[17] L. Kautz, D. Meynard, A. Monnier et al., "Iron regulates phosphorylation of Smad1/5/8 and gene expression of Bmp6, Smad7, Id1, and Atoh8 in the mouse liver," *Blood*, vol. 112, no. 4, pp. 1503–1509, 2008.

[18] U. Merle, E. Fein, S. G. Gehrke, W. Stremmel, and H. Kulaksiz, "The iron regulatory peptide hepcidin is expressed in the heart and regulated by hypoxia and inflammation," *Endocrinology*, vol. 148, no. 6, pp. 2663–2668, 2007.

[19] G. Simonis, K. Mueller, P. Schwarz et al., "The iron-regulatory peptide hepcidin is upregulated in the ischemic and in the remote myocardium after myocardial infarction," *Peptides*, vol. 31, no. 9, pp. 1786–1790, 2010.

[20] L. Zhang, D. Lu, W. Zhang et al., "Cardioprotection by Hepc1 in cTnTR141W transgenic mice," *Transgenic Research*, vol. 21, no. 4, pp. 867–878, 2012.

[21] Y. P. Hsieh, C. H. Huang, C. Y. Lee, C. Y. Lin, and C. C. Chang, "Silencing of hepcidin enforces the apoptosis in iron-induced human cardiomyocytes," *Journal of Occupational Medicine and Toxicology*, vol. 9, no. 1, p. 11, 2014.

[22] S. Lakhal-Littleton, M. Wolna, C. A. Carr et al., "Cardiac ferroportin regulates cellular iron homeostasis and is important for cardiac function," *Proceedings of the National Academy of Sciences*, vol. 112, no. 10, pp. 3164–3169, 2015.

[23] S. Lakhal-Littleton, M. Wolna, Y. J. Chung et al., "An essential cell-autonomous role for hepcidin in cardiac iron homeostasis," *Elife*, vol. 5, 2016.

[24] A. H. Koeppen, R. L. Ramirez, A. B. Becker et al., "The pathogenesis of cardiomyopathy in Friedreich ataxia," *PLoS One*, vol. 10, no. 3, article e0116396, 2015.

[25] Y. Wu and R. M. Brosh, "DNA helicase and helicase-nuclease enzymes with a conserved iron-sulfur cluster," *Nucleic Acids Research*, vol. 40, no. 10, pp. 4247–4260, 2012.

[26] A. S. Fleischhacker and P. J. Kiley, "Iron-containing transcription factors and their roles as sensors," *Current Opinion in Chemical Biology*, vol. 15, no. 2, pp. 335–341, 2011.

[27] K. J. Thompson, M. G. Fried, Z. Ye, P. Boyer, and J. R. Connor, "Regulation, mechanisms and proposed function of ferritin translocation to cell nuclei," *Journal of Cell Science*, vol. 115, Part 10, pp. 2165–2177, 2002.

[28] S. Michael, S. V. Petrocine, J. Qian et al., "Iron and iron-responsive proteins in the cardiomyopathy of Friedreich's ataxia," *Cerebellum*, vol. 5, no. 4, pp. 257–267, 2006.

[29] A. Y. Tsou, E. K. Paulsen, S. J. Lagedrost et al., "Mortality in Friedreich ataxia," *Journal of the Neurological Sciences*, vol. 307, no. 1-2, pp. 46–49, 2011.

[30] V. Campuzano, L. Montermini, M. D. Molto et al., "Friedreich's ataxia: autosomal recessive disease caused by an intronic GAA triplet repeat expansion," *Science*, vol. 271, no. 5254, pp. 1423–1427, 1996.

[31] M. Pandolfo, "Iron metabolism and mitochondrial abnormalities in Friedreich ataxia," *Blood Cells, Molecules and Diseases*, vol. 29, no. 3, pp. 536–547, 2002.

[32] K. Takahashi and S. Yamanaka, "Induction of pluripotent stem cells from mouse embryonic and adult fibroblast cultures by defined factors," *Cell*, vol. 126, no. 4, pp. 663–676, 2006.

[33] X. Lian, J. Zhang, S. M. Azarin et al., "Directed cardiomyocyte differentiation from human pluripotent stem cells by modulating Wnt/β-catenin signaling under fully defined conditions," *Nature Protocols*, vol. 8, no. 1, pp. 162–175, 2012.

[34] P. M. Abruzzo, M. Marini, A. Bolotta et al., "Frataxin mRNA isoforms in FRDA patients and normal subjects: effect of

tocotrienol supplementation," *BioMed Research International*, vol. 2013, Article ID 276808, 9 pages, 2013.

[35] K. J. Livak and T. D. Schmittgen, "Analysis of relative gene expression data using real-time quantitative PCR and the 2(-delta delta C(T)) method," *Methods*, vol. 25, no. 4, pp. 402–408, 2001.

[36] M. W. Pfaffl, "A new mathematical model for relative quantification in real-time RT-PCR," *Nucleic Acids Research*, vol. 29, no. 9, pp. 45e–445, 2001.

[37] S. Kosugi, M. Hasebe, N. Matsumura et al., "Six classes of nuclear localization signals specific to different binding grooves of importin α," *Journal of Biological Chemistry*, vol. 284, no. 1, pp. 478–485, 2008.

[38] N. C. Dubois, A. M. Craft, P. Sharma et al., "SIRPA is a specific cell-surface marker for isolating cardiomyocytes derived from human pluripotent stem cells," *Nature Biotechnology*, vol. 29, no. 11, pp. 1011–1018, 2011.

[39] S. L. Ross, K. Biswas, J. Rottman et al., "Identification of antibody and small molecule antagonists of ferroportin-hepcidin interaction," *Frontiers in Pharmacology*, vol. 8, p. 838, 2017.

[40] A. Hick, M. Wattenhofer-Donze, S. Chintawar et al., "Neurons and cardiomyocytes derived from induced pluripotent stem cells as a model for mitochondrial defects in Friedreich's ataxia," *Disease Models & Mechanisms*, vol. 6, no. 3, pp. 608–621, 2013.

[41] H. Puccio, D. Simon, M. Cossée et al., "Mouse models for Friedreich ataxia exhibit cardiomyopathy, sensory nerve defect and Fe-S enzyme deficiency followed by intramitochondrial iron deposits," *Nature Genetics*, vol. 27, no. 2, pp. 181–186, 2001.

[42] Y.-K. Lee, P. W.-L. Ho, R. Schick et al., "Modeling of Friedreich ataxia-related iron overloading cardiomyopathy using patient-specific-induced pluripotent stem cells," *Pflügers Archiv - European Journal of Physiology*, vol. 466, no. 9, pp. 1831–1844, 2014.

[43] A. Raha, R. Vaishnav, R. Friedland, A. Bomford, and R. Raha-Chowdhury, "The systemic iron-regulatory proteins hepcidin and ferroportin are reduced in the brain in Alzheimer's disease," *Acta Neuropathologica Communications*, vol. 1, no. 1, p. 55, 2013.

[44] M. L.-H. Huang, E. M. Becker, M. Whitnall, Y. S. Rahmanto, P. Ponka, and D. R. Richardson, "Elucidation of the mechanism of mitochondrial iron loading in Friedreich's ataxia by analysis of a mouse mutant," *Proceedings of the National Academy of Sciences*, vol. 106, no. 38, pp. 16381–16386, 2009.

[45] M. Perdomini, A. Hick, H. Puccio, and M. A. Pook, "Animal and cellular models of Friedreich ataxia," *Journal of Neurochemistry*, vol. 126, Supplement 1, pp. 65–79, 2013.

[46] X. B. Liu, F. Yang, and D. J. Haile, "Functional consequences of ferroportin 1 mutations," *Blood Cells, Molecules, and Diseases*, vol. 35, no. 1, pp. 33–46, 2005.

[47] A. Fernandes, G. C. Preza, Y. Phung et al., "The molecular basis of hepcidin-resistant hereditary hemochromatosis," *Blood*, vol. 114, no. 2, pp. 437–443, 2009.

[48] J. B. Jordan, L. Poppe, M. Haniu et al., "Hepcidin revisited, disulfide connectivity, dynamics, and structure," *Journal of Biological Chemistry*, vol. 284, no. 36, pp. 24155–24167, 2009.

[49] E. S. Henle, Z. Han, N. Tang, P. Rai, Y. Luo, and S. Linn, "Sequence-specific DNA cleavage by Fe2+-mediated Fenton reactions has possible biological implications," *Journal of Biological Chemistry*, vol. 274, no. 2, pp. 962–971, 1999.

[50] J. B. Schulz, T. Dehmer, L. Schols et al., "Oxidative stress in patients with Friedreich ataxia," *Neurology*, vol. 55, no. 11, pp. 1719–1721, 2000.

[51] P. A. Harvey and L. A. Leinwand, "The cell biology of disease: cellular mechanisms of cardiomyopathy," *The Journal of Cell Biology*, vol. 194, no. 3, pp. 355–365, 2011.

[52] M. Seddon, Y. H. Looi, and A. M. Shah, "Oxidative stress and redox signalling in cardiac hypertrophy and heart failure," *Heart*, vol. 93, no. 8, pp. 903–907, 2007.

[53] D. B. Sawyer, "Oxidative stress in heart failure: what are we missing?," *The American Journal of the Medical Sciences*, vol. 342, no. 2, pp. 120–124, 2011.

[54] H. Tsutsui, S. Kinugawa, and S. Matsushima, "Oxidative stress and heart failure," *American Journal of Physiology-Heart and Circulatory Physiology*, vol. 301, no. 6, pp. H2181–H2190, 2011.

5

Quantile Regression Analysis of Depression and Clinical Symptom Degree in Chinese Patients with Spinocerebellar Ataxia Type 3

Xiaoping Chen, Lihui Zheng⑩, and Jianqi Yao

Department of Statistics, College of Mathematics and Informatics & FJKLMAA, Fujian Normal University, Fuzhou 350000, China

Correspondence should be addressed to Lihui Zheng; fbx20180024@yjs.fjnu.edu.cn

Academic Editor: Chenxi Huang

Spinal cerebellar ataxia type 3 is a common SCA subtype in the world. It is a neurodegenerative disease characterized by ataxia. Patients exhibit common neuropsychological symptoms such as depression and anxiety. Some patients have suicidal tendencies when they are severely depressed. So, it is very important to study the severity of depression and clinical symptoms (SARA), to find out the patient's psychological state in time and to help patients actively respond to treatment. A total of 97 Chinese SCA3 patients were enrolled in the study. The Beck Depression Scale was used to investigate the prevalence of depression in the confirmed patients. The distribution of depression data in these patients was investigated. Then, the quantifier was used to model the depression status of Chinese SCA3 patients. An analysis was conducted to identify the key factors affecting depression under different quantiles. Studies have shown that SARA and gender are important factors affecting depression; the effect of initial SARA is small, then the degree of influence increases, and the degree of influence decreases in the later period, but it is always positively correlated with depression; the development of women's SARA is gentler than that of men, and the degree of depression is lower than that of men.

1. Introduction

Machado–Joseph disease or spinocerebellar ataxia 3 (MJD/SCA3) is a clinically heterogeneous, neurodegenerative disorder characterized by varying degrees of ataxia, ophthalmoplegia, peripheral neuropathy, pyramidal dysfunction, and movement disorder. MJD/SCA3 is caused by a CAG repeat expansion mutation in the protein coding region of the ATXN3 gene located at chromosome 14q32.1 [1]. So far, the pathogenesis and pathological effects of such diseases have not been clarified, and there was no effective treatment. Conventional treatment can only improve the clinical symptoms.

Previous studies on SCA3 focused the pathogenesis of SCA3, CAG mutation amplification, and ethnic differences. In the study of the role of the proteasome in the pathogenesis of SCA3/MJD, it was found that the proteasome plays a direct role in suppressing polyglutamine aggregation in disease. Also, the result suggested that modulating proteasome activity is a potential approach to altering the progression of this and other polyglutamine diseases [2]. The CAG repeat amplified in the SCA3 gene caused the patient's restless legs syndrome (RLS) and sleep impairment, and impaired sleep in SCA3 was associated with older age, longstanding disease, and brainstem involvement [3]. There were significant differences in predominant spinopontine atrophy, lack of dystonic features, and larger CAG repeat expansion between families with spinal cord ataxia 3 in two different ethnic origins in the United States [4]. The frequency of trinucleotide repeats in different ataxic categories in Chinese patients was studied to find that the frequency of SCA3/MJD is substantially higher than that of SCA1 and SCA2 in patients with autosomal dominant SCA from Chinese kindreds, who are non-Portuguese. Dementia and hyporeflexia were more frequent in patients with SCA2, while spasticity, hyperreflexia, and Babinski signs were more frequent in patients with SCA3/MJD, and those might be helpful in clinical work to primarily distinguish patients with

SCA3/MJD and SCA2 from others with different types of SCA [5].

SCA3 not only affected patients' ataxia and cognitive ability but also led to depression or anxiety with the development of the disease, seriously affecting patients' physical and mental health. Foreign studies, namely, the study of stuneuropsychological and neurobehavioral characteristics of SCA3 patients and the degree of emotional dysfunction of patients, found that, in addition to anxiety and depression, SCA3 patients also showed the development of increased apathy [6]. The research on the influence between SCAs depression and ataxia found that depression was very common in SCA and would not develop in 2 years. The suicidal ideation of SCA3 patients was significantly higher than that of other types, and there were differences in the suicidal ideation of SCA patients in different regions (North America and Europe). The effect of depression on the progression of ataxia varies by the SCA type [7]. Depression in patients with SCA3 has also been studied in China. Through the establishment of multiple linear equations, it was found that depression is caused by the movement disorder caused by ataxia. In addition, the two had interaction, and gender and ICARS were important factors affecting depression [8].

In summary, domestic and foreign scholars have conducted a large number of in-depth studies on the factors affecting the incidence of SCA3 and other related content. However, there are a few studies on depression in Chinese SCA3 patients, and the main method is linear regression. There are a few studies combining the quantile regression method with the influencing factors of depression in Chinese SCA3 patients. Considering the quantile, regression can effectively avoid the heteroscedasticity and nonnormal distribution of the data, and with the change of the quantile used, it can more accurately describe the influence of independent variables on dependent variables and characterize the conditional distribution. Therefore, it is necessary to study the factors affecting the quantile regression in SCA3 patients with depression.

2. Objects and Methods

2.1. Study Subjects. Participants in this study included 97 patients with confirmed SCA3, all of whom over 18 years of age. This study was approved by the ethics committee of the first affiliated hospital of Fujian Medical University. Written informed consent forms were signed by all subjects.

2.2. Observation Method. Beck depression inventory (BDI) was used to evaluate the severity of depression in SCA3 patients. There were 21 questions in the whole scale, and each question was divided into different grades. According to the total score of the scale, the severity of depressive symptoms can be evaluated. In this study, a BDI score greater than or equal to 19 was defined as clinically related depression [8].

The severity of the patient was assessed using the ataxia rating scale (SARA). SARA is a semiquantitative neurologic functional assessment scale that describes and quantitatively evaluates symptoms of cerebellar ataxia.

2.3. Statistical Analyses. Firstly, the data set was descriptively analyzed. The K-S discriminant method was used to analyze the normal distribution of data variables, and the mean and median values of the variables in the nondepressive group and the depression group were calculated.

Secondly, using univariate and multivariate quantile regression, different vacancies were taken, and the significance and correlation of each variable were judged according to the test P value. The density function maps of depression and SARA were plotted, as well as the density function maps by gender. The density function maps of depression BDI scores at 10% and 90% of the SARA were plotted. The dependent variable was the depression BDI score (Beck), and the independent variables were the gender, SARA score, disease duration, age of onset, small CAG, and large CAG.

Quantile regression [9] was a modeling method to estimate the relationship between regression variable x and dependent variable y at any probability level. Suppose the distribution function of the random variable was $F(y) = \text{Prob}(Y \leq y)$, and define the τ quantile of y to be

$$Q(\tau) = \inf\{y: F(y) \geq \tau\}, \quad 0 < \tau < 1. \quad (1)$$

When τ was equal to 1/2, that was the median. In the quantile regression model, the loss function was defined as a piecewise linear function:

$$\rho_\tau(u) = (\tau - I(u < 0))u, \quad u = y_i - \widehat{\xi}, \quad (2)$$

where $\widehat{\xi}$ was the expectation $E(y)$ of the dependent variable and I was the indicator function. The basic idea of regression analysis was to minimize the distance between the sample value and the fitting value, so the optimization problem from the loss function expectation can be converted to another form:

$$\min \sum_{i=1}^{n} \rho_\tau(y_i - \widehat{\xi}). \quad (3)$$

Given the information set x and condition $Q_\tau(\varepsilon \mid x) = 0$, the conditional quantile function of y can be expressed as $Q_y(\tau \mid x) = x'\beta_\tau$.

The software tool was the R 3.5.1 version. Model results were significant at $P < 0.05$ and were statistically significant.

3. Result

3.1. Variable Descriptive Statistics. Of the 97 patients with SCA3, 41 were nondepressed and 56 were depressed. The depression rate was 57.73%, and SCA3 patients had a higher depression rate. The mean course of the patients with depression (9.259 ± 8.0) was significantly larger than that of the nondepressed group (6.329 ± 6); SARA (13.22 ± 13) was higher than that of nondepressed patients (8.085 ± 7). The depression degree (33.21 ± 32) in the depression group was 4 times higher than that in the nondepression group

TABLE 1: Descriptive statistics of variables.

	Distribution	Nondepressed group	Depression group
Number	——	41	56
Gender (M/F)	——	19/22	35/21
CAG small	Skewed	20.9 ± 20	21.57 ± 14
CAG large	Normal	74.34 ± 74.34	74.84 ± 75
Age at onset (years)	Normal	35.24 ± 34	33.59 ± 34.5
Disease duration	Skewed	6.329 ± 6	9.259 ± 8.0
SARA	Skewed	8.085 ± 7	13.22 ± 13
BDI score	Normal	8.878 ± 9	33.21 ± 32

TABLE 2: Univariate regression results.

	OLS	$Q_\tau(0.1 \mid X)$	$Q_\tau(0.25 \mid X)$	$Q_\tau(0.5 \mid X)$	$Q_\tau(0.75 \mid X)$	$Q_\tau(0.9 \mid X)$
CAG small	-0.005	$1.202e - 17$	0.233	-0.116	0.071	-0.02
CAG large	0.032	0.333	0.75	0.25	-0.833	$-1.33 ** (0.00092)$
Age at onset (years)	0.059	0	-0.154	-0.2	0.36	$0.429 ** (0.0005)$
Disease duration	$0.924 ** (0.00101)$	0.538	$1.190 * (0.012)$	$1.333 ** (0.00036)$	$0.9375 * (0.012)$	$0.571 ** (0.005)$
SARA	$0.952 ** (3.25e - 06)$	$0.727 ** (0.0043)$	$0.868 ** (0.0024)$	$1.273 ** (3.044e - 05)$	$0.765 ** (0.004)$	$0.647 ** (0.00057)$

Note. (1) If the P value is less than 0.01, it is considered that the effect of the independent variable is highly significant, which is represented by "$**$." (2) If the P value is less than 0.05, it is considered that the effect of the independent variable is significant, which is indicated by "$*$."

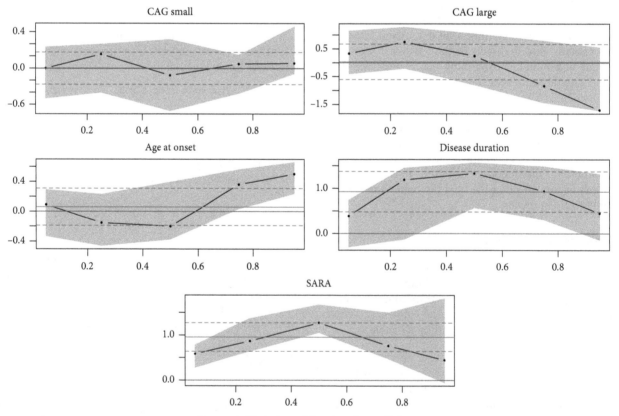

FIGURE 1: Variation of the quantile coefficient.

(8.878 ± 9), and the depression degree was relatively deep. In the data, the small CAG, the disease duration, and SARA were skewed. The large CAG, the age of onset, and Beck were normally distributed. Therefore, it is more appropriate to use the quantile regression relative least squares regression (the data are shown in Table 1).

TABLE 3: Estimated values of each quantile parameter.

	OLS		$Q_\tau(0.05 \mid X)$		$Q_\tau(0.1 \mid X)$		$Q_\tau(0.25 \mid X)$	
	Estimated value	P	Estimated value	P	Estimated value	P	Estimated value	P
(Intercept)	14.223	$2.15e{-}07$	-3.26	0.189	0.2	0.920	4.143	0.170
Gender (F)	$-6.196*$	0.0181	$-6.282*$	0.038	-3.4	0.296	-4.143	0.184
SARA	$1.036**$	$4.48e{-}07$	$1.026**$	$1.098e{-}07$	$0.8**$	$4.08e{-}07$	$0.905**$	$7.7e{-}4$
	$Q_\tau(0.5 \mid X)$		$Q_\tau(0.6 \mid X)$		$Q_\tau(0.75 \mid X)$		$Q_\tau(0.9 \mid X)$	
	Estimated value	P	Estimated value	P	Estimated value	P	Estimated value	P
(Intercept)	11.571	$3.3e{-}03$	31.795	0.58844	24	$5.0e{-}09$	34	$1.25e{-}10$
Gender (F)	-6.0	0.102	$-10.506**$	0.00049	$-9*$	0.019	-5	0.18
SARA	$1.238**$	$3.1e{-}06$	$1.010**$	0.00000	$1*$	$1.48e{-}05$	$0.67*$	0.02

Note. (1) If the P value is less than 0.01, it is considered that the effect of the independent variable is highly significant, which is represented by "$**$." (2) If the P value is less than 0.05, it is considered that the effect of the independent variable is significant, which is indicated by "$*$."

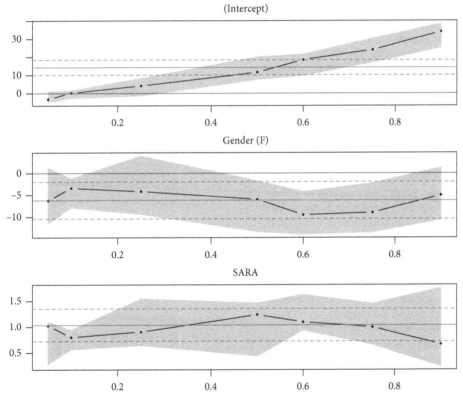

FIGURE 2: Variation of the quantile coefficient.

3.2. Univariate Regression Analysis. The Beck depression score was used as the dependent variable, and the CAG small, CAG large, age of onset, course of disease, and SARA were used as independent variables. Quantile regression and OLS regression were used to model the variables. The results were as shown in Table 2. From the regression results of the OLS model, it can be seen that in the linear regression model, the duration of disease, and SARA have a significant positive effect on depression. The longer the duration of disease is, the greater will be the SARA score and the more severe the depression will be. However, the CAG small, CAG large, and age of onset had no effect on depression.

The OLS model required that all variables obey normal distribution, but some of the data were biased. The validity of

the OLS model fitting was limited, while the quantile regression did not require normal distribution. Columns 3–7 showed the quantile regression coefficients, and P values in parentheses. Compared with the regression coefficients of the OLS model, the quantile regression coefficients changed. The variation of the coefficients is shown in Figure 1, where the red horizontal line represents the OLS regression coefficient and the curve represents variation of the quantile regression coefficient.

In the quantile regression, the CAG was not significant at each quantile. The CAG and the onset age were not significant at other quantile, and only had an effect on depression at 90%. At this time, CAG was negatively correlated (-1.33). The age of onset was positively correlated (0.429). From the low quantile to the high quantile, the CAG large coefficient symbol changed from positive to negative, and the onset age coefficient symbol changed from negative to positive.

SARA was significant at each quantile. The course of the disease was 10%, and the others were significant. The two variables were positively correlated with depression and the same as the univariate linear regression coefficient. When considering the univariate influence on depression, SARA and disease duration were important variables.

3.3. Multivariate Quantile Regression. In the establishment of multiple quantile regression, variable modeling with higher significance should be selected as far as possible. So, the course of disease and SARA were selected as independent variables. In the study of Lin et al. [8], gender was found to be an important factor affecting depression. So, gender was also selected as an independent variable. Through preliminary modeling, it was found that the disease course coefficient is not significant. Therefore, the disease course was excluded, and only the quantile model of SARA and gender was established.

The *R* software was used to conduct quantile regression on SCA3 patient data. Table 3 lists the parameter estimation, *P* value, and significance results of different quantile points $\tau = (0.05, 0.1, 0.25, 0.5, 0.6, 0.75, 0.9)$ in quantile regression.

Comparing the results of parameter estimation under 7 quantiles, it can be seen that SARA has always played a significant role, and the gender was significant when the quantile was 0.05, 0.6, and 0.75. Figure 2 is the parameter estimation chart of each variable under each quantile. In the figure, it can be seen that although the coefficients of the SARA points that have a significant effect on depression are changing, they were always positive, indicating a positive correlation with depression. When the quantile was small, it can be seen that the SARA coefficient has a decreasing trend. It showed that the effect of SARA on depression was small in the initial period of time. With the increase of SARA, the degree of depression will be aggravated, and the decrease in the coefficient value indicated that the development of SARA to the later stage has a reduced impact on depression.

Gender (female) was negatively correlated with depression, and only became significant when the coefficient value was less than about −6. When the depression score was used as the dependent variable, gender and SARA were used as independent variables to establish linear multiple regression. The coefficient of gender (female) was −6.196, the quantile at this time was between about 0.5 and 0.8, and the degree of depression in women was lower than that in men.

3.4. Density Function Diagram. Furthermore, the density function diagram of BDI scores and SARA, as well as the density function diagram of male and female, was drawn. From Figure 3, it can be more intuitively seen that the BDI score distribution was close to the normal distribution, and SARA presented a skewed distribution. The peak BDI scores of women and men were different, about 10 for women and

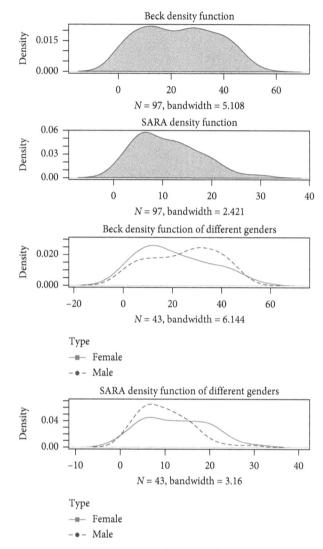

FIGURE 3: BDI score and the SARA density function.

35 for men. The distribution of the SARA density function was relatively flat for women and steep for men.

In order to study the effect of SARA on depression, the effects of clinical symptom severity on low and high scores were compared, and the comparison of BDI scores at 10% and 90% of SARA was drawn (90% is the blue dotted line). From Figure 4, it can be found that the BDI scores of SARA at different points were significantly different. The higher the value of SARA, the higher the BDI score. The right figure reflected the density image of the BDI score in the case of a large SARA value and small SARA value. The larger SARA value was, the larger the BDI score was. The BDI score with a small SARA value was concentrated around 5, while the BDI score with a large SARA value was concentrated around 40.

4. Discussion

In this study, SCA3 patients had a higher rate of depression, and SARA had a significant effect on depression. In the early stage of development, SARA had less effect on depression. At this time, the patient's depressive symptoms were not

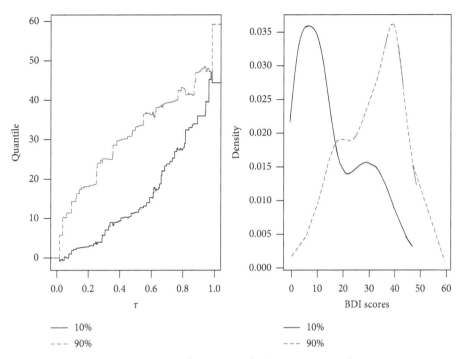

FIGURE 4: BDI score density map for SARA at 10% and 90%.

obvious. With the aggravation of clinical symptoms, depression of patients will be more affected and may be accompanied by anxiety, apathy, and other manifestations. By the end of the disease, SARA still had an effect on depression, but the degree of influence was reduced. Lo et al. [7] mentioned in their study that depression was very common in SCA and will not develop in 2 years. Therefore, it was speculated that the initial period when SARA has a small impact on depression may be 2 years. After 2 years, we need to pay attention to the impact of SARA on patients' depression. Some SCA3 patients in this article were also accompanied by suicidal tendencies, lethargy, fatigue, etc, which seriously affected the quality of life and physical health of patients. From the early stage of the disease, it was necessary to pay attention to the depressive symptoms and psychological state of SCA3 patients. The treatment of depressive symptoms may be beneficial to improve the clinical symptoms of patients and reduce the risk of suicide.

Gender was also an important factor affecting patients' depression. In this study, the depression degree of women was lower than that of men. Considering that the graph of SARA density function of women presents a relatively flat state and that of men was rather steep, the difference in SARA development between men and women may be the reason for the difference in depression. Therefore, SARA

development of SCA3 patients of different genders can be considered in subsequent studies and targeted treatment programs for depression.

Acknowledgments

The authors sincerely thank the participants for their help and willingness to participate in this study. This study was supported by the National Natural Science Foundation of China (11601083 and U1805263), the Program for Probability and Statistics: Theory and Application (IRTL1704), and Innovative Research Team in Science and Technology in Fujian Province University (IRTSTFJ).

References

[1] A. D'Abreu, M. C. França, H. L. Paulson et al., "Caring for Machado–Joseph disease:Current under-standing and how to help patients," *Parkinsonism and Related Disorders*, vol. 16, no. 1, pp. 2–7, 2010.

[2] Y. Chai, S. L. Koppenhafer, S. J. Shoesmith, M. K. Perez, and H. L. Paulson, "Evidence for proteasome involvement in polyglutamine disease: localization to nuclear inclusions in SCA3/MJD and suppression of polyglutamine aggregation in vitro," *Human Molecular Genetics*, vol. 8, no. 4, pp. 673–682, 1999.

[3] L. Schols, J. Haan, O. Riess, G. Amoiridis, and H. Przuntek, "Sleep disturbance in spinocerebellar ataxias: is the SCA3

mutation a cause of restless legs syndrome?" *Neurology*, vol. 51, no. 6, pp. 1603–1607, 1998.

[4] J. J. Higgins, L. E. Nee, O. Vasconcelos et al., "Mutations in American families with spinocerebellar ataxia (SCA) type 3: SCA3 is allelic to Machado-Joseph disease," *Neurology*, vol. 46, no. 1, pp. 208–213, 1996.

[5] B. Tang, C. Liu, L. Shen et al., "Frequency of SCA1, SCA2, SCA3/MJD, SCA6, SCA7, and DRPLA CAG trinucleotide repeat expansion in patients with hereditary spinocerebellar ataxia from Chinese kindreds," *Archives of Neurology*, vol. 57, no. 4, pp. 540–544, 2000.

[6] T. M. Zawacki, J. Grace, J. H. Friedman, and L. Sudarsky, "Executive and emotional dysfunction in Machado-Joseph disease," *Movement Disorders*, vol. 17, no. 5, pp. 1004–1010, 2002.

[7] R. Y. Lo, K. P. Figueroa, S. M. Pulst et al., "Depression and clinical progression in spinocerebellar ataxias," *Parkinsonism & Related Disorders*, vol. 22, pp. 87–92, 2016.

[8] M.-T. Lin, J.-S. Yang, P.-P. Chen et al., "Bidirectional connections between depression and ataxia severity in spinocerebellar ataxia type 3 patients," *European Neurology*, vol. 79, no. 5-6, pp. 266–271, 2018.

[9] L. Hao and D. Q. Naiman, *Quantile Regression*, pp. 40–52, SAGE Publications Inc, Thousand Oaks, CA, USA, 2007.

6

Analysis of Residual DSBs in Ataxia-Telangiectasia Lymphoblast Cells Initiating Apoptosis

Teresa Anglada, Mariona Terradas, Laia Hernández, Anna Genescà, and Marta Martín

Departament de Biologia Cel·lular, Fisiologia i Immunologia, Universitat Autònoma de Barcelona, Edifici C, Bellaterra, 08193 Cerdanyola del Vallès, Spain

Correspondence should be addressed to Marta Martín; marta.martin@uab.cat

Academic Editor: Yi-Xiang Wang

In order to examine the relationship between accumulation of residual DNA double-strand breaks (DSBs) and cell death, we have used a control and an ATM (Ataxia-Telangiectasia Mutated) defective cell line, as Ataxia-Telangiectasia (AT) cells tend to accumulate residual DSBs at long times after damage infliction. After irradiation, AT cells showed checkpoint impairment and a fraction of cells displayed an abnormal centrosome number and tetraploid DNA content, and this fraction increased along with apoptosis rates. At all times analyzed, AT cells displayed a significantly higher rate of radiation-induced apoptosis than normal cells. Besides apoptosis, 70–85% of the AT viable cells (TUNEL-negative) carried ≥10 γH2AX foci/cell, while only 12–27% of normal cells did. The fraction of AT and normal cells undergoing early and late apoptosis were isolated by flow cytometry and residual DSBs were concretely scored in these populations. Half of the γH2AX-positive AT cells undergoing early apoptosis carried ≥10 γH2AX foci/cell and this fraction increased to 75% in late apoptosis. The results suggest that retention of DNA damage-induced γH2AX foci is an indicative of lethal DNA damage, as cells undergoing apoptosis are those accumulating more DSBs. Scoring of residual γH2AX foci might function as a predictive tool to assess radiation-induced apoptosis.

1. Introduction

Following DNA double-strand breaks (DSBs) generation by ionizing radiation (IR), the cell undergoes an Ataxia-Telangiectasia Mutated (ATM) dependent p53 activation of the DNA damage response (DDR) cascade to activate the cell checkpoints in order to gain time for DNA repair [1–3]. If the DNA damage cannot be repaired during checkpoint arrest, cells are driven to undergo an irreversible fate by apoptosis or senescence [4, 5]. Sensing of the DNA damage involves the extensive phosphorylation of histone H2AX molecules at both sides of the DNA break [6]. Phosphorylated H2AX forms foci immediately after DNA damage induction by IR. These γH2AX IRIF (Ionizing Radiation-Induced Foci) are detectable with immunostaining or cytometry techniques as soon as 3 minutes afterwards, and the maximum number of foci is detected 30–60 minutes after irradiation [7]. The number of γH2AX foci has been found to closely correlate with the number of radiation-induced DSBs [8, 9]. Very soon after irradiation, γH2AX foci are numerous and small and

they disappear along with resolution of DNA damage [8]. Nonetheless, several results have shown that radiosensitive cell lines retain γH2AX foci longer than radioresistant cell lines after exposure to radiation [10–12]. The fraction of tumor cells that retain γH2AX foci 24 hours after irradiation has been correlated with the fraction of cells that fail to divide and form colonies [13, 14], suggesting that the H2AX assay can be used as an indicator of cell death. However, there are also negative studies that found no correlation between γH2AX and clonogenic cell survival [15, 16], demonstrating that it is yet unclear whether residual DSBs are ultimately related with apoptosis triggering.

Recently, apoptosis and mitotic catastrophe (MC) have been functionally linked [17, 18]. MC has been defined as an oncosuppressive mechanism resulting from a combination of deficient cell cycle checkpoints, persistence of DNA damage and mitotic failure, which can ultimately lead to cell death during mitosis or alternatively by apoptosis or senescence. This mechanism mainly operates in a cell-cycle-specific kinases-dependent and p53-dependent way to avoid accumulation of genomic instability and is prevalent in cancer cells that exhibit genomic instability and are devoid of proper checkpoint control [17, 19, 20].

The goal of this study was to examine the relationship between DNA damage accumulation and apoptosis. In radiosensitive ATM deficient cells, the defects in triggering the whole DDR following IR lead to checkpoint failure and to the accumulation of unresolved DSBs [1, 3], thus being an ideal model to study this relationship. Our results show that AT and normal lymphoblastoid cell lines undergoing apoptosis accumulate a higher number of γH2AX foci than those belonging to the viable fraction. Specifically, AT lymphoblasts accumulate a higher fraction of residual DSBs and undergo significantly higher levels of IR-induced apoptosis at all postirradiation (pIR) times analyzed. Also AT lymphoblasts display a strong G2/M arrest and tetraploidization, suggesting that MC contributes to apoptosis in ATM deficient cells.

2. Results and Discussion

2.1. AT Lymphoblasts Efficiently Trigger a p53-Dependent Apoptotic Response and Undergo High Levels of Radiation-Induced Apoptosis. In order to determine a relationship between persistent radiation-induced DSBs and apoptosis, we had to first determine the ability to undergo apoptosis in AT and normal lymphoblastoid cell lines (LCLs). To this end, Annexin-V (An) and propidium iodide (PI) incorporation in cells was measured by flow cytometry, and cells were analyzed at 0, 24, 48, and 72 hours after 5 Gy irradiation. Loss of plasma membrane asymmetry by exposing phosphatidylserine in the outer leaflet is an early event in the apoptotic process, previous to loss of membrane integrity and to DNA fragmentation. Thereby, cells positive for Annexin-V and negative for PI staining (An+/PI−) are considered to be undergoing early stages of apoptosis (EA) [21–23]. Later in this process, cells lose membrane integrity, allowing PI staining. Therefore, cells that are An+/IP+ are considered to be in late apoptosis (LA), although necrotic cells can also be found in this fraction [21, 24].

As shown in Figure 1(a), the fraction of An+/PI− cells is higher in AT LCL at all times analyzed, even before irradiation. AT cells undergoing early apoptosis reach 8.0% and 12.5% at 24 hours and 48 hours pIR, respectively, while the fraction of normal cells An+/PI− during these time points is always lower than 5%. The overall fraction of Annexin-positive cells (sum of An+/PI− and An+/PI+ cells) reaches its maximum at 48 hours after irradiation, being 12.3% in normal LCL and 31.8% in AT LCL. At later time points, An+/PI− and An+/PI+ cells start to slowly decline, although they are still significantly higher in AT cells and far from the basal levels in both cell lines. These results demonstrate that this AT LCL not only efficiently triggers apoptosis, but also undergoes higher rates of radiation-induced apoptosis than its normal counterpart.

Because several works have reported contradictory results regarding apoptosis induction in AT cells [25–31], we aimed to confirm the previous results obtained with Annexin-V/PI by analyzing radiation-induced apoptosis

using TUNEL methodology. One characteristic feature of the later stages of apoptosis is the internucleosomal fragmentation of DNA into ~180 bp repeats often referred to as DNA laddering [32]. TUNEL allows the detection of these DNA fragments by labeling their 3′-OH end with a fluorescent molecule. AT and normal lymphoblasts were irradiated at the same dose of γ-rays (5 Gy), and apoptosis levels were analyzed at the same time points previously described. TUNEL was performed on slides and quantitation of TUNEL-positive cells was performed with an epifluorescence microscope. The majority of TUNEL-positive cells also displayed characteristic morphological features of apoptosis, such as nuclei shrinkage, DNA compaction, and nuclear fragmentation. All these features combined with TUNEL staining allowed certain detection of apoptotic cells (Figure 1(b)).

As shown in Figure 1(a), the levels of spontaneous apoptosis measured with TUNEL were higher in AT than in normal cells. Higher rates of spontaneous apoptosis in AT lymphoblasts have been described before [33] and are confirmed by the results obtained in the present study with both apoptotic cell detection assays (total Annexin-V-positive cells before irradiation: 5.2% in normal cells versus 10.9% in AT cells; χ^2 test, $p < 0.0001$; TUNEL: 3.7% in AT cells versus 1.7% in normal cells; χ^2 test, $p < 0.0072$). At early postirradiation times, the fraction of TUNEL-positive cells remains low in both cell lines, but they increase at 48 hours pIR and reach maximum levels at 72 hours pIR, being of 17.2% in normal and 32.4% in AT cells (χ^2 test, $p < 0.0001$). Although both Annexin-V/PI and TUNEL methodologies measure apoptosis, they seem to detect correlative stages of this process. At twenty-four hours after irradiation, there has been an increase of cells undergoing EA and evolving to a LA stage compared to unirradiated cells, while yet very few cells are positive for TUNEL staining. EA and LA fractions reach a *plateau* level at 48 hours pIR, while at this time there is an increasing frequency of TUNEL-positive events. Because TUNEL methodology detects extensive DNA fragmentation, TUNEL-positive cells might undergo a later apoptotic stage than those signaled with Annexin. In this way, the combination of the results obtained with the Annexin-V/PI and the TUNEL procedures renders a dynamic picture of the apoptotic process in the lymphoblast cells analyzed.

Lymphocytes are removed, both physiologically and after irradiation, by a p53- and caspase-dependent apoptotic pathway that leads to DNA cleavage [19, 34, 35]. The role of the ATM protein in triggering this IR-induced apoptotic response has been examined using different experimental systems in AT lymphoblasts, AT lymphoblastoid cell lines (LCLs), and Atm$^{-/-}$ mouse thymocytes with conflicting results. Lymphocytes from AT patients were found to have an increased spontaneous apoptotic level [33]. Also, a normal apoptotic response after IR was demonstrated in Atm$^{-/-}$ mouse cells [26] and in lymphocytes from AT patients [27]. Variable results have been described in AT LCLs, although most of them displayed a normal apoptotic response to IR [28, 36]. To ultimately determine p53 status, we analyzed p53 presence and its activation after IR. Levels of p21, a p53 effector involved in cell cycle arrest at G1 and S phases

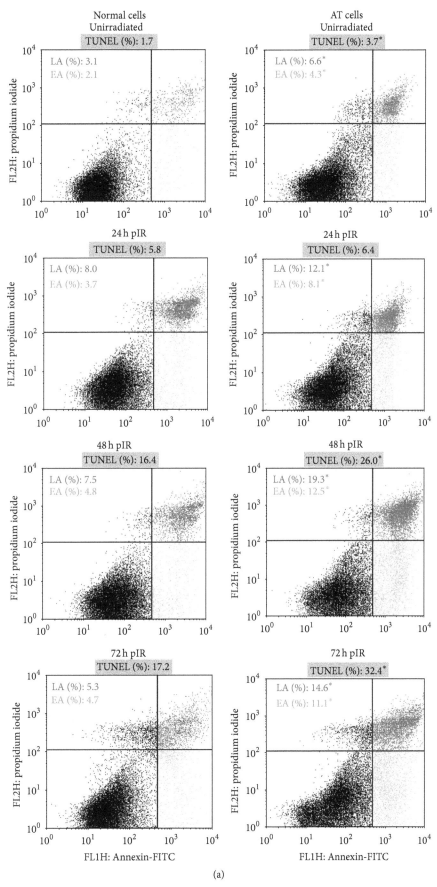

(a)

FIGURE 1: Continued.

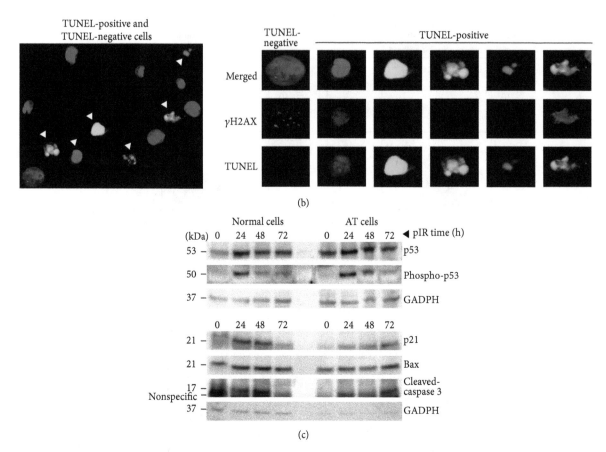

FIGURE 1: (a) Radiation-induced apoptosis measured by means of Annexin-V/PI and TUNEL methodologies. Cytometry plots were used for gating cells stained using Annexin-V (An) and propidium iodide (PI) before and after irradiation. In all plots, the lower left quadrant corresponds to the viable, nonapoptotic cell population (An–/PI–). The lower right quadrant corresponds to the cell population An+PI–, which is undergoing early apoptosis (EA) and is shown in green. The upper right quadrant corresponds to the cell population An+PI+, which is undergoing late apoptosis (LA) and is shown in red. Frequencies of EA and LA are shown in each graph at 0, 24, 48, and 72 hours after irradiation in normal and AT cells and they correspond to the mean of 3 different experiments with two replicas each. A minimal number of 10000 cells were analyzed in each experiment. The asterisks indicate statistical differences in the apoptotic levels between AT and normal cells when comparing the EA fraction, the LA fraction, and the sum of Annexin-V-positive cells (EA + LA). In all cases, χ^2 test was applied and the p values were <0.005. Frequencies of TUNEL-positive cells for each cell type at 0, 24, 48, and 72 hours pIR are shown over each cytometry plot. The asterisks indicate statistical differences between AT and normal cells (χ^2 test; p values < 0.007). The values for TUNEL were obtained after scoring 1000 cells for each time point and each cell line using an epifluorescence microscope. (b) Scoring of TUNEL-positive cells. On the left, a general view under the microscope (40x) showing irradiated cells in which a combination of TUNEL staining (green) and γH2AX immunofluorescence (red) has been applied. DNA is stained with DAPI (blue). TUNEL-positive cells (white arrowheads) depict intense TUNEL staining and they show the morphological features of apoptotic cells (right panel): smaller nuclei with highly condensed chromatin—intensely stained with blue—undergoing variable levels of nuclear fragmentation. Also, TUNEL-positive cells could depict a pan-nuclear γH2AX staining but never had γH2AX foci. (c) Western blot detection of apoptotic markers. Normal and AT cells were irradiated with 5 Gy of γ-rays and expression of p53, its activated form phospho-p53 (Ser15), and other p53 targets such as p21, Bax, and the cleaved fraction of caspase 3 were analyzed at 0, 24, 48, and 72 hours after irradiation. Proteins were detected in two different experiments and GADPH was used as the housekeeping gene.

after DNA damage induction [37], have also been analyzed. As shown in Figure 1(c), despite ATM absence, p53 was effectively induced in normal and AT cells at 24 hours pIR, when the fraction of apoptotic cells starts to increase. Consistent with greater apoptotic induction, levels of activated p53 are still high in AT cells at 48 hours pIR. Induction of p21 is observed in both cell lines although higher expression is observed in normal than in AT cells. In this regard, it has been suggested that ATM regulates distinct p53-dependent pathways that selectively trigger checkpoint arrest

or apoptosis. For example, effective p53 induction coupled with checkpoint failure and a normal apoptotic response after IR has been described in ATM deficient cells [26, 28, 38, 39]. In agreement with these works, normal cells efficiently arrest at G1 after irradiation while the AT lymphoblastoid cell line tested in this study undergoes high apoptosis rates along with G1 checkpoint failure (see Section 2). Bax, another p53 target involved in activation of caspases, shows a similar expression in both LCLs. The cleaved fragment of caspase 3 is detected only after irradiation in both cell lines but in

AT cells its expression is still visible at 72 hours, consistent with higher frequency of apoptotic AT cells at this time point. Altogether, our results are in agreement with a role for ATM selectively activating p53 to regulate cell-cycle checkpoint but not apoptosis. In this regard, ATM- and Rad3-related (ATR), Chk2 and DNA-PKcs have been proposed as candidates to regulate IR-induced apoptosis in AT cells [38–40].

2.2. Radiation-Induced Mitotic Catastrophe Is a More Relevant Cell Death Process in AT Lymphoblasts Than in Its Normal Counterparts. We proceeded by analyzing cell cycle progression after irradiation. As shown in Figure 2(a), normal lymphoblasts are efficiently arrested at G1, as demonstrated by a diminution of the S fraction at 24 h pIR that prevails up to 72 h. As expected, impairment of proper G1 arrest in the AT LCL was demonstrated by no noticeable decrease in the S fraction at 24 hours pIR, and later decreases were low when compared to normal cells. These results are consistent with the Western blot results showing a weak induction of p21 in AT cells after irradiation (Figure 1(c)) and are in agreement with the ATM deficiency cell phenotype, which is characterized by impairment of G1 and intra-S checkpoint activation upon DNA damage infliction. This leads to cell cycle progression of cells bearing unresolved DNA damage [3, 41]. These cells are efficiently arrested in G2 [42] unless the DNA damage has been inflicted during G2 phase, in which case ATM deficient cells proceed into mitosis [43]. In any case, damaged cells that surpass G1 and/or G2 checkpoints become later arrested in mitosis (M) because of spindle anaphase checkpoint (SAC). In this work, cells were irradiated during their exponential growth, implying that many AT cells will surpass G1 and intra-S checkpoints and will be arrested at G2, while those AT cells irradiated during G2 phase will surpass the G2 checkpoint and arrest in M by SAC. Remarkably, our results show that AT lymphoblasts significantly accumulate at G2/M after irradiation at all times analyzed (Figure 2(a)), suggesting that, besides cells arrested at G2 checkpoint, some of them might remain in M phase.

Persistent arrest at G2/M boundaries after DNA damage infliction is a first indicator of mitotic catastrophe (MC), so we aimed to analyze the possibility that MC contributes to cell death in AT cells. MC has been described as an oncosuppressive mechanism that, in order to avoid accumulation of genomic instability, senses this mitotic failure and responds to it by driving the cell to death during mitosis [20]. Sometimes, some of these cells do not die during mitosis and eventually overcome SAC signaling and "slip" into the next interphase without dividing. These cells may reenter the cell cycle and reduplicate its DNA content, turning into the accumulation of tetraploid cells within the population. Indeed, AT lymphoblasts showed an increasing frequency of cells with a 4N DNA content that reached 5.6% at 72 hours after irradiation (Figures 2(a) and 2(b)). Although small, this fraction was higher than in normal lymphoblasts, whose tetraploid population was lower than 0.7% at all times analyzed. To further confirm these results, we quantified the centrosome number, as cells that skip mitosis and reenter the cell cycle will reduplicate their centrosomes along with DNA.

Centrosomes were scored by means of immunofluorescent pericentrin detection and cells were classified into those having a normal number of centrosomes (1 centrosome in interphase and 2 centrosomes in S, G2, and M phases) or an aberrant number of centrosomes (more than 2). As shown in Figure 2(b), the basal frequency of AT cells with >2 centrosomes was very low, but it strikingly increased at 48 hours after irradiation, when it reached almost 3% of the cell population and correlated with the appearance of a 4N cell population (Figure 2(b)). In contrast, the fraction of normal lymphoblasts with an abnormal number of centrosomes did not reach 1% of the population during the 48 h analyzed (χ^2 test, $p < 0.002$). Thus, some AT cells are able to reach mitosis despite defective repair. Eventually, some of them skip M phase, giving raise to the appearance of a tetraploid population together with an increasing population of cells with an abnormal centrosome number. Polyploid cells with extra centrosomes are prone to form transient multipolar mitotic spindles, which can either directly trigger mitotic death or result in the generation of aneuploid daughter cells. A small fraction of these cells might survive and enter a mitotic round that is also likely to be catastrophic [20]. Because the MC mechanism can ultimately culminate in apoptotic cell death [20], we propose that this mechanism contributes to the radiation-induced apoptotic levels detected in AT lymphoblasts.

2.3. Viable AT Lymphoblasts Display Higher Levels of Radiation-Induced DNA Damage and Delayed DSB Repair at Long Times after Irradiation. We next aimed to examine the levels of radiation-induced DNA damage in both lymphoblast cell lines. To this end, we analyzed γH2AX foci corresponding to radiation-induced DSBs in viable cells—those negative for TUNEL (Figure 3(a)). Figure 3(b) shows that, 24 h after irradiation, 64.1% of the normal lymphoblasts have γH2AX foci, a 3.2-fold increase compared to unirradiated cells. Within the same time interval, viable AT lymphoblasts displayed a 7-fold increase, as 87% of them showed γH2AX foci (χ^2 test, $p = 0.0135$). At 72 h pIR normal cells have repaired most of their DSBs and only 22.2% of them have γH2AX foci, while this fraction is still around 50% in AT lymphoblasts (χ^2 test, $p < 0.0001$). All together, these results reflect the DNA repair impairment of AT cells, which repair most of the DSBs in a fast and efficient way, while a subset of breaks remains unrepaired for long times, even days, after DNA damage infliction [3, 10–12, 44]. In agreement with that, our results show that AT cells, despite showing an initial decline in the fraction of cells displaying γH2AX foci, are unable to efficiently proceed to further diminish this population and accumulate high numbers of residual DSBs, even at very long times after DNA damage has been induced.

After that, we scored the number of γH2AX foci in the TUNEL-negative cells and classify them into two groups: cells with less than 10 γH2AX foci and cells with 10 or more γH2AX foci (Figure 3(b)). Only a small fraction of the normal cells accumulated 10 or more γH2AX foci, reaching a peak of ~18% at 24 hours pIR and declining thereafter. On the contrary, most of the irradiated AT cells accumulated 10 or

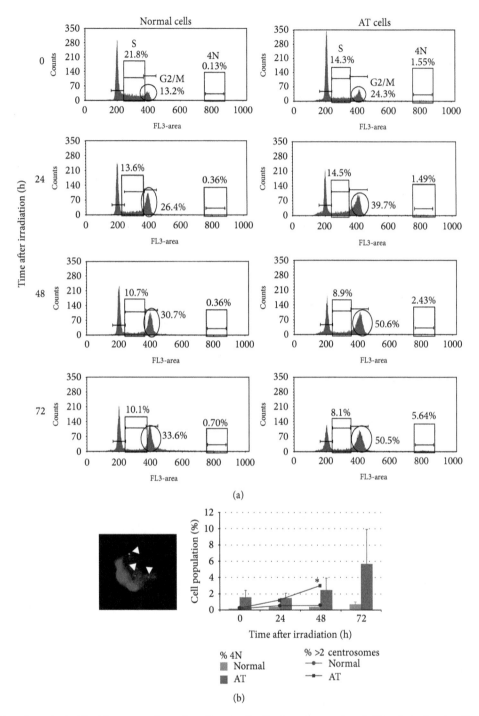

(a)

(b)

FIGURE 2: (a) Cell cycle analysis. The histograms show the cell cycle distribution of normal and AT cells before irradiation and at 24, 48, and 72 hours after irradiation. Cell cycle distribution was obtained by means of PI staining, which measures DNA content. The frequency of cells entering in S-phase for each cell type and each time point is shown, evidencing lack of IR-induced G1 checkpoint arrest in AT cells. The fraction of cells arrested in G2/M after irradiation and the tetraploid population (4N) arising after irradiation have also been highlighted. The frequencies displayed are the mean of two independent experiments in which a minimum number of 10000 cells were analyzed. (b) Tetraploidization and centrosome number. The image shows an AT lymphoblast (probably a metaphase) with 3 pericentrin signals (green; white arrowheads). The DNA is stained with DAPI and the red staining corresponds to α-tubulin. The bars in the graph show the fraction of tetraploid cells scored in AT and normal lymphoblasts before and after irradiation. The values are the mean of two experiments, and the error bars show the standard deviation. The lines in the graph depict the fraction of cells with an abnormal centrosome number (>2) within the same time points. The values for centrosome number were obtained after analyzing a minimal number of 400 cells for each cell type and each time point. The asterisk indicates statistical differences between normal and AT lymphoblasts in the frequency of cells with more than 2 centrosomes (χ^2 test; p values < 0.002).

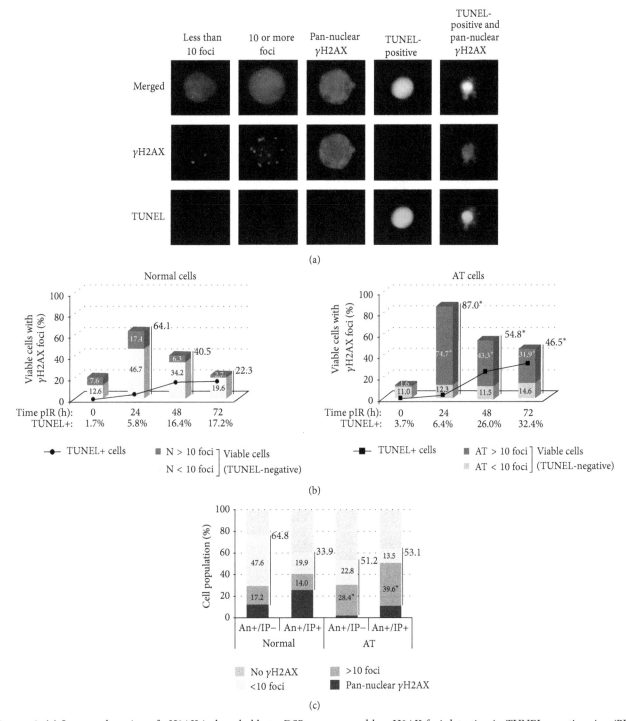

FIGURE 3: (a) Immunodetection of γH2AX in lymphoblasts. DSBs were scored by γH2AX foci detection in TUNEL-negative, An+/PI−, and An+/PI+ cells. Pan-nuclear γH2AX staining was scored in TUNEL-negative, An+/PI−, and An+/PI+ and in TUNEL-positive cells. (b) γH2AX-labeling in viable (TUNEL-negative) cells. The number and frequency of viable cells with γH2AX foci are reflected in the bars. Within this fraction, the frequency of cells with <10 foci or with ≥10 foci is shown inside the bars. The asterisks indicate statistical differences between normal and AT lymphoblasts in the fraction of cells with γH2AX foci or in the fraction of cells with ≥10 γH2AX foci (χ^2 test; p values from $p = 0.0270$ to $p < 0.0001$). The frequencies for each category are calculated over the total number of TUNEL-negative scored cells. A minimal number of 350 TUNEL-negative cells were analyzed for each cell type and each time point. The apoptotic rate measured with TUNEL is depicted in the graph as a continuous line. Values for TUNEL-positive cells are given under the x-axis and are those corresponding to Figure 1(a). (c) γH2AX-labeling in Annexin-positive cells. AT and normal cells were irradiated and fractions corresponding to EA and LA were isolated by cell sorting. An+/PI− and An+/PI+ cells were classified into those with or without γH2AX foci and those with pan-nuclear γH2AX staining. The frequency of cells with γH2AX foci is depicted next to the bar. Within this fraction, the frequency of cells with less than 10 foci (light pink) or with 10 or more foci (pink) is shown inside the bars. The asterisks indicate statistical differences between normal and AT lymphoblasts in the frequency of cells with ≥10 γH2AX foci (χ^2 test; p values from $p = 0.0020$ to $p < 0.0001$). The frequencies are calculated over the total number of An+/PI− and An+/PI+ sorted cells. A minimal number of 400 cells were analyzed for each cell type and each time point.

more γH2AX foci, reaching a maximum of around 75% at 24 hours pIR (χ^2 test, $p < 0.0001$). From 24 to 72 hours after irradiation, 85 to 70% of the γH2AX-positive AT cells carry 10 or more DSBs while this frequency is much lower in normal cells (27 to 12%). Thus, after irradiation, AT cells accumulate more cells with DSBs and more DSBs/cell than their normal counterparts.

The results presented here suggest that DSB repair might be inversely correlated with apoptosis induction. Indeed, at 48 hours pIR, the percentage of normal cells with $\geq$10 γH2AX foci is low (6.3%) and it coincides with the stabilization of the TUNEL-positive rate (around 17%). On the other hand, at 48 hours pIR, still most of AT cells have $\geq$10 γH2AX foci (43.3%) and TUNEL rates continue to increase at 72 hours pIR (from 26 to 32%; Figure 3(b)). In agreement with that, recent studies have revealed that some residual 53BP1, Rad51, and γH2AX foci remain in cells for a relatively long time after irradiation and have indicated an inverse correlation between the number of residual foci and the surviving fraction of cells [45–49]. Similarly, a correlation between a higher rate of foci loss and a higher clonogenic surviving fraction in ten different cancer cell lines has been described [50]. Finally, it is worth noting that the fraction of AT cells with less than 10 γH2AX foci remains stable before and after irradiation and is hardly changed along with the apoptotic rate (Figure 3(b)), thus discarding this subpopulation of cells as that with more probabilities of undergoing IR-induced apoptosis. This result is in agreement with other studies describing that low background levels of foci (<3 foci per cell) scored at 24 hours after irradiation were correlated with cell survival [14, 51].

2.4. Apoptotic AT Cells Accumulate More Residual DSBs Than Normal Lymphoblasts. To further analyze this possibility, we proceeded to analyze radiation-induced DSBs in normal and AT lymphoblasts undergoing apoptosis. The characteristic DSB-signaling processes of the DDR, such as phosphorylation of histone H2AX forming visible foci, are eventually abolished in cells undergoing last stages of apoptosis, probably due to DNA condensation [52]. Consequently, no γH2AX foci were scored in TUNEL-positive cells (Figure 3(a)). We reasoned that earlier apoptotic stages, such as those detected with Annexin-V/PI methodology, would better allow the detection of radiation-induced DSBs. To this end, AT and normal lymphoblasts were irradiated and enriched populations of early apoptotic (An+/PI−) and late apoptotic/necrotic (An+/PI+) cells were obtained by flow sorting at 48 hours after irradiation. Immediately after sorting, cells were fixed on slides and γH2AX immunofluorescence was performed. This procedure resulted in the loss of Annexin-V and PI staining, allowing for reliable identification of γH2AX signaling. In all the populations analyzed we found a fraction of cells displaying a pan-nuclear γH2AX staining (Figure 3(a)). This kind of staining has been related to apoptosis induced by several DNA damaging agents and is concurrent with the initiation of DNA fragmentation resulting from the apoptotic process [53, 54]. This fraction of cells was taken into account when calculating the percentages shown in the figures. At the time point selected after

irradiation (48 hours), the fraction of cells undergoing early and late apoptosis was at its maximum in both cell lines. Cells undergoing early apoptosis (An+/PI−) were 4.8% in normal and 12.5% in AT cells, while those undergoing late apoptosis (An+/PI+) were 7.5% and 19.3% in normal and AT LCL, respectively (Figure 1(a)).

Within the above mentioned fraction of cells undergoing early apoptosis (An+/PI−), most of them had γH2AX foci— 64.8% of the normal lymphoblasts and 51.2% of the AT cells (Figure 3(c)). Nonetheless, most of the cells undergoing early apoptosis had less than 10 γH2AX foci/cell in normal cells (47.6%) but $\geq$10 γH2AX foci/cell in AT cells (28.4%), demonstrating that also the AT cells that initiate apoptosis (An+/PI−) accumulate a significantly higher number of DSBs than normal cells (χ^2 test; $p < 0.0001$). As normal lymphoblasts enter in later apoptotic/necrotic stages (An+/PI+), the frequency of cells with less than 10 γH2AX foci is sharply reduced (from 47.6% to 19.9%; 2.4-fold reduction), while the fraction of cells with $\geq$10 γH2AX foci is more or less maintained (14%). Similarly, the frequency of AT lymphoblasts undergoing later apoptotic stages (An+/PI+) that present less than 10 γH2AX foci is reduced, while the population of cells with $\geq$10 γH2AX foci is increased with respect to early apoptosis and to normal cells (75% of the γH2AX-positive AT lymphoblasts). Thus, AT lymphoblasts accumulate more DSBs/cell than their normal counterparts, also while undergoing apoptosis (χ^2 test; $p = 0.0020$).

It is important to note that An+/PI− cells might be considered viable, as early apoptosis is believed to be reversible if the conditions inducing apoptosis are removed [55–57]. Moreover, it has been suggested that DNA repair is involved in this reversibility [58]. Thus, while undergoing early apoptosis, cells might be able to perform some degree of DSB repair that leads to reduction of γH2AX foci-positive cells in later apoptotic stages. Most probably, cells that carry a larger amount of DSBs have a lower probability of eventually performing successful repair; thus cells with $\geq$10 γH2AX foci accumulate at later stages of apoptosis. In this work, cells undergoing late apoptosis are those accumulating more DSBs, and the cell line with impaired repair activity is the one carrying more residual DSBs and displaying higher rates of cell death. Similar results have been very recently described in which cells carrying Rad51 foci at 24 hours pIR are the ones more likely to die [44]. It cannot be concluded that accumulation of $\geq$10 γH2AX foci signals cells to undergo apoptosis, as γH2AX foci dose-response may depend on cell type, time allowed after irradiation, and the cell cycle phase in the moment of irradiation among other factors. Nonetheless, these results support the notion that persistence of residual DSBs signals those cells that are more likely to undergo cell death.

3. Conclusions

Annexin-V/PI and TUNEL methodologies have been used to analyze IR-induced apoptosis. These methodologies seem to detect subtle differences in apoptotic frequencies that might correspond to progressive apoptotic stages, as maximum levels of Annexin-V-positive cells are reached earlier than maximum levels of TUNEL-positive cells. Annexin-V/PI allows discrimination between cells undergoing early and late apoptosis as well as fast scoring of more cells. TUNEL detection on slides and subsequent microscope analysis allows the combination of TUNEL and protein immunodetection—like γH2AX—and the analysis of these events in the apoptotic and the healthy fraction at the same time.

The results in this work show that AT LCL efficiently undergoes IR-induced apoptosis to a higher level than its normal counterpart at all times analyzed. Along with accumulation of residual DSBs, indicators of mitotic catastrophe such as prolonged G2/M arrest and DNA and centrosomes reduplication are found in irradiated AT cells, which also contribute to the apoptotic levels scored. In these cells, apoptosis is accompanied with p53 induction and cleavage of caspase 3, while they show low levels of p21 induction that correlate with impairment of G1 and intra-S checkpoint activation after irradiation. These results agree with a role for ATM selectively activating p53 to regulate apoptosis and not cell cycle checkpoint. Accumulation of radiation-induced unrepaired DSBs contributes to cell death. For this reason, viable cells that are undergoing apoptosis (Annexin-positive) have been isolated in both cell lines and γH2AX foci have been scored. The results show that these are the cells accumulating more DSBs per cell. As cells progress from EA to LA, the fraction of cells with fewer γH2AX foci decreases in both AT and normal cells, while cells with more than 10 γH2AX foci accumulate in LA, especially in AT cells—consistent with their DNA repair defect. These results support the notion that persistence of residual DSBs signals those cells that are more likely to undergo cell death and that scoring of γH2AX foci might function as a predictive tool to assess radiation-induced apoptosis.

4. Material and Methods

4.1. Cell Culture and γ-Irradiation. EBV-transformed human lymphoblastoid cell lines (LCLs) GM08436A (derived from a child suffering from Ataxia-Telangiectasia) and GM09622 (derived from a sex and age matched control) were obtained from the Coriell Cell Culture Repositories. Cells were grown in suspension in RPMI 1640 medium with GlutaMAX-I (Life Technologies, CA, USA) supplemented with 15% fetal bovine serum and kept in the incubator at 37°C and 5% CO_2 atmosphere. When indicated, cells were irradiated with 5 Gy γ-rays using an IBL-437C R-137 Cs irradiator, with a dose rate of 5.10 Gy/min.

4.2. Apoptosis Detection

4.2.1. Annexin-V-Fluorescein Assay. The Annexin-V/propidium iodide (PI) assay was performed following the manufacturer's instructions (Annexin-V-FLUOS Staining Kit, Roche, Switzerland). Briefly, lymphoblast cells were collected, centrifuged, and washed in 1xPBS. The cell pellet was resuspended in freshly prepared Annexin-V-FLUOS labeling solution with PI and incubated for 15 minutes (min) at

room temperature, in the dark. Cells were analyzed on a FACSCalibur flow cytometer (Becton-Dickinson, CA, USA) using 488 nm excitation and 530/30 nm band pass filter for fluorescein detection and a FL2 photomultiplier and band pass filter 585/42 nm for PI detection after electronic compensation. Flow cytometry analysis was done with the CellQuest software (Becton-Dickinson, CA, USA). Cells were classified into the following fractions: (a) viable cells (An−/PI−) were impermeable for PI and also did not bind Annexin-V (An); (b) early apoptotic cells (An+/PI−) bound An and were PI impermeable; (c) late apoptotic or, also called, secondary necrotic cells (An+/PI+) bound An and were PI permeable; (d) primary necrotic cells (An−/PI+) only displayed PI staining. When indicated, cell sorting of enriched populations of An+/PI− and An+/PI+ cells was performed with a FACS Aria SORP sorting cytometer (Becton-Dickinson Biosciences, CA, USA) using a 488 nm excitation laser and 525 nm band pass filter for fluorescein detection and a 350 nm excitation UV laser and 660/400 nm band pass filter for PI detection. Cells obtained after sorting were dropped on poly-L-lysine coated slides and allowed to attach for 3 min before proceeding with immunofluorescence.

4.2.2. TUNEL Assay. The TUNEL assay was performed following the manufacturer's instructions (In Situ Cell Death Detection Kit, Fluorescein, Roche, Switzerland). Briefly, lymphoblasts were centrifuged, washed with 1xPBS, and dropped on poly-L-lysine coated slides. Cells were then fixed with 2% paraformaldehyde for 20 min at room temperature and permeabilized with 0.1% Triton-X100 and 0.1% sodium citrate in 1xPBS for 5 min in ice. The TUNEL mix was applied to the cells following the manufacturer's instructions and allowed to be incubated at 37°C for 40 minutes. Before analysis, Vectashield Mounting Medium for fluorescence (Vector Laboratories Inc., CA, USA) supplemented with 4′,6-diamino-2-phenylindole (DAPI) was applied. TUNEL analysis was performed with an Olympus BX41TF epifluorescence microscope equipped with an Olympus U-TVIX digital camera using the Isis v5.4.9 software (MetaSystems, Germany).

4.3. Cell Cycle Analysis. Lymphoblasts were washed in 1xPBS, centrifuged, and kept in 70% ethanol at −20°C until analysis. Cells were then centrifuged, washed with 1xPBS, and resuspended in 1 mL of freshly prepared PI/Triton/RNAsa solution: 0.1%Triton-X100, 2 mg RNAsa A (DNAsa free), and 200 μL of 1 mg/mL PI. After 15 min incubation at 37°C, DNA content was measured on a FACSCalibur flow cytometer (Becton-Dickinson, CA, USA). Red fluorescence of PI-stained nuclei was excited at 488 nm with an argon laser and was collected through a 670 nm long pass filter detection into the FL3 photomultiplier tube on a linear scale, at a flow rate of 12 mL/min (low). Cell cycle analysis of the DNA histograms of integrated red fluorescence was performed with CellQuest software (Becton-Dickinson, CA, USA).

4.4. Immunofluorescence. Immunodetection of γH2AX was performed on the same samples previously analyzed for

TUNEL or sorted after Annexin-V/PI staining. Pericentrin detection was performed on newly obtained samples of irradiated lymphoblasts allowed to attach onto poly-L-lysine slides. Cells were fixed for 15 min in 4% paraformaldehyde and permeabilized in 1xPBS-0.5% Triton-X100 solution for 15 min. After 30 minutes of blocking with 0.1% Tween20 and 5% FBS, mouse anti-γH2AX (Ser139) (Upstate/Millipore, MA, USA) or rabbit anti-pericentrin (Abcam, UK) was applied at a 1:1000 concentration and allowed to incubate for 1 hour at room temperature. Anti-mouse Cy3 (Amersham Biosciences/GE Healthcare, NJ, USA) and anti-rabbit A488 (Invitrogen/Molecular Probes, OR, USA) secondary antibodies were applied at 1:1000 final concentration for 45 minutes at room temperature, followed by extensive washing. Before analysis, Vectashield Mounting Medium for fluorescence (Vector Laboratories Inc., CA, USA) supplemented with DAPI was applied. Slides were analyzed using an Olympus BX41TF epifluorescence microscope equipped with an Olympus U-TVIX digital camera using the Isis v5.4.9 software (MetaSystems, Germany).

4.5. Western Blotting. Cells were collected by centrifugation, washed with PBS, treated with RIPA lysis buffer, and sonicated. Whole-cell extracts were loaded onto a 10% SDS-polyacrylamide gel that was run at 150 V for 50 minutes in a Bio-Rad mini-gel system. Proteins were transferred to a nitrocellulose membrane (30 V, 90 minutes) and blocked for 1 h at room temperature in 5% BSA brought to 37°C or with nonfat milk at 4°C. Primary antibodies used were mouse monoclonal anti-p53 (Santa Cruz Biotechnology, Inc., TX, USA), rabbit monoclonal anti-phospho-p53 (Ser15) (Thermo Fisher Scientific, MA, USA), rabbit monoclonal anti-p21 (Abcam, UK), rabbit monoclonal anti-Bax (Abcam, UK), rabbit polyclonal anti-active caspase 3 (Abcam, UK), and mouse anti-GAPDH (Abcam, UK). Membranes were washed with TTBS (Tris 10 mM, NaCl 150 mM, and 0.005% Tween20) and incubated for 1 hour at room temperature with secondary antibody, goat anti-rabbit or goat anti-mouse, conjugated to horseradish peroxidase (Upstate/Millipore, MA, USA). Proteins were visualized using Immobilon Western kit (Upstate/Millipore, MA, USA) and the signal was captured with ChemiDoc XRS (Bio-Rad, CA, USA).

4.6. Statistical Analysis. The statistical analysis was performed using GraphPad InStat version 3.05 (GraphPad Software Inc., CA, USA).

Disclosure

The funders had no role in study design, data collection and analysis, decision to publish, or preparation of the paper.

Authors' Contribution

Marta Martín and Anna Genescà developed the study concept and design. Testing and data collection and analysis

were performed by Teresa Anglada, Marta Martín, Mariona Terradas, and Laia Hernández. Marta Martín and Anna Genescà wrote the paper and approved its final version for submission.

Acknowledgments

This work was funded by grants from Consejo de Seguridad Nuclear (CSN 2012-0001) and EURATOM (Dark.Risk GA 323216). Anna Genescà Laboratory is supported by Generalitat de Catalunya (2009SGR-282). Laia Hernández is supported by the Universitat Autònoma de Barcelona Ph.D. programme fellowship. The authors would like to thank Dr. Dik van Gent and Dr. Humberto Sánchez for their valuable comments. They also thank the Radiological Protection Unit at Universitat Autònoma de Barcelona for sample irradiation and the Cytometry Service from the Centres Científics i Teconològics (CCiT), Universitat de Barcelona (UB), for cell sorting.

References

[1] C. J. Bakkenist and M. B. Kastan, "Initiating cellular stress responses," *Cell*, vol. 118, no. 1, pp. 9–17, 2004.

[2] E. U. Kurz and S. P. Lees-Miller, "DNA damage-induced activation of ATM and ATM-dependent signaling pathways," *DNA Repair*, vol. 3, no. 8-9, pp. 889–900, 2004.

[3] Y. Shiloh, "ATM and related protein kinases: safeguarding genome integrity," *Nature Reviews Cancer*, vol. 3, no. 3, pp. 155–168, 2003.

[4] A. Di Leonardo, S. P. Linke, K. Clarkin, and G. M. Wahl, "DNA damage triggers a prolonged p53-dependent G1 arrest and long-term induction of Cip1 in normal human fibroblasts," *Genes & Development*, vol. 8, no. 21, pp. 2540–2551, 1994.

[5] M. B. Kastan, O. Onyekwere, D. Sidransky, B. Vogelstein, and R. W. Craig, "Participation of p53 protein in the cellular response to DNA damage," *Cancer Research*, vol. 51, no. 23, pp. 6304–6311, 1991.

[6] E. P. Rogakou, D. R. Pilch, A. H. Orr, V. S. Ivanova, and W. M. Bonner, "DNA double-stranded breaks induce histone H2AX phosphorylation on serine 139," *The Journal of Biological Chemistry*, vol. 273, no. 10, pp. 5858–5868, 1998.

[7] E. P. Rogakou, C. Boon, C. Redon, and W. M. Bonner, "Megabase chromatin domains involved in DNA double-strand breaks in vivo," *The Journal of Cell Biology*, vol. 146, no. 5, pp. 905–916, 1999.

[8] M. Löbrich, A. Shibata, A. Beucher et al., "γH2AX foci analysis for monitoring DNA double-strand break repair: strengths, limitations and optimization," *Cell Cycle*, vol. 9, no. 4, pp. 662–669, 2010.

[9] O. A. Sedelnikova, E. P. Rogakou, I. G. Panyutin, and W. M. Bonner, "Quantitative detection of 125IdU-induced DNA double-strand breaks with gamma-H2AX antibody," *Radiation Research*, vol. 158, no. 4, pp. 486–492, 2002.

[10] M. Kühne, E. Riballo, N. Rief, K. Rothkamm, P. A. Jeggo, and M. Löbrich, "A double-strand break repair defect in ATM-deficient

cells contributes to radiosensitivity," *Cancer Research*, vol. 64, no. 2, pp. 500–508, 2004.

[11] M. Martín, M. Terradas, G. Iliakis, L. Tusell, and A. Genescà, "Breaks *invisible* to the DNA damage response machinery accumulate in ATM-deficient cells," *Genes Chromosomes and Cancer*, vol. 48, no. 9, pp. 745–759, 2009.

[12] E. Riballo, M. Kühne, N. Rief et al., "A pathway of double-strand break rejoining dependent upon ATM, Artemis, and proteins locating to γ-H2AX foci," *Molecular Cell*, vol. 16, no. 5, pp. 715–724, 2004.

[13] J. P. Banáth, S. H. MacPhail, and P. L. Olive, "Radiation sensitivity, H2AX phosphorylation, and kinetics of repair of DNA strand breaks in irradiated cervical cancer cell lines," *Cancer Research*, vol. 64, no. 19, pp. 7144–7149, 2004.

[14] D. Klokov, S. M. MacPhail, J. P. Banáth, J. P. Byrne, and P. L. Olive, "Phosphorylated histone H2AX in relation to cell survival in tumor cells and xenografts exposed to single and fractionated doses of X-rays," *Radiotherapy and Oncology*, vol. 80, no. 2, pp. 223–229, 2006.

[15] H. Mahrhofer, S. Bürger, U. Oppitz, M. Flentje, and C. S. Djuzenova, "Radiation induced DNA damage and damage repair in human tumor and fibroblast cell lines assessed by histone H2AX phosphorylation," *International Journal of Radiation Oncology, Biology, Physics*, vol. 64, no. 2, pp. 573–580, 2006.

[16] T. Yoshikawa, G. Kashino, K. Ono, and M. Watanabe, "Phosphorylated H2AX foci in tumor cells have no correlation with their radiation sensitivities," *Journal of Radiation Research*, vol. 50, no. 2, pp. 151–160, 2009.

[17] M. Castedo, J.-L. Perfettini, T. Roumier, K. Andreau, R. Medema, and G. Kroemer, "Cell death by mitotic catastrophe: a molecular definition," *Oncogene*, vol. 23, no. 16, pp. 2825–2837, 2004.

[18] H. Vakifahmetoglu, M. Olsson, and B. Zhivotovsky, "Death through a tragedy: mitotic catastrophe," *Cell Death and Differentiation*, vol. 15, no. 7, pp. 1153–1162, 2008.

[19] L. Galluzzi, I. Vitale, J. M. Abrams et al., "Molecular definitions of cell death subroutines: recommendations of the Nomenclature Committee on Cell Death 2012," *Cell Death and Differentiation*, vol. 19, no. 1, pp. 107–120, 2012.

[20] I. Vitale, L. Galluzzi, M. Castedo, and G. Kroemer, "Mitotic catastrophe: a mechanism for avoiding genomic instability," *Nature Reviews. Molecular cell biology*, vol. 12, no. 6, pp. 385–392, 2011.

[21] R. W. Bailey, T. Nguyen, L. Robertson et al., "Sequence of physical changes to the cell membrane during glucocorticoid-induced apoptosis in S49 lymphoma cells," *Biophysical Journal*, vol. 96, no. 7, pp. 2709–2718, 2009.

[22] A. Hochreiter-Hufford and K. S. Ravichandran, "Clearing the dead: apoptotic cell sensing, recognition, engulfment, and digestion," *Cold Spring Harbor Perspectives in Biology*, vol. 5, no. 1, Article ID a008748, 2013.

[23] I. Vermes, C. Haanen, H. Steffens-Nakken, and C. Reutelingsperger, "A novel assay for apoptosis Flow cytometric detection of phosphatidylserine expression on early apoptotic cells using fluorescein labelled Annexin V," *Journal of Immunological Methods*, vol. 184, no. 1, pp. 39–51, 1995.

[24] Z. Bacso and J. F. Eliason, "Measurement of DNA damage associated with apoptosis by laser scanning cytometry," *Cytometry*, vol. 45, no. 3, pp. 180–186, 2001.

[25] J. B. P. Barber, C. M. L. West, A. E. Kiltie, S. A. Roberts, and D. Scott, "Detection of individual differences in radiation-induced apoptosis of peripheral blood lymphocytes in normal individuals, ataxia telangiectasia homozygotes and heterozygotes, and breast cancer patients after radiotherapy," *Radiation Research*, vol. 153, no. 5, pp. 570–578, 2000.

[26] C. Barlow, K. D. Brown, C.-X. Deng, D. A. Tagle, and A. Wynshaw-Boris, "Atm selectively regulates distinct p53-dependent cell-cycle checkpoint and apoptotic pathways," *Nature Genetics*, vol. 17, no. 4, pp. 453–456, 1997.

[27] D. G. Bebb, P. J. Warrington, G. De Jong et al., "Radiation induced apoptosis in ataxia telangiectasia homozygote, heterozygote and normal cells," *Mutation Research/Fundamental and Molecular Mechanisms of Mutagenesis*, vol. 476, no. 1-2, pp. 13–20, 2001.

[28] M. Fernet, S. Angele, T. Dörk, and J. Hall, "Variation in radiation-induced apoptosis in ataxia telangiectasia lymphoblastoid cell lines," *International Journal of Radiation Biology*, vol. 79, no. 3, pp. 193–202, 2003.

[29] B. Humar, H. Müller, and R. J. Scott, "Elevated frequency of p53-independent apoptosis after irradiation increases levels of DNA breaks in ataxia telangiectasia lymphoblasts," *International Journal of Radiation Biology*, vol. 72, no. 3, pp. 257–269, 1997.

[30] A. E. Meijer, B. Zhivotovsky, and R. Lewensohn, "Epstein-Barr virus-transformed lymphoblastoid cell lines of ataxia telangiectasia patients are defective in X-ray-induced apoptosis," *International Journal of Radiation Biology*, vol. 75, no. 6, pp. 709–716, 1999.

[31] Y.-Q. Shi, L. Li, O. Sanal et al., "High levels of delayed radiation-induced apoptosis observed in lymphoblastoid cell lines from ataxia-telangiectasia patients," *International Journal of Radiation Oncology Biology Physics*, vol. 49, no. 2, pp. 555–559, 2001.

[32] G. R. Bicknell, R. T. Snowden, and G. M. Cohen, "Formation of high molecular mass DNA fragments is a marker of apoptosis in the human leukaemic cell line, U937," *Journal of Cell Science*, vol. 107, no. 9, pp. 2483–2489, 1994.

[33] E. Duchaud, A. Ridet, D. Stoppa-Lyonnet, N. Janin, E. Moustacchi, and F. Rosselli, "Deregulated apoptosis in ataxia telangiectasia: association with clinical stigmata and radiosensitivity," *Cancer Research*, vol. 56, no. 6, pp. 1400–1404, 1996.

[34] C. G. Proud, "Regulation of mammalian translation factors by nutrients," *European Journal of Biochemistry*, vol. 269, no. 22, pp. 5338–5349, 2002.

[35] A. Strasser, "Life and death during lymphocyte development and function: evidence for two distinct killing mechanisms," *Current Opinion in Immunology*, vol. 7, no. 2, pp. 228–234, 1995.

[36] A. E. Meijer, J. Ekedahl, B. Joseph et al., "High-LET radiation induces apoptosis in lymphoblastoid cell lines derived from ataxia-telangiectasia patients," *International Journal of Radiation Biology*, vol. 77, no. 3, pp. 309–317, 2001.

[37] A. L. Gartel and S. K. Radhakrishnan, "Lost in transcription: p21 repression, mechanisms, and consequences," *Cancer Research*, vol. 65, no. 10, pp. 3980–3985, 2005.

[38] A. Hirao, A. Cheung, G. Duncan et al., "Chk2 is a tumor suppressor that regulates apoptosis in both an ataxia telangiectasia mutated (ATM)-dependent and an ATM-independent manner," *Molecular and Cellular Biology*, vol. 22, no. 18, pp. 6521–6532, 2002.

[39] S. Wang, M. Guo, H. Ouyang et al., "The catalytic subunit of DNA-dependent protein kinase selectively regulates p53-dependent apoptosis but not cell-cycle arrest," *Proceedings of the National Academy of Sciences of the United States of America*, vol. 97, no. 4, pp. 1584–1588, 2000.

[40] B. Vogelstein and K. W. Kinzler, "Cancer genes and the pathways they control," *Nature Medicine*, vol. 10, no. 8, pp. 789–799, 2004.

[41] K. K. Khanna, M. F. Lavin, S. P. Jackson, and T. D. Mulhern, "ATM, a central controller of cellular responses to DNA damage," *Cell Death and Differentiation*, vol. 8, no. 11, pp. 1052–1065, 2001.

[42] D. Scott, A. R. Spreadborough, and S. A. Roberts, "Radiation-induced G2 delay and spontaneous chromosome aberrations in ataxia-telangiectasia homozygotes and heterozygotes," *International Journal of Radiation Biology*, vol. 66, no. 6, pp. S157–S163, 1994.

[43] H. Beamish and M. F. Lavin, "Radiosensitivity in ataxia-telangiectasia: anomalies in radiation-induced cell cycle delay," *International Journal of Radiation Biology*, vol. 65, no. 2, pp. 175–184, 1994.

[44] M. Gatei, B.-B. Zhou, K. Hobson, S. Scott, D. Young, and K. K. Khanna, "Ataxia telangiectasia mutated (ATM) kinase and ATM and Rad3 related kinase mediate phosphorylation of Brca1 at distinct and overlapping sites. In vivo assessment using phospho-specific antibodies," *Journal of Biological Chemistry*, vol. 276, no. 20, pp. 17276–17280, 2001.

[45] J. P. Banáth, D. Klokov, S. H. MacPhail, C. A. Banuelos, and P. L. Olive, "Residual γH2AX foci as an indication of lethal DNA lesions," *BMC Cancer*, vol. 10, article 4, 2010.

[46] E. Dikomey, I. Brammer, J. Johansen, S. M. Bentzen, and J. Overgaard, "Relationship between DNA double-strand breaks, cell killing, and fibrosis studied in confluent skin fibroblasts derived from breast cancer patients," *International Journal of Radiation Oncology Biology Physics*, vol. 46, no. 2, pp. 481–490, 2000.

[47] H. D. Halicka, X. Huang, F. Traganos, M. A. King, W. Dai, and Z. Darzynkiewicz, "Histone H2AX phosphorylation after cell irradiation with UV-B: relationship to cell cycle phase and induction of apoptosis," *Cell Cycle*, vol. 4, no. 2, pp. 339–345, 2005.

[48] H. Kunogi, T. Sakanishi, N. Sueyoshi, and K. Sasai, "Prediction of radiosensitivity using phosphorylation of histone H2AX and apoptosis in human tumor cell lines," *International Journal of Radiation Biology*, vol. 90, no. 7, pp. 587–593, 2014.

[49] A. Menegakis, A. Yaromina, W. Eicheler et al., "Prediction of clonogenic cell survival curves based on the number of residual DNA double strand breaks measured by γH2AX staining," *International Journal of Radiation Biology*, vol. 85, no. 11, pp. 1032–1041, 2009.

[50] S. H. Macphail, J. P. Banáth, T. Y. Yu, E. H. M. Chu, H. Lambur, and P. L. Olive, "Expression of phosphorylated histone H2AX in cultured cell lines following exposure to X-rays," *International Journal of Radiation Biology*, vol. 79, no. 5, pp. 351–358, 2003.

[51] P. L. Olive and J. P. Banáth, "Kinetics of H2AX phosphorylation after exposure to cisplatin," *Cytometry Part B: Clinical Cytometry*, vol. 76, no. 2, pp. 79–90, 2009.

[52] E. Marková, J. Torudd, and I. Belyaev, "Long time persistence of residual 53BP1/γ-H2AX foci in human lymphocytes in relationship to apoptosis, chromatin condensation and biological dosimetry," *International Journal of Radiation Biology*, vol. 87, no. 7, pp. 736–745, 2011.

[53] E. P. Rogakou, W. Nieves-Neira, C. Boon, Y. Pommier, and W. M. Bonner, "Initiation of DNA fragmentation during apoptosis induces phosphorylation of H2AX histone at serine 139," *The Journal of Biological Chemistry*, vol. 275, no. 13, pp. 9390–9395, 2000.

[54] B. Mukherjee, C. Kessinger, J. Kobayashi et al., "DNA-PK phosphorylates histone H2AX during apoptotic DNA fragmentation in mammalian cells," *DNA Repair*, vol. 5, no. 5, pp. 575–590, 2006.

[55] F. J. Geske, A. C. Nelson, R. Lieberman, R. Strange, T. Sun, and L. E. Gerschenson, "DNA repair is activated in early stages of p53-induced apoptosis," *Cell Death and Differentiation*, vol. 7, no. 4, pp. 393–401, 2000.

[56] A. K. Hammill, J. W. Uhr, and R. H. Scheuermann, "Annexin V staining due to loss of membrane asymmetry can be reversible and precede commitment to apoptotic death," *Experimental Cell Research*, vol. 251, no. 1, pp. 16–21, 1999.

[57] H. L. Tang, K. L. Yuen, H. M. Tang, and M. C. Fung, "Reversibility of apoptosis in cancer cells," *British Journal of Cancer*, vol. 100, no. 1, pp. 118–122, 2009.

[58] F. J. Geske, R. Lieberman, R. Strange, and L. E. Gerschenson, "Early stages of p53-induced apoptosis are reversible," *Cell Death and Differentiation*, vol. 8, no. 2, pp. 182–191, 2001.

7

Partial Body Weight-Supported Treadmill Training in Spinocerebellar Ataxia

Laura Alice Santos de Oliveira [1,2] **Camilla Polonini Martins,**[1]
Carlos Henrique Ramos Horsczaruk,[1] **Débora Cristina Lima da Silva,**[1]
Luiz Felipe Vasconcellos [3] **Agnaldo José Lopes** [1]
Míriam Raquel Meira Mainenti,[4] **and Erika de Carvalho Rodrigues**[1,5]

[1]*Post-Graduation Program in Rehabilitation Sciences, Augusto Motta University Center (UNISUAM), Rio de Janeiro, RJ, Brazil*
[2]*School of Physiotherapy, Federal Institute of Rio de Janeiro, Rio de Janeiro, RJ, Brazil*
[3]*Institute of Neurology Deolindo Couto, Federal University of Rio de Janeiro (UFRJ), Rio de Janeiro, RJ, Brazil*
[4]*Physical Education College of the Brazilian Army (EsEFEx), Rio de Janeiro, RJ, Brazil*
[5]*D'Or Institute for Research and Education (IDOR), Rio de Janeiro, RJ, Brazil*

Correspondence should be addressed to Laura Alice Santos de Oliveira; lauraoliveira.ft@gmail.com

Academic Editor: Velio Macellari

Background and Purpose. The motor impairments related to gait and balance have a huge impact on the life of individuals with spinocerebellar ataxia (SCA). Here, the aim was to assess the possibility of retraining gait, improving cardiopulmonary capacity, and challenging balance during gait in SCA using a partial body weight support (BWS) and a treadmill. Also, the effects of this training over functionality and quality of life were investigated. *Methods.* Eight SCA patients were engaged in the first stage of the study that focused on gait training and cardiovascular conditioning. From those, five took part in a second stage of the study centered on dynamic balance training during gait. The first and second stages lasted 8 and 10 weeks, respectively, both comprising sessions of 50 min (2 times per week). *Results.* The results showed that gait training using partial BWS significantly increased gait performance, treadmill inclination, duration of exercise, and cardiopulmonary capacity in individuals with SCA. After the second stage, balance improvements were also found. *Conclusion.* Combining gait training and challenging tasks to the postural control system in SCA individuals is viable, well tolerated by patients with SCA, and resulted in changes in capacity for walking and balance.

1. Introduction

Spinocerebellar ataxia (SCA) comprises a family of autosomal dominant inherited disorders that result from progressive degeneration of the cerebellum and its associated systems [1]. Besides cerebellar deterioration, SCA is often accompanied by degeneration of other sites of the nervous system, leading to noncerebellar signs such as pyramidal and extrapyramidal losses, which are uncommon in ataxia of other etiologies and that can worsen the impairments of people with SCA [2].

Among the motor deficits prompted by SCA, those related to gait and balance are the most common [3]. Gait in SCA is usually described as uncoordinated, unsteady, wide-based, and highly variable [4–6]. In turn, balance abnormalities in SCA are characterized by an increased postural sway and poor balance control during both static and dynamic tasks [7]. It is noteworthy that both the balance and gait impairments in SCA are strongly associated with an increased number of fall episodes [8, 9] and can favor physical inactivity, adversely affecting cardiorespiratory fitness [10]. Together, these problems can impair mobility, deteriorate general health, and yield physical and social consequences for these individuals [7].

Despite the huge recent advances in neurogenetic research, an effective pharmacological approach to face this condition is still unknown [11, 12]. Indeed, with the exception of a few kinds of hereditary ataxia (e.g., Niemann–Pick disease type C, cerebrotendinous xanthomatosis, coenzyme Q-10 responsive ataxia, or ataxia with vitamin E deficiency), no specific treatments exist for hereditary ataxia, including SCA (for a review, see Jayadev and Bird [13]). In this context, rehabilitation strategies could represent an alternative to improve the physical condition and to reduce the impairments of these individuals. But, sadly, clinical trials testing the effects of physical therapy approaches in ataxia are scarce and the few existing studies include cerebellar ataxias of different etiologies, beyond SCA (for a review, see Martins et al. [14]) [15, 16]. As the natural course and prognosis are different between SCA and cerebellar ataxias of other etiologies it could be artificial to generalize the results from the available clinical trials to the SCA population, especially considering the peculiarity of the progressive degeneration found in SCA. In this context, it is relevant to advance strategies of rehabilitation that could benefit SCA individuals.

One strategy suggested to improve gait in ataxic individuals is to attach weights to their ankles or trunk. Although widely used in everyday physiotherapy practice, there is no consensus about the efficacy of this compensatory approach [17–20]. More recently it was proposed that alleviating the weight of cerebellar ataxic individuals during gait training could represent a perspective to improve this activity [21–23]. The neuromuscular impairments from ataxia could favor physical inactivity that can lead to additional neuromuscular and cardiopulmonary disturbances affecting overall functionality and quality of life [10, 24].

One alternative that has been successfully employed to improve gait performance in people with motor impairments is partial body weight support associated with gait training on a treadmill (PBWSTT). It consists of using an overhead harness to support a percentage of body weight while walking. The advantages of using PBWSTT are to provide task-oriented training; to allow several repetitions of a supervised gait pattern with an almost null fall risk; to enable an increasing pace of effort and postural control demands; and to make possible improvements of cardiopulmonary capacity [25–28]. Some case reports describe successful use of PBWSTT for gait and balance problems of non-SCA individuals [21–23]. Although providing promising results the feasibility and general effects of this strategy have not yet been tested in SCA individuals.

Studies based on dynamic balance training of SCA individuals are less scarce but also include cerebellar ataxia of other etiologies [16, 17]. Recently, our group tested the effectiveness of a modified version of an exercise program proposed by Ilg et al. [16] to improve coordination and balance [24]. Exercises for static and dynamic balance were applied exclusively to people with SCA and seem to be safe, with improvements in fall risk and balance in the sample of individuals studied [24]. Likewise, challenging balance during dynamic tasks such as gait training in SCA individuals will probably have an important impact on functionality since walking is an everyday activity that allows independence and autonomy in various other activities and individuals' social roles.

Until now, there has been no consensus in the literature about the best way to cope with the gait and balance problems presented by people with SCA. Therefore, the aim of the present pilot study was to assess the possibility of retraining gait, recovering/improving cardiopulmonary capacity, and challenging balance during gait in people with SCA using a partial body weight support device associated with a treadmill and to observe its effects on functionality and quality of life.

2. Materials and Methods

This was a pretest-posttest quasi-experimental open-label uncontrolled study design. It began with a set of assessments, followed by a PBWSTT protocol performed in 2 stages (gait/conditioning and dynamic balance training) followed by another set of assessments at the end of each stage. This study was approved by the local ethics committee (process number 17754813.0.0000.5235) and was carried out according to the Declaration of Helsinki. Written consent was obtained from all participants.

2.1. Participants. Twenty-five individuals with ambulatory movement disorders from a local neurological hospital that had positive genetic testing for any SCA subtype were invited to participate. Ten refused participation. Fifteen accepted the invitation and underwent an interview to search for eligibility criteria. Inclusion criteria were having received a diagnosis of SCA from a neurologist; answering "no" to all questions of the PAR-Q (a questionnaire that determines the possible risk of exercising for an individual based on the answers to specific health history questions [29]); and being able to walk 10 meters with or without a device. Exclusion criteria included being at "stage 0" (no gait difficulties) of ataxia disease [30] and the presence of vertigo, hypertension, postural hypotension, heart or coronary disease, epilepsy, or orthopedic problems that could limit gait. Five participants were excluded because of these criteria, 1 who was not able to ambulate and 4 because they were at "stage 0" of ataxia. Thus, 10 participants matched the exclusion/inclusion criteria and began the protocol of intervention. During the study, 2 participants dropped out of the protocol due to personal problems. Eight individuals (5 male) aged 27 to 58 (43 ± 11 years) participated in this pilot study. All of them gave informed written consent. Table 1 summarizes the personal characteristics of the participants.

2.2. Intervention Procedures. Firstly, all participants underwent 2 sessions of assessment, with 1 week of interval between them. One aimed to evaluate cardiopulmonary capacity during exercise and the other functionality and quality of life (see below). Immediately after the last evaluation, participants started the PBWSTT protocol. Before and after each session of PBWSTT, participants had their blood pressure measured. During the session they also had their heart rate monitored. PBWSTT was implemented using a Biodex 500 harness (Biodex; Shirley, New York) with the capacity to lift up to 82 kg. Each participant was attached to the harness apparatus with a set of straps and fittings, by which he/she was fastened

TABLE 1: Sample personal characteristics.

Participant	Sex	Age (yrs)	Weight (Kg)	Body height (m)	BMI (Kg/m^2)	SCA type	Disease course (yrs)
1	F	32	84.2	1.68	29.83	2	12
2	M	27	56.3	1.76	18.18	3	4
3	M	31	54.9	1.71	18.78	3	7
4	M	58	64.2	1.70	22.21	3	8
5	M	44	113.2	1.73	37.82	3	6
6	F	47	43.5	1.66	15.79	7	4
7	F	52	53.9	1.66	19.56	3	7
8	M	54	85	1.72	28.57	3	12

F = female; M = male; Yrs = years; Kg = kilograms; m = meters; BMI = body mass index; Kg/m^2 = weight in kilograms divided by height in meters squared; SCA = spinocerebellar ataxia.

to the PBWSTT device. The support vest was secured tightly around the lower trunk of the participant, allowing hip flexion and extension. After that, the participant was invited to climb onto the treadmill (Ecafix EG 700.2). Participants started the program with 30% of their body weight alleviated by the device.

In the first stage of the PBWSTT program (gait/conditioning training), the main goals were (i) to progressively reduce body support to zero and (ii) to progressively increase velocity to the "maximal" for each individual. In this context, "maximal" was considered the highest speed the patient could achieve during the treadmill training without running. In the second stage (dynamic balance training), the main goal was challenging balance during gait. The first and second stages lasted 8 and 10 weeks each, respectively, both comprising a 50 min duration session with a frequency of 2 times per week.

As mentioned, in the gait/conditioning training stage, participants started walking on a treadmill with 30% of their body weight alleviated by the device. In this stage the participants were free to hold onto the handrails. The sessions were divided as follows: the first 10 min was dedicated to cardiovascular system warm-up by increasing the speed until reaching the maximal velocity (as described above) for that individual without running or losing coordination. For the next 30 min, the participant walked at this maximal speed. Their perceived effort was monitored every 5 min (Borg modified scale—0 to 10 [31]). Finally, in the course of the last 10 min, the speed was gradually decreased to zero to allow the heart rate to slow down and breathing to return to normal levels. The maximal speed during treadmill training was increased individually over the course of the 8 weeks, varying depending on participant ability and capacity. Additionally, the percentage of corporeal weight supported by the device was gradually decreased until the participant was able to walk attached to the support but without any body weight alleviated. At the end of the 8 weeks of this first stage, cardiopulmonary capacity, functional capacity, and quality of life of the participants were evaluated again.

After the evaluation, the dynamic balance training stage began. In this second stage, participants walked attached to the body weight support device without any weight alleviated, at the maximal velocity that they had reached at the end of

stage 1. The first and last 10 min of training were also dedicated to warm-up and cool-down of participants. During the middle 30 min, participants were stimulated to progressively walk without any hand support. About 2 weeks after that, the participant's balance started to be challenged by throwing and catching a ball to the individual while walking on the treadmill, at intervals of 5 min, intercalated by 1 min of rest. At the end of this stage, the functional capacity and quality of life, but not cardiopulmonary capacity, of the participants were evaluated again. Figure 1 summarizes all procedures.

2.3. Outcome Measures. Physiotherapists and a physician expert in the instruments employed in this study performed all evaluations.

2.3.1. Cardiopulmonary Performance. The cardiopulmonary performance during exercise was assessed through cardiopulmonary exercise testing (CPET). Respiratory gas exchange was sampled from a mouthpiece connected to a medium flow pneumotachograph (Medgraphics, Minnesota, USA) and a gas analyzer (VO2000, Medgraphics, Minnesota, USA), calibrated before each test with gas standards of known concentrations [oxygen (O_2) = 12.0%; carbon dioxide (CO_2) = 5.3%]. The ventilation flow and O_2 and CO_2 expired fractions were measured breath by breath. A nose clip was used to avoid gas escape. The CPET was performed on a treadmill (FE 700.2, Ecafix, São Paulo, Brazil) using a modified version of the Naughton protocol [32]. Participants were instructed to hold their hands on the treadmill bars during the entire test to avoid falls. Before the test, the participants underwent a familiarization period of about 1 min of walking on the treadmill (low velocity, no inclination). After that, the test began with an initial speed of 1.6 km/h with one increment to 3.2 km/h after 3 min. Increments were performed only in graduation, with a rise of 3.5° every 3 min. All participants were informed about the test interruption criteria: chest pain, systolic blood pressure (SBP) > 220 mmHg, diastolic blood pressure (DBP) > 115 mmHg, a drop in SBP despite an increase in workload, dizziness, physical manifestations of extreme fatigue, ECG changes, and the subject's request to stop and when the maximal grade was achieved [29]. The Borg perception effort scale was used to check the degree of perceived effort at every step of the test [31].

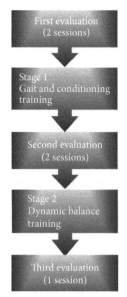

First evaluation
(2 sessions)

(i) Assessment of cardiopulmonary capacity
    during exercise, functionality, and quality of life

Stage 1
Gait and conditioning
training

(i) Walking on a treadmill with hands on handrails
(ii) Starting with 30% of the body weight alleviated and gradually decreasing to 0%
(iii) Speed increased individually in each session

Second evaluation
(2 sessions)

(i) Assessment of cardiopulmonary capacity
    during exercise, functionality, and quality of life

Stage 2
Dynamic balance
training

(i) Participants walk attached to the device with no weight alleviated
(ii) Progressively walking without hand support
(iii) Balance challenged by throwing and catching a ball

Third evaluation
(1 session)

(i) Assessment of functionality and quality of life

FIGURE 1: The experimental protocol.

The relative oxygen consumption (VO_2; mL/kg/min) and minute ventilation (VE; L/min) variables were considered at the peak of the exercise. The peak VO_2 was considered as the highest VO_2 reached in the final minute of the effort. Other variables analyzed included the duration of the CPET and the maximum inclination achieved on the treadmill during this test.

2.3.2. Functional Capacity and Quality of Life. Functional capacity was assessed in respect of balance, gait, and severity of ataxia. Balance was assessed with the Brazilian Portuguese validated version of the Berg balance scale (BBS) [33], in which scores range from 0 to 56 [34]. The higher the score in the BBS, the better the postural control. Chiu et al. [35] suggested that BBS scores equal to or less than 45 points indicate an increased fall risk. Here, the same criterion was used. The participants' ability to respond to demands during walking was assessed with the dynamic gait index (DGI), in which scores range from 0 (high risk of falls) to 24 (low risk of fall) [36]. Scores equal to or less than 19 are associated with an increased risk of falling. To assess the severity of ataxia we used both the scale for the assessment and rating of ataxia (SARA) score, a standardized clinical measure of neurologic manifestations of cerebellar ataxia in which scores range from 0 (no ataxia symptoms) to 40 (most severe ataxia) [37], and the brief ataxia rating scale (BARS), with a total score of 30 points (most severe ataxia) [38]. Quality of life was assessed by means of the Katz index of independence in activities of daily living (Katz ADL), an instrument to assess functional status by measuring an individual's ability to perform activities of daily living independently, in which scores vary from 6 (patient independent) to 0 (patient very dependent) [39].

2.4. Statistics. Results were expressed as the median, minimum and maximum value ranges. Given the nonnormal distribution of the data (Kolmogorov–Smirnov), a Wilcoxon matched-pairs test was applied for comparisons of outcome

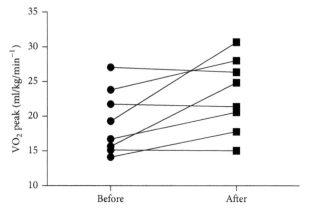

FIGURE 2: VO_2 Peak values for each participant before and after the gait/conditioning stage.

measures of functional capacity, quality of life, and cardiopulmonary capacity obtained before and after gait/conditioning training stages. A Wilcoxon matched-pairs test was also used for comparisons between functional capacity and quality of life before and after the dynamic balance training. A significance level of 5% was used. The statistical analyses were performed using Statistica 7 software.

3. Results

Eight SCA individuals participated in the first stage (gait/conditioning) of this study. From those, 5 also took part in the second stage (dynamic balance training). After the gait/conditioning stage the participants showed significant improvements in CPET duration ($P < 0.01$) and the maximal treadmill inclination achieved during the test ($P < 0.01$; see Table 2). The VE Peak ($P = 0.050$) and VO_2 Peak did not show statistical significance ($P = 0.093$) after intervention. Despite the nonsignificance, however, from Figure 2 it is

TABLE 2: Outcome measures before and after the gait/conditioning stage.

Outcome measure	Before	After	P value
Duration			
Median/range	9.4/2.15–22.4	20.9/3.08–22.9	**0.04***
Inclination %			
Median/range	5.25/0–10.5	21/0–21	**0.04***
VE Peak L/min			
Median/range	26.6/17.3–54.1	32.1/23.3–56.5	0.05
Borg peak			
Median/range	17/15–20	15/11–20	0.55
DGI			
Median/range	13/1–21	16.5/8–24	**0.03***
BBS			
Median/range	48.5/28–54	48/16–54	0.89
SARA			
Median/range	13.5/8–18.5	9/7–19.5	0.08

Values are median or range (minimum–maximum) of 8 individuals with SCA. VE Peak = minute ventilation for the peak of effort; DGI = dynamic gait index; BBS = Berg balance scale; SARA = scale for the assessment and rating of ataxia. ∗ = statistically significant in the Wilcoxon matched-pairs test.

TABLE 3: Outcome measures before and after the dynamic balance training stage.

Outcome measure	Before	After	P value
DGI			
Median/range	21/12–24	22/16–23	0.36
BBS			
Median/range	48/44–54	54/47–55	**0.04***
SARA			
Median/range	7.5/7–12	9/5–13	0.90

Values are median and range (minimum–maximum) of 5 individuals with SCA. DGI = dynamic gait index; BBS = Berg balance scale; SARA = scale for the assessment and rating of ataxia. ∗ = statistically significant in the Wilcoxon matched-pairs test.

possible to see that a few SCA individuals benefit from training, as 5 individuals presented an increment while 3 show a slight decrement of VO_2 Peak.

The gait/conditioning training also had an impact on postural demands during walking, as observed in the DGI scores compared with before the intervention (Table 2).

The dynamic balance training stage brought significant improvements in balance as measured by the BBS scores when this parameter was compared before and after the intervention (Table 3), but without further changes in DGI scores.

SARA and Katz ADL scores did not show any changes after the intervention (Tables 2 and 3).

4. Discussion

This study is the first, to our knowledge, to investigate the feasibility and consequences of the association of gait training and balance challenges using PBWSTT on functionality, cardiopulmonary capacity, and quality of life in SCA individuals. The results demonstrated that the training was feasible and well tolerated by people with SCA. Trends of improvements were found after the gait/conditioning training using PBWSTT in the capacity for walking by increasing the gait performance and the cardiopulmonary capacity of the sample of individuals studied. The dynamic balance training also brought statistically significant improvements in balance.

At the end of the gait/conditioning training stage, as expected, improvements were found in gait as measured by DGI. SCA participants were also capable of walking with higher inclination of the treadmill for longer periods of time in the CPET. Probably, several mechanisms play a role in these improvements. The use of task-oriented training and increasing the pace of effort may have been relevant [25–27]. Additionally, the majority of studies with PBWSTT attribute the gait improvements observed to changes in the central pattern generator in different conditions such as Parkinson's disease, spinal cord injury, and stroke (e.g., Wickelgren [40] and Miyai et al. [41]). Although there was no statistical difference between the VO_2 Peak after and before the gait/conditioning training stage it was observed that, in 5 of 8 participants tested, there was a VO_2 Peak increment. It was expected since treadmill training has already been associated with cardiopulmonary capacity improvement after stroke and in individuals with coronary artery disease [42, 43]. Moreover, the level of intensity of CPET increased for the group (as suggested by treadmill inclination and CPET duration increments), suggesting an increased correspondent effort during its execution. It may explain the absence of VO_2 Peak and Borg improvement for some individuals.

As expected, after the dynamic balance training stage, an improvement of balance was observed as measured by BBS. In this stage the strategy was to challenge balance by throwing and catching a ball to the individual during treadmill training. Keeping the patient attached to the body weight device even without alleviating weight helped to avoid falls, providing the possibility of performing exercises that otherwise would be very dangerous to SCA individuals. In fact, it is already known that SCA is strongly associated with an increased number of fall episodes [8, 9]. In a one-year period, 73.6% of 228 SCA patients reported at least one fall; from these, 74% related a high rate of fall-related injuries [8]. Another study showed that, from 113 SCA patients that recorded their falls in a diary during one year, 84.1% reported at least one fall. One method to measure fall status can be through the BBS score [36]. Here the increment of BBS scores indicates a decrease in participants' fall risk, which is very relevant, due to the impact of falls on morbidity and mortality in this population [4]. It is already known that balance perturbations during walking improve balance in healthy older people and individuals who have suffered a stroke [44, 45]. A case study about a patient with progressive supranuclear palsy during walk training, balance perturbation, and step training using a PBWSTT also found improvements of gait and balance [46]. However, the exact mechanisms responsible for the balance improvement remain unclear. Given that SCA is a progressive disease that affects multiple central nervous system sites and the cerebellum that is essential in motor learning, this becomes even more challenging [2]. Finally, it is important to remember that, in this study, the individuals were not able to walk on the treadmill without holding onto handrails. So, without previous training of gait and improvement of cardiovascular conditioning, the dynamic balance training stage of exercises would not have been possible.

In respect of quality of life, the absence of change after the accomplishment of both stages of this study may be due to a ceiling effect. In fact, the major part of participants of this study was considered independent according to the Katz ADL index even during the first evaluation. Similarly, there are insufficient data to show that individuals after stroke, with Parkinson disease and spinal cord injury, improved their quality of life after PBWSTT [47–57].

The results relative to SARA scale were not as significant as expected. This may indicate that the progression of the disease had not changed in the course of this study, maybe due to its short duration.

The PBWSTT is largely used in the rehabilitation of patients with various neurological conditions beyond SCA, including Parkinson's disease, stroke, and spinal cord injury [47–57]. For example, in individuals with Parkinson's disease, PBWSTT was able to improve gait velocity, cadence, and step length, besides improving the weight distribution between lower limbs during walking [47–49]. Regarding the use of PBWSTT after stroke, there are reports of improvement related to the affected side: increases in step length, longer stance phase, larger swing phase, and a bigger distance traveled in the six-minute walk test [50–54]. Finally, the use of PBWSTT in spinal cord injury was being able to improve gait speed and backward gait speed, 6-minute walk distance, stride length. and mobility [55–57].

On the other hand, due to the novelty of the training protocol proposed here, contrasts with previous studies that involved cerebellar ataxic individuals are complex. Moreover, the studies available employed locomotor training strategies to improve gait in cerebellar ataxic individuals with non-SCA etiologies. For instance, Vaz et al. [21] reported promising evidence with treadmill training only, more strong in 1 of 2 participants with traumatic brain injury (TBI) and ataxic gait. There were gains in cadence, walking speed, step length, mobility, and balance. Two studies employed PBWSTT. Freund et al. [22] reported some gains in balance and gait in 1 ataxic individual by TBI that attained a program of exercises with PBWSTT. Cernak et al. [23] reported a single case of a 13-year-old girl who had a cerebellar/brainstem infarct and performed locomotor training with PBWSTT. She reached modified independence for transfers, supervision for walking, and minimal assistance for stairs after 6 months of intervention. Additionally, the studies proposing programs of exercise for gait and balance in ataxia did not include only people with SCA, highlighting the importance of the present study (for a review, see Martins et al. [14]) [15–17, 41].

The results of the present study are pioneering in suggesting that PBWSTT could be effective in improving both cardiopulmonary exercise capacity and balance during gait in SCA individuals, but some limitations need to be considered. The lack of a control group and the small sample size are the major constraints of the present study. We request that interpretation of the results should be done with caution, but it is important to keep in mind that SCA is considered a rare disease and its impairments make the mobility of outpatients difficult by limiting their participation in studies that require urban displacement. Another limitation is that although participants started the program with about 30% of their body weight alleviated by the device, these values are referred to a very heterogeneous sample of patients in terms of BMI, as it was indicated in the sample personal characteristics table. Finally, it would have been useful to quantify changes between pre- and posttraining by using instrumental tools (i.e., kinematic, kinetic, and EMG analysis) and range of motions, muscle behaviors, reaction forces, and internal moments specially because the experimental setup was based on gait and balance training.

We concluded that combining gait and conditioning training with dynamic balance training using a PBWSTT device is feasible and well tolerated by people with SCA. Additionally, it resulted in trends of improvement in capacity for walking and balance. A larger sample of SCA individuals is necessary to confirm these results by means of a randomized controlled clinical trial. Also, future studies would include more qualitative measures related to movement to evaluate the impact of this approach on gait.

References

[1] L. Schöls, P. Bauer, T. Schmidt, T. Schulte, and O. Riess, "Autosomal dominant cerebellar ataxias: clinical features, genetics, and pathogenesis," *The Lancet Neurology*, vol. 3, no. 5, pp. 291–304, 2004.

[2] K. Seidel, S. Siswanto, E. R. P. Brunt, W. den Dunnen, H.-W. Korf, and U. Rüb, "Brain pathology of spinocerebellar ataxias," *Acta Neuropathologica*, vol. 124, no. 1, pp. 1–21, 2012.

[3] S. M. Morton and A. J. Bastian, "Cerebellar control of balance and locomotion," *The Neuroscientist*, vol. 10, no. 3, pp. 247–259, 2004.

[4] M. Serrao, G. Chini, C. Casali et al., "Progression of Gait Ataxia in Patients with Degenerative Cerebellar Disorders: a 4-Year Follow-Up Study," *The Cerebellum*, vol. 16, no. 3, pp. 629–637, 2017.

[5] M. Serrao, F. Pierelli, A. Ranavolo et al., "Gait pattern in inherited cerebellar ataxias," *The Cerebellum*, vol. 11, no. 1, pp. 194–211, 2012.

[6] G. Martino, Y. P. Ivanenko, M. Serrao et al., "Locomotor patterns in cerebellar ataxia," *Journal of Neurophysiology*, vol. 112, no. 11, pp. 2810–2821, 2014.

[7] S. M. Morton and A. J. Bastian, "Mechanisms of cerebellar gait ataxia," *The Cerebellum*, vol. 6, no. 1, pp. 79–86, 2007.

[8] E. M. R. Fonteyn, T. Schmitz-Hübsch, C. C. Verstappen et al., "Falls in spinocerebellar ataxias: Results of the EuroSCA fall study," *The Cerebellum*, vol. 9, no. 2, pp. 232–239, 2010.

[9] E. M. R. Fonteyn, T. Schmitz-Hübsch, C. C. P. Verstappen et al., "Prospective analysis of falls in dominant ataxias," *European Neurology*, vol. 69, no. 1, pp. 53–57, 2013.

[10] L. A. S. Oliveira, E. D. C. Rodrigues, A. G. Sancho et al., "Functional capacity, cardiorespiratory fitness and quality of life in spinocerebellar ataxia: Implications for rehabilitation," *European Journal of Physiotherapy*, vol. 17, no. 4, pp. 176–182, 2015.

[11] A. Matilla-Dueñas, M. Corral-Juan, V. Volpini, and I. Sanchez, "The spinocerebellar ataxias: Clinical aspects and molecular genetics," *Advances in Experimental Medicine and Biology*, vol. 724, pp. 351–374, 2012.

[12] W. Ilg, A. J. Bastian, S. Boesch et al., "Consensus paper: Management of degenerative cerebellar disorders," *The Cerebellum*, vol. 13, no. 2, pp. 248–268, 2014.

[13] S. Jayadev and T. D. Bird, "Hereditary ataxias: Overview," *Genetics in Medicine*, vol. 15, no. 9, pp. 673–683, 2013.

[14] C. Martins, E. Rodrigues, and L. Oliveira, "Physical therapy approach to spinocerebellar ataxia: a systematic review," *Fisioter e Pesqui*, vol. 20, pp. 293–298, 2013.

[15] Y. Shiga, T. Tsuda, Y. Itoyama et al., "Transcranail magnetic stimulation alleviates truncal ataxia in spinocerebellar degeneration," *Journal of Neurology, Neurosurgery & Psychiatry*, vol. 72, no. 1, pp. 124–126, 2002.

[16] W. Ilg, M. Synofzik, D. Brötz, S. Burkard, M. A. Giese, and L. Schöls, "Intensive coordinative training improves motor performance in degenerative cerebellar disease," *Neurology*, vol. 73, no. 22, pp. 1823–1830, 2009.

[17] M. Dias, F. Toti, S. Regina, M. Almeida, and T. Oberg, "Efeito do peso para membros inferiores no equilíbrio estático e dinâmico nos portadores de ataxia," *Acta Fisiátrica*, vol. 16, pp. 3–7, 2009.

[18] S. D. Lucy and K. C. Hayes, "Postural sway profiles: normal subjects and subjects with cerebellar ataxia," *Physiotherapy Canada*, vol. 37, pp. 140–147, 1985.

[19] T. J. Folz and M. Sinaki, "A nouveau aid for posture training in degenerative disorders of the central nervous system," *Journal of Musculoskeletal Pain*, vol. 3, no. 4, pp. 69–74, 1995.

[20] N. Clopton, D. Schultz, C. Boren, J. Porter, and T. Brillbart, "effects of axial weight loading on gait for subjects with cerebellar ataxia: preliminary findings," *Neurology Report*, vol. 27, no. 1, pp. 15–21, 2003.

[21] D. V. Vaz, R. D. C. Schottino, T. R. R. de Castro, V. R. Teixeira, S. R. C. Furtado, and E. de Mello Figueiredo, "Treadmill training for ataxic patients: a single-subject experimental design," *Clinical Rehabilitation*, vol. 22, no. 3, pp. 234–241, 2008.

[22] J. E. Freund and D. M. Stetts, "Use of trunk stabilization and locomotor training in an adult with cerebellar ataxia: A single system design," *Physiotherapy Theory and Practice*, vol. 26, no. 7, pp. 447–458, 2010.

[23] K. Cernak, V. Stevens, R. Price, and A. Shumway-Cook, "Locomotor training using body-weight support on a treadmill in conjunction with ongoing physical therapy in a child with severe cerebellar ataxia," *Physical Therapy in Sport*, vol. 88, no. 1, pp. 88–97, 2008.

[24] L. A. Santos De Oliveira, C. P. Martins, C. H. R. Horsczaruk et al., "Decreasing fall risk in spinocerebellar ataxia," *Journal of Physical Therapy Science*, vol. 27, no. 4, pp. 1223–1225, 2015.

[25] S. Hesse, C. Bertelt, M. T. Jahnke et al., "Treadmill training with partial body weight support compared with physiotherapy in nonambulatory hemiparetic patients," *Stroke*, vol. 26, no. 6, pp. 976–981, 1995.

[26] H. Barbeau and M. Visintin, "Optimal outcomes obtained with body-weight support combined with treadmill training in stroke subjects," *Archives of Physical Medicine and Rehabilitation*, vol. 84, no. 10, pp. 1458–1465, 2003.

[27] A. L. Behrman, M. G. Bowden, and P. M. Nair, "Neuroplasticity after spinal cord injury and training: an emerging paradigm shift in rehabilitation and walking recovery," *Physical Therapy in Sport*, vol. 86, no. 10, pp. 1406–1425, 2006.

[28] A. Behrman, A. Lawless-Dixon, S. Davis et al., "Locomotor training progression and outcomes after incomplete spinal cord injury," *Physical Therapy in Sport*, vol. 85, pp. 135–137, 2005.

[29] G. F. Fletcher, P. A. Ades, P. Kligfield et al., "Exercise standards for testing and training: a scientific statement from the American heart association," *Circulation*, vol. 128, no. 8, pp. 873–934, 2013.

[30] T. Klockgether, R. Lüdtke, B. Kramer et al., "The natural history of degenerative ataxia: A retrospective study in 466 patients," *Brain*, vol. 121, no. 4, pp. 589–600, 1998.

[31] G. Borg, *Borg's Perceived Exertion and Pain Scales*, Human Kinetics, Champaign, Ill, USA, 1998.

[32] K. Wasserman, J. Hansen, D. Sue et al., *Principles of Exercise Testing and Interpretation*, Lea and Febiger, Philadelphia, Penn, USA, 1987.

[33] S. T. Miyamoto, I. Lombardi Jr., K. O. Berg, L. R. Ramos, and J. Natour, "Brazilian version of the Berg balance scale," *Brazilian Journal of Medical and Biological Research*, vol. 37, no. 9, pp. 1411–1421, 2004.

[34] K. Berg, S. Wood-Dauphinee, and J. Williams, "The Balance Scale: reliability assessment for elderly residents and patients with an acute stroke," *Scandinavian Journal of Rehabilitation Medicine*, vol. 27, pp. 27–36, 1995.

[35] A. Y. Chiu, S. S. Au-Yeung, and S. K. Lo, "A comparison of four functional tests in discriminating fallers from non-fallers in older people," *Disability & Rehabilitation*, vol. 25, no. 1, pp. 45–50, 2003.

[36] A. Shumway-Cook, M. Baldwin, N. L. Polissar, and W. Gruber, "Predicting the probability for falls in community-dwelling older adults," *Physical Therapy in Sport*, vol. 77, no. 8, pp. 812–819, 1997.

[37] T. Schmitz-Hübsch, S. du Montcel, L. Baliko et al., "Scale for the assessment and rating of ataxia: development of a new clinical scale," *Neurology*, vol. 66, pp. 1717–1720, 2006.

[38] J. D. Schmahmann, R. Gardner, J. MacMore, and M. G. Vangel, "Development of a brief ataxia rating scale (BARS) based on a modified form of the ICARS," *Movement Disorders*, vol. 24, no. 12, pp. 1820–1828, 2009.

[39] Y. Duarte, C. de Andrade, and M. Lebrão, "Katz Index on elderly functionality evaluation," *Revista Da Escola De Enfermagem Da USP*, vol. 41, pp. 317–325, 2007.

[40] I. Wickelgren, "Teaching the spinal cord to walk," *Science*, vol. 279, no. 5349, pp. 319–321, 1998.

[41] I. Miyai, M. Ito, N. Hattori et al., "Cerebellar ataxia rehabilitation trial in degenerative cerebellar diseases," *Neurorehabilitation and Neural Repair*, vol. 26, no. 5, pp. 515–522, 2012.

[42] R. F. Macko, F. M. Ivey, L. W. Forrester et al., "Treadmill exercise rehabilitation improves ambulatory function and cardiovascular fitness in patients with chronic stroke: a randomized, controlled trial," *Stroke*, vol. 36, no. 10, pp. 2206–2211, 2005.

[43] S. Marzolini, P. I. Oh, and D. Brooks, "Effect of combined aerobic and resistance training versus aerobic training alone in individuals with coronary artery disease: A meta-analysis," *European Journal of Preventive Cardiology*, vol. 19, no. 1, pp. 81–94, 2012.

[44] A. Shapiro and I. Melzer, "Balance perturbation system to improve balance compensatory responses during walking in old persons," *Journal of NeuroEngineering and Rehabilitation*, vol. 7, no. 1, pp. 32–38, 2010.

[45] A. Mansfield, E. L. Inness, J. Komar et al., "Training rapid stepping responses in an individual with stroke," *Physical Therapy in Sport*, vol. 91, no. 6, pp. 958–969, 2011.

[46] M. Suteerawattananon, B. MacNeill, and E. J. Protas, "Supported treadmill training for gait and balance in a patient with progressive supranuclear palsy," *Physical Therapy in Sport*, vol. 82, no. 5, pp. 485–495, 2002.

[47] I. Miyai, Y. Fujimoto, H. Yamamoto et al., "Long-term effect of body weight-supported treadmill training in Parkinson's disease: a randomized controlled trial," *Archives of Physical Medicine and Rehabilitation*, vol. 83, no. 10, pp. 1370–1373, 2002.

[48] M. H. Rose, A. Løkkegaard, S. Sonne-Holm, and B. R. Jensen, "Effects of training and weight support on muscle activation in Parkinson's disease," *Journal of Electromyography & Kinesiology*, vol. 23, no. 6, pp. 1499–1504, 2013.

[49] M. Ganesan, T. N. Sathyaprabha, A. Gupta, and P. K. Pal, "Effect of partial weight-supported treadmill gait training on balance in patients with Parkinson disease," *PM&R : The Journal of Injury, Function, and Rehabilitation*, vol. 6, no. 1, pp. 22–33, 2014.

[50] K. Kim, S. Lee, and K. Lee, "Effects of progressive body weight support treadmill forward and backward walking training on stroke patients' affected side lower extremity's walking ability," *Journal of Physical Therapy Science*, vol. 26, no. 12, pp. 1923–1927, 2014.

[51] L. Ada, C. M. Dean, and R. Lindley, "Randomized trial of treadmill training to improve walking in community-dwelling people after stroke: The AMBULATE trial," *International Journal of Stroke*, vol. 8, no. 6, pp. 436–444, 2013.

[52] H. J. Lee, K. H. Cho, and W. H. Lee, "The effects of body weight support treadmill training with power-assisted functional electrical stimulation on functional movement and gait in stroke patients," *American Journal of Physical Medicine & Rehabilitation*, vol. 92, no. 12, pp. 1051–1059, 2013.

[53] M. MacKay-Lyons, A. McDonald, J. Matheson, G. Eskes, and M.-A. Klus, "Dual effects of body-weight supported treadmill training on cardiovascular fitness and walking ability early after stroke: a randomized controlled trial," *Neurorehabilitation and Neural Repair*, vol. 27, no. 7, pp. 644–653, 2013.

[54] J. Mehrholz, S. Thomas, and B. Elsner, "Treadmill training and body weight support for walking after stroke," *Cochrane Database of Systematic Reviews*, no. 8, article CD002840, 2017.

[55] M. B. Gardner, M. K. Holden, J. M. Leikauskas, and R. L. Richard, "Partial body weight support with treadmill locomotion to improve gait after incomplete spinal cord injury: A single-subject experimental design," *Physical Therapy in Sport*, vol. 78, no. 4, pp. 361–374, 1998.

[56] H. Foster, L. DeMark, P. M. Spigel, D. K. Rose, and E. J. Fox, "The effects of backward walking training on balance and mobility in an individual with chronic incomplete spinal cord injury: A case report," *Physiotherapy Theory and Practice*, vol. 32, no. 7, pp. 536–545, 2016.

[57] S. L. Stevens, J. L. Caputo, D. K. Fuller, and D. W. Morgan, "Effects of underwater treadmill training on leg strength, balance, and walking performance in adults with incomplete spinal cord injury," *The Journal of Spinal Cord Medicine*, vol. 38, no. 1, pp. 91–101, 2015.

8

Ataxia Telangiectasia Mutated Protein Kinase: A Potential Master Puppeteer of Oxidative Stress-Induced Metabolic Recycling

Marguerite Blignaut ⓘ, **Sarah Harries** ⓘ, **Amanda Lochner** ⓘ, and **Barbara Huisamen** ⓘ

Centre for Cardio-Metabolic Research in Africa (CARMA), Division of Medical Physiology, Department of Biomedical Sciences, Faculty of Medicine and Health Sciences, Stellenbosch University, South Africa

Correspondence should be addressed to Marguerite Blignaut; mblignaut@sun.ac.za

Academic Editor: Jon D. Lane

Ataxia Telangiectasia Mutated protein kinase (ATM) has recently come to the fore as a regulatory protein fulfilling many roles in the fine balancing act of metabolic homeostasis. Best known for its role as a transducer of DNA damage repair, the activity of ATM in the cytosol is enjoying increasing attention, where it plays a central role in general cellular recycling (macroautophagy) as well as the targeted clearance (selective autophagy) of damaged mitochondria and peroxisomes in response to oxidative stress, independently of the DNA damage response. The importance of ATM activation by oxidative stress has also recently been highlighted in the clearance of protein aggregates, where the expression of a functional ATM construct that cannot be activated by oxidative stress resulted in widespread accumulation of protein aggregates. This review will discuss the role of ATM in general autophagy, mitophagy, and pexophagy as well as aggrephagy and crosstalk between oxidative stress as an activator of ATM and its potential role as a master regulator of these processes.

1. Introduction

Ataxia Telangiectasia Mutated protein kinase (ATM) derives its name from the severe, recessive autosomal disease Ataxia-Telangiectasia (A-T). Although this neurodegenerative disease was initially identified in 1926 [1] and described as a clinical entity in 1958 [2], the gene and protein responsible for the disease were only characterized in the early 90's [3–5]. Null mutations in the *Atm* gene that cause the loss of functional ATM, a 370 kDa protein, results in severe characteristic cerebral ataxia and dilated blood vessels present in the conjunctivae of the eyes, also known as telangiectasia [6]. Moreover, nonfunctional ATM has been associated with an increased risk for cancer, radiation sensitivity, endocrine disruption, progressive neurodegeneration, premature ageing, and chromosomal instability (most recently reviewed by Shiloh [7]). The degree of disease severity is dependent on the type of mutation in the *Atm* gene (single or bi-allelic) and heterozygous patients, which make up as much as 1.4-2% of the general population, also exhibit a high incidence of ischaemic heart disease and insulin resistance [8, 9].

Constant oxidative stress is a common denominator in many of the A-T clinical and cellular phenotypes [10]. The loss of functional ATM results in prolonged activation of stress response pathways in the cerebellum but not in the cerebrum or liver [11]. More importantly, this suggests a cytoplasmic role for ATM. The protein resides predominantly in the nucleus of dividing cells [12], where it acts as a transducer in the DNA damage response pathway (DDR), but ATM is mainly found in the cytoplasm of nondividing neuronal cells where it maintains basal metabolic flux [13]. In these cell types, ATM maintains autophagy, a catabolic process that delivers cytoplasmic components for degradation to the lysosome, as well as redox homeostasis, rather than genomic stability and apoptosis. Moreover, it has been suggested that these divergent pathways could be a result of ATM's subcellular localization, as well as different mechanisms of activation and cell survival outcomes [13]. The seminal study of Guo et al. [14] demonstrated for the first time that ATM can be activated in the cytosol in response to exogenous hydrogen peroxide (H_2O_2) independently of DNA damage response, through the formation of a reversible disulphide bond at the only cysteine site within the protein kinase domain, Cys^{2991}. Low levels of ROS are sufficient to activate ATM at this residue, independently of the DNA damage response pathway [15], and these distinct activation mechanisms allow ATM to respond to different stresses as well as control different cytoplasmic pathways [16]. More recently, studies showed that ATM can be activated by endogenous ROS including peroxisomal reactive oxygen species (ROS) induced by clofibrate treatment [17] and mitochondrial superoxide induced by low doses of the redox-cycling chemical, menadione [18]. Both peroxisomal and mitochondrial ROS activation of ATM increase autophagy through the activation of AMPK that results in mTOR suppression in the cytosol [19]. Taken together, this suggests that ATM can directly modulate the rate of autophagy in a ROS dependent manner [20] and will be discussed in further detail.

ATM acts as an important sensor of oxidative stress in cells and regulates defences against redox stress [14] by rerouting of glycolysis to the pentose phosphate pathway (PPP) [21] (reviewed more extensively by Blignaut [22]). ATM also regulates mitochondrial biogenesis and DNA content [23] and can lead to mitochondrial dysfunction when absent [24, 25]. Antioxidative treatment that targets the mitochondria in the absence of ATM can decrease the metabolic syndrome, which supports the notion that A-T might be a mitochondrial disease [26, 27]. Importantly, ATM also contributes to glucose homeostasis [28] and is required for the phosphorylation of the insulin-dependent protein kinase, Akt [29, 30].

This review will focus on crosstalk between ROS as an activator of ATM and autophagy as a regulatory mechanism of protein aggregation and oxidative stress in the context of nondividing cells.

2. ATM and Oxidative Stress

ATM is a relatively large protein of 370 kDA, consists of approximately 3056 residues and is part of the PI-3 kinase-like protein kinase (PIKKs) family [31]. The catalytic function of ATM identifies with the mechanisms mostly found in serine-threonine proteins that phosphorylate downstream proteins on the hydroxyl group of the serine or threonine residues [32].

The most common function of ATM is to respond to double strand DNA breaks in the nucleus, where the protein is autophosphorylated at Ser^{1996}, followed by monomerization of the dimer, and activated in response to DNA damage [33–35]. Upon activation, ATM is responsible for the phosphorylation and activation of downstream proteins, including the Mre11, Rad50, and Nbs1 complex (MRN complex), which aid in DNA repair [35].

Alternatively, ATM can be activated in response to oxidative stress and hypoxic conditions [36, 37], but the question remained whether this can be achieved independently of the DDR pathway. This was answered in a groundbreaking study that reported the direct activation of ATM by hydrogen peroxide (H_2O_2) as an inducer of oxidative stress [14]. This study investigated ATM activation under oxidative stress conditions generated with H_2O_2 and double strand DNA

breaks (DSBs) with bleomycin, a well-known genotoxic agent, in human fibroblasts. Although p53 was phosphorylated at Ser^{15} and Thr^{68} in response to H_2O_2 and bleomycin, in an ATM-specific manner, the histone variant, H2AX, as a marker of DNA repair, was only phosphorylated in response to the latter treatment. Inhibition of ATM ablated the phosphorylation of the DNA damage-specific proteins p53, ATM, and Chk2 in the presence of H_2O_2, whilst activation of ATM by H_2O_2 was inhibited in the presence of the strong hydroxyl scavenger, N-acetylcysteine (NAC). They reported that oxidation resulted in a conformational change in ATM but not the monomerization observed in response to DNA damage. The study found that ATM forms a reversible disulphide bond at the cysteine site, Cys^{2991}, and mutation of this site from Cys^{2991} to Ala^{2991}, resulted in a construct that can be activated in the presence of DSBs but not oxidative stress. Although ATM contains several disulphide bonds, it is the covalent disulphide bond at Cys^{2991} through which ROS modulates its effects.

However, it should be noted that the interplay between oxidized ATM and DSB-activated ATM is complicated: Guo et al. [14] suggested that oxidative stress disrupts DNA binding at the complex responsible for ATM recruitment to the damaged site and can therefore inhibit ATM activation by DSBs, resulting in the oxidation of ATM under high ROS conditions. A more recent study showed that excess endogenous ROS represses ATM-dependent homologous DNA repair in cells obtained from ataxia patients with oculomotor apraxia type 3 (AOA3 cells) which has implications for both neurodegeneration and tumorigenesis [38]. Irrespective of the lack of consensus with regard to the oxidation of ATM under either high or low ROS conditions, many of the ATM substrates identified with proteomic analyses, implicate ATM in metabolic signalling pathways [39].

Under normal physiological conditions, ROS act as signalling intermediates in many cellular processes to induce redox homeostasis. On the other hand, elevated ROS levels, aptly described as oxidative stress, have been linked with over 150 diseases, most notably atherosclerosis, diabetes, and cancer [19]. It has therefore been suggested that A-T might, in essence, be an oxidative stress disorder [40]. In order to understand how ATM contributes towards the maintenance of basal metabolic flux and redox homeostasis, a short overview of oxidants and their cellular targets is required.

Briefly, ROS derive from the reduction of molecular oxygen which most notably includes oxygen ($O_2^{\bullet-}$), hydroxyl ($^{\bullet}OH$), peroxyl ($RO_2\bullet$), and alkoxyl ($RO\bullet$), as well as certain nonradicals that are either oxidizing agents or can be converted into radicals such as hypochlorous acid (HOCl), ozone (O_3), single oxygen ($^1O_2$), and H_2O_2 [41]. Metabolism of nitric oxide (NO) results in the formation of reactive nitrogen species (RNS) that can either contribute to oxidation, nitrosation, or nitration [42]. The enzymatic action of nitric oxide synthase (NOS) results in the formation of nitric oxide (NO) but can also produce $O_2^{\bullet-}$ under the right circumstances. A rapid reaction between NO and $O_2^{\bullet-}$ results in the formation of peroxynitrite (ONOOH) which is involved in oxidation, nitrosation, and nitration. In the case of nitration, nitrotyrosine can be formed and alter cell signalling pathways. For example, nitrite together with HOCl has been detected in diseased human vascular tissue and drives the formation of artherogenic LDL which is implicated in atherosclerosis [43].

There are numerous sources of endogenous ROS including the cytoplasm, where $O_2^{•-}$, generated by either mitochondria or the NOX-family (nicotinamide adenine dinucleotide phosphate (NADPH) oxidases), is converted to H_2O_2, as well as the production of H_2O_2 by the endoplasmic reticulum (ER) as a byproduct of protein oxidation and as an end product in several peroxisomal oxidation pathways including β-oxidation of long-chain fatty acids [44, 45]. NOX1, -2, -4, and -5 transport electrons across biological membranes in order to reduce oxygen to superoxide and are expressed throughout the cardiovascular system, brain, and cerebrovascular tissue (extensively reviewed by [41]). This protein family is one of the best known sources of cytoplasmic ROS, which in itself has been described as the cornerstone of cellular signalling and disease pathophysiology [46–48]. The broad impact of ROS is made possible by the large number of molecules that ROS can interact with, including small organic molecules, proteins, lipids, carbohydrates, and nucleic acids. These interactions can either destroy or irreversibly change the function of the target molecule and accordingly contribute towards pathogenesis [41].

Most redox reactions, however, occur through the reversible reduction and oxidation of crucial reactive cysteine residues that form thiolate anions at a physiological pH [49]. Oxidation of this residue, as is the case for ATM at Cys^{2991}, results in a sulfenic residue (SOH), which is further modified to form an intramolecular disulphide bond. As mentioned previously, the addition of exogenous H_2O_2 in vitro forms an active ATM dimer of two covalently-linked monomers. Possible in vivo sources of oxidants, that can reduce thiol and oxidizing disulphide bonds, are generated by the membrane bound NOX-family of NADPH oxidases. These enzymes produce anions that can be dismutated into H_2O_2 which selectively re-enters the cell through aquaporin channels [44].

NOX-4, which is located in close proximity of the nucleus in a wide range of human cells, produces ROS innately and is elevated in A-T cells [50]. Specific inhibition of both NOX-4 and NOX-2 alleviates increased cancer risk in A-T null mice, whilst the inhibition of ATM increased NOX-4 expression in normal cells. NOX-4 is thus potentially a critical mediator of ROS and in the development of A-T.

Most recently, Zhang et al. [18] reported that ATM acts as a redox-sensor in response to endogenous mitochondrial ROS (H_2O_2) and serves as a critical juncture in the regulation of carbohydrate metabolism. The study showed that glutathione production, which is also an endogenous antioxidant, is increased in cells expressing an ATM Cys^{2991}Ala mutant construct and suggests that this is an attempt to compensate for a lower glucose flux through the PPP, thus decreasing the availability of NADPH.

Taken together, ATM can be activated in response to exogenous (H_2O_2) and endogenous ROS (mitochondrial) as well as through NADPH-oxidases, allowing it to respond as a redox-sensor for the PPP [16]. However, ATM has also

been shown to mediate autophagy in response to oxidative stress, which will be discussed in the following section.

3. ATM-Mediated Autophagy

Autophagy is a highly regulated catabolic process that literally translates to "self-eating"; this general term describes the delivery of cytoplasmic components, including parts of the cytosol and large protein complexes, within a double membrane vesicle (autophagosome) to the lysosome for degradation [51]. Basal physiological autophagy ensures cellular homeostasis and protein recycling within all eukaryotic cells [52] but can also be stimulated in response to cellular stress, including but not limited to, oxidative stress, hypoxia, nutrient starvation, DNA damage, and protein aggregation [53]. The ubiquitin-proteosome system (UPS) targets only individual, short lived, or misfolded proteins for degradation, whilst autophagy recycles larger components such as damaged organelles, excessive, or toxic byproducts and larger protein complexes and aggregates [54]. This diverse but specific degradation response is enabled by three types of autophagy, namely, macroautophagy, microautophagy, and chaperone-mediated autophagy, which differ with regard to their targeted substrate and sequestration mechanism [55]. This review will focus on the role of ATM in ROS-induced macroautophagy.

The initiation of macroautophagy occurs in the cytoplasm via the activation of adenosine $5'$-monophosphate-(AMP-) activated protein kinase (AMPK) in response to nutrient starvation and hypoxia [56]. Moreover, AMPK activation results in the inhibition of lipid and glycogen synthesis, whilst concurrently activating free fatty acid oxidation and glycolysis [56]. Moreover, the activation of AMPK phosphorylates and activates TSC2 (tuberous sclerosis complex 2) resulting in the repression of mTOR complex 1 (mechanistic target of rapamycin complex 1), which is a negative regulator of autophagy [57]. AMPK activation can also phosphorylate the mTOR-binding partner, raptor, and induces 14-3-3 binding to raptor, which is required for the inhibition of mTORC1 [58], as well as phosphorylate mTORC1 directly at Thr^{2446} [59]. Once mTORC1 is repressed, unc-51-like kinase (ULK1) is dephosphorylated and consequently activated. Under starvation conditions, AMPK promotes autophagy through the direct phosphorylation of ULK1 at Ser^{317} and Ser^{777}, whereas sufficient nutrients promote mTOR activity and prevents ULK1 activation through phosphorylation at Ser^{757}, consequently disrupting the interaction between ULK1 and AMPK [60]. ULK1, together with Atg1, form one of at least five core molecular components that is required for the formation of the autophagosome membrane [61]. The other core molecular components include the Beclin1/class III PI3K complex; the transmembrane proteins, Atg9 and vacuole membrane protein 1 (VMP1); and two ubiquitin-like protein conjugation systems, Atg12 and Atg8/LC3 [62]. Once the formation of a phagophore is initiated, the vesicle expands sequentially and engulfs the cytosolic cargo, in either a selective or nonselective manner, to form the autophagosome [63]. The formation of the autophagosome is driven by the Atg (AuTophagy related) proteins and has been reviewed extensively [63, 64].

Selectivity of the targeted cargo is conferred by receptors that recognize and interact with lipidated ATG8 family proteins, which are located on the concave side of the developing autophagosome [65]. This interaction is enabled by LC3 interacting regions (LIR) that bind to the LIR docking sites of ATG8 family proteins [65]. The ATG8 family consists of the LC3/GABARAP protein family and includes the microtubule-associated protein 1 light chain 3 (MAP1LC3A-B and C) or γ-aminobutyric acid (GABA) type A receptor–associated protein (GABARAP and GABARAP-like 1 and -2) [66]. Of these proteins, the best-studied protein is LC3B, which confers selectivity, together with the GABARAP proteins, for pexophagy and mitophagy through interaction with adapter proteins [66]. LC3B associates with the forming autophagosomal membrane through the formation of a covalent bond to phosphatidylethanol (PE) enabled by a ubiquitination-like sequence of enzymatic events where ATG7 acts as the LC3 activating enzyme and ATG 3 as the conjugating enzyme that transfer LC3 to PE to form lipidated LC3-PE/LC3-II [67, 68].

Autophagy adapter proteins interact directly with the ATG8 proteins and share the ability to interact simultaneously with the autophagosome through interaction of their LIR motif with LC3 as well as the cargo substrate, which is often ubiquitylated [67]. These receptors include, amongst others, p62/SQSTM1, BNIP3 (BCL2/adenovirus E1B 19 kDa interacting protein), FUNDC1 (Fun14 domain containing 1), NBR1 (neighbour of BRCA1), NDP52 (nuclear dot protein of 52 kDa), and optineuron, of which many have a ubiquitin-binding domain (UBD) that can interact with different ubiquitin chain linkages associated with the targeted cargo and in doing so, provide selectivity [67]. Once the cargo is tethered to the forming autophagosome, LC3B and the GABARAP subfamily promote the elongation and fusion (closure) of the autophagosome [66], which can then fuse with the lysosome to form an autolysosome and results in pH changes to occur in the lumen of the lysosome [69]. The change in lysosomal pH is essential for successful protein degradation as the hydrolyses responsible for cargo breakdown are activated in an acidic environment [70]. The process of autophagosome maturation, trafficking, and lysosomal fusion as well as the proteins involved in this process has recently been reviewed extensively [71].

In view of the oxidative stress induced activation of ATM, as well as the pathophysiology associated with elevated ROS in ATM-deficient cells, Alexander et al. [19] reported that the activation of oxidized ATM increases autophagy through the activation of TSC2 via the liver kinase B1 (LKB1)/AMPK pathway, resulting in the repression of mTORC1. Moreover, inhibition of mTORC1 with rapamycin results in the concomitant improvement of ROS levels in ATM$^{-/-}$ mice. The authors found that low concentrations of H_2O_2 rapidly induced mTORC1 repression that could, in turn, be rescued by the addition of NAC or pretreatment with catalase. Of relevance as well, is that chemical mitochondrial uncoupling which depletes the antioxidant, glutathione, also repressed mTORC1 signalling, indicating that both exogenous and endogenous ROS activation of ATM can induce mTORC1 repression.

The same research group found that nitrosative stress (nitric oxide (NO)) also activates ATM and results in the phosphorylation of AMPK through LKB1, activation of the TSC2 complex and consequent repression of mTORC1 [72]. ATM-mediated repression of mTORC1 decreased phosphorylation of direct target proteins of mTORC1 such as 4E-BP1 (4E-binding protein 1), S6K (ribosomal S6 kinase), and ULK1 (Unc-51 like autophagy activating kinase). Consequently, nitrosative stress-mediated activation of ATM can increase autophagy by decreasing mTORC1 mediated phosphorylation of ULK1 at Ser^{757} and increasing ULK1-phosphorylation at Ser^{317} by AMPK. However, the precise mechanism through which NO activates ATM is still unknown. Induction of autophagy by NO also resulted in decreased cell viability, which suggests a cytotoxic response.

LKB1 can be phosphorylated directly at Thr^{366} by active ATM in response to ionising radiation (IR) [73] as well as through oxidative stress as discussed above, consequently activating AMPK directly to modulate apoptosis [74] or autophagy in the event of energetic stress.

On the other hand, one of the key roles of AMPK in cardiac tissue is the response to hypoxia/ischaemia, which is also under the direct control of LKB1; in the absence of LKB1, mouse hearts show increased mTORC1 signalling and protein synthesis that can lead to hypertrophy [75]. Interestingly, Emerling et al. [76] showed that the hypoxic activation of AMPK in mouse fibroblasts is dependent on mitochondrial oxidative stress that is generated by the ETC and not the cytosolic adenosine monophosphate (AMP)/adenosine triphosphate (ATP) ratio. Although they did not evaluate the role of ATM in their study, it supports the notion that the oxidative activation of ATM, due to increased mitochondrial dysfunction, can potentially mediate the activation of AMPK in response to hypoxic stress.

In a nutshell, autophagy is a catabolic process responsible for the degradation and recycling of damaged organelles and is central to the maintenance of cellular homeostasis. The activation of ATM through ROS and NO places ATM directly upstream of AMPK, which in turn, drives the inhibition of mTORC1 and upregulation of autophagy through ULK1. This allows cells to eliminate damaged organelles that can drive increased oxidative stress and recycle these components to maintain nutrient and energy homeostasis, but this process can also be mediated independently of ATM. ROS-induced autophagy can be induced by either $O_2^{\bullet-}$ [77] or H_2O_2 [78] that is produced in response to either glucose or nutrient starvation and can cause mitochondrial energetic stress due to decreased ATP availability [52]. Both redox balance and ROS formation can be regulated by changes in the autophagy rate and consequently either directly regulate mitochondrial homeostasis or indirectly regulate mitochondrial function [79].

Key to effective autophagy, which is also responsible for the degradation of ATM [80], is the fusion of the autophagosome to lysosomes, in order to form an autolysosome where the targeted content is degraded. Recent observations in ATM$^{-/-}$ neurons showed upregulated autophagic flux of lysosomes with a more acidic pH and led to the finding that the ATPase, H$^+$ transporting lysosomal V1 subunit A

(ATP6V1A proton pump) is a target of ATM [80]. The absence of ATM results in the peri-nuclear accumulation of lysosomes which suggests that this could be due to a physical interaction between ATM and the retrograde transport motor protein, dynein. Lysosomal dynein accumulates in ATM $^{-/-}$ mouse brains indicating that ATM inhibits axonal transport through dynein motor proteins. Similarly, the study found that the loss of ATM resulted in the impaired glucose uptake due to the inhibition of the translocation of the SLC2A4/GLUT4 (solute carrier family 4 (facilitated glucose transporter) 4) to the plasma membrane, and increased trafficking to lysosomes instead [80]. This observation further supports previous reports that decreased ATM activity is associated with metabolic syndrome [81] and insulin resistance [82]. The importance of ATM in autophagy is highlighted by the accumulation of lysosomes, as well as increased oxidative stress in the cerebellum of ATM-null mice [83].

Increased oxidative stress and a weakened antioxidant defence due to dysfunctional autophagy can induce cellular damage and result in neuronal cell death, which is the major causative factor in the development of Parkinson's disease, which predominantly affects aged individuals above 60 [71]. Increasing age results in a decline in autophagy as well as an increase in protein misfolding and oxidative stress [67] and can lead to the disruption of cellular homeostasis [68]. Similarly, age-associated decreases in ATM protein levels [84] may result in the development of metabolic syndrome, lysosomal accumulation, and protein aggregation that are associated with age-related neuronal diseases [85] and the development of cardiac dysfunction including fibrosis and hypertrophy [86].

4. ATM and Aggrephagy

Protein aggregates develop when proteins are misfolded due to mutations, incomplete translation, inappropriate protein modifications, oxidative stress, and ineffective assembly of protein complexes [87]. The accumulation of misfolded and dysfunctional protein aggregates, often due to oxidative stress [88, 89] or downregulated or disrupted autophagy [90], can be toxic to the cell and cause a disruption of cellular homeostasis that is detrimental to cellular survival in many diseases, and in particular, neurodegenerative diseases [91]. Aggregation is driven by exposed hydrophobic patches in misfolded proteins that sequester other proteins. Misfolding can be repaired by molecular chaperones, but if the damage is too great, the misfolded proteins are guided by chaperone complexes for degradation by either the ubiquitin-proteosome system (UPS) or the lysosome through chaperone mediated autophagy or aggrephagy [87]. The latter process specifically refers to the selective sequestration of protein aggregates by macroautophagy and will be the discussed further.

Protein aggregation is classically associated with neurodegeneration but has been observed in nearly every cardiometabolic disease [92]. The accumulation of proteins and dysfunctional organelles contributes to the development of pathology in almost all tissues and thus requires a very fine

balance between apoptosis and autophagy [93]. There seems to be synergistic roles for ATM and p53 with regard to the regulation of autophagy, where ATM regulates mitochondrial homeostasis and oxidative stress in order to prevent cells from undergoing apoptosis in response to nongenotoxic p53 activation [94]. Genetic or pharmacological loss of ATM kinase activity blocks autophagy and increases ROS, which is sufficient to commit cells to apoptosis in response to Nutlin 3 treatment, an inhibitor of the p53 E3 ubiquitin ligase MDM2 that activates p53 [94].

Most recently, it has been shown that the loss of function mutation that blocks ATM activation by oxidative stress, but not genotoxic stress, results in widespread protein aggregation, especially when cells are exposed to low levels of ROS, and includes polypeptides mainly implicated in DNA metabolism and gene expression [95]. This implicates a role for ATM in protein homeostasis. Moreover, protein aggregation is very relevant to neurodegeneration, especially with regard to the loss of function of Purkinje neuronal cells, which is a hallmark of A-T [96].

Proteasomal degradation is also required for the maintenance of autophagy at physiological levels as is the case with ULK1; it is specifically ubiquitinated by the E3 ligase NEDD44 that marks it for proteasomal degradation, whilst still being actively translated and transcribed [75]. The transcription of ULK1 is in turn inhibited by mTOR during prolonged autophagy and allows for the maintenance of ULK1 protein at basal levels within the cell.

It is also possible that ATM can play a more active role in ULK1 phosphorylation through p32. Although p32 was first recognized as a novel substrate of ATM in cardiac DNA damage [97], it has recently been identified as a regulator of ULK1 stability [98]. In a study that investigated the cardiotoxicity and genotoxic effect of chemotherapeutic agents that induce cell death through the ATM-mediated phosphorylation of p53, the protein, p32 (CIQBP/HABP1), was identified as an endogenous substrate in mouse hearts [97]. The protein is phosphorylated at Ser^{148} by ATM in response to genotoxic stress, but the authors did not comment on the physiological effect thereof [97]. However, p32 has been found to be essential for maintaining the activity and stability of ULK1 [98]. The study found that the ablation of p32 results in increased proteolysis of ULK1, that consequently impaired starvation-induced autophagic flux as well as the clearance of damaged (uncoupled) mitochondria, and highlights the importance of p32 for ULK1 activity. The phosphorylation of ULK1 by AMPK also regulates the translocation of ULK1 to mitochondria in response to hypoxia [99] where it phosphorylates the autophagy cargo receptor, FUNDC1 [100], and regulates mitophagy [101]. Although ATM was not investigated in this context, it is tempting to hypothesize that ATM could influence ULK1 potentially through the phosphorylation of p32 in the heart.

5. ATM Mediates Selective Autophagy

Constitutive autophagy plays a protective role in mitochondrial rich cardiomyocytes, where accumulation of abnormal proteins and organelles, especially mitochondria, may directly cause cardiac dysfunction [102]. Mitophagy, a specialized mechanism of autophagy that specifically aims to degrade and maintain mitochondrial quality, is central to maintaining cellular integrity and cellular homeostasis [103]. The process of mitophagy is known to decrease during ageing, thus resulting in mitochondrial dysfunction [104].

Classically, depolarized mitochondria initiate the accumulation of (PTEN-) induced kinase 1 (PINK1) on the outer mitochondrial membrane [105]. PINK1 is degraded in healthy mitochondria but accumulate on the outer mitochondrial membrane of damaged mitochondria that, in turn, drives the recruitment and translocation of Parkin [85] to the mitochondria. Parkin is an E3 ubiquitin ligase which is phosphorylated by PINK1, stimulating its translocation to the mitochondria where it ubiquinates several outer mitochondrial membrane proteins. This promotes further PINK1 phosphorylation and the formation of ubiquitin chains that localizes mitophagy receptors that contain UBDs to Parkin-ubiquitylated mitochondria, including p62 (SQSTM1), NBR1, and optineurin [106] that can attach to autophagosomal membranes and envelop the damaged mitochondria (reviewed by Nguyen et al. [107]) for degradation [108].

PINK1 also phosphorylates the fusion protein, mitofusin 2 (Mfn2), which can serve as a mitochondrial receptor for Parkin, promoting its ubiquitination [88]. The loss of Mfn2 prevents the translocation of Parkin in depolarized mitochondria and suppresses mitophagy, which drives the accumulation of dysfunctional mitochondria and decreased mitochondrial respiration in mouse cardiomyocytes [88]. Alternatively, mitophagy can be mediated by mitophagy receptors. Mitochondrial receptor-mediated autophagy is mediated by the pro-apoptotic proteins, BNIP3 and NIX, that localize to the outer mitochondrial membrane and act as receptors for targeting autophagosomes through direct interaction of conserved LC3-interacting regions (LIRs) with LC3 on the autophagosome, often in response to hypoxia [109] and in the absence of mitochondrial membrane permeabilization [110]. FUNDCI is an outer mitochondrial membrane protein that has been implicated in hypoxia-mediated mitophagy in mammalian cells [111]. Similar to BNIP3 and NIX, FUNDC1 acts as a receptor for the autophagosomal membrane and interacts directly with LC3 through LIR. The serine/threonine protein phosphatase, PGAM5, dephosphorylates FUNDC1 during hypoxia or mitochondrial membrane depolarization and promotes interaction with LC3 with consequent mitophagy [112].

More recently, a direct link between ATM and PINK1/-Parkin recruitment was shown, as ATM was able to initiate the accumulation of PINK1 and translocation of Parkin in the presence of spermidine and lead (Pb) initiating mitophagy [113, 114]. Spermidine is a natural polyamine involved in several biological processes including cell proliferation and apoptosis and tends to decline with age [115]. Spermidine also elicits mitochondrial depolarization that causes the formation of mitophagosomes and mitochondrial targeted lysosomes, which has been suggested to occur via ATM-dependent activation of the PINK1/Parkin mitophagy pathway [114]. Spermidine-induced mitochondrial depolarization is abrogated in the presence of the chemical ATM

inhibitor, KU55933. Moreover, spermidine promotes the colocalization of phosphorylated ATM and PINK1 on the outer mitochondrial membrane, which, together with the translocation of Parkin, can be blocked by the ATM inhibitor. The authors suggest a model whereby activated ATM drives PINK1 accumulation as well as Parkin translocation with consequent mitophagy in response to spermidine treatment (Figure 1).

ATM may therefore be central to mitophagy by directly activating the pathway or by indirectly activating autophagy in response to oxidative stress. Thus, if pathological ATM signalling occurs, mitophagy could be affected, predisposing the cell to mitochondrial oxidative stress [22]. ATM is also activated by nitrosative stress and contribute to sustained mitophagy of damaged mitochondria through the newly characterized ATM-denitrosylase S-nitrosoglutathione reductase (GSNOR) axis [116].

The chronic oxidative stress observed in A-T has led to the suggestion that A-T might be a mitochondrial disease [40] and has also been linked with intrinsic mitochondrial dysfunction [24]. The latter study found that lymphoblastoid cells from A-T patients contain an increased population of mitochondria with a decreased membrane potential, when compared to control cells. Proteins with specific roles in mitochondrial DNA damage and/or ROS scavenging, including mnSOD, peroxiredoxin 3, and mitochondrial topoisomerase, were also elevated in these cells. Indeed, the decreased membrane potential translated into decreased respiratory activity in the A-T cells compared to the wild type controls. Concomitantly, the authors showed that the *in vivo* loss of *ATM* in mice resulted in mitochondrial dysfunction in thymocytes that was accompanied by increased mitochondrial content and mitochondrial ROS due to a decrease in mitophagy. Interestingly, they observed a significant decrease in complex I activity as well as ATP production and an increase in oxygen consumption. The study also found that autophagy was not affected by the absence of ATM and suggested that changes in mitochondrial dynamics such as fission and fusion could contribute towards defective mitophagy. The authors concluded that the observed defects in the absence of ATM suggest that ATM might localize directly to mitochondria. Fractionation studies in cells revealed that the mitochondrial fraction of HepG2 cells was enriched with ATM and activated ATM in response to H_2O_2 treatment [117]. In contrast to previous observations that ATM associated with the peroxisomal fraction [118], Morita et al. [117] detected almost no ATM in this fraction. This reverberates with the suggestion [119] that both the cell type and culture conditions of immortalized A-T cells can affect mitochondrial homeostasis and autophagic responses which explain the differences in mitochondrial content reported in A-T deficient cell lines.

Mitochondrial respiration inhibition can also lead to increased mitochondrial ROS production. Treatment of HeLa cells with either rotenone or Antimycin C failed to increase mitochondrial hydrogen peroxide production although it did increase mitochondrial superoxide production [18]. Superoxide itself failed to drive ATM dimerization and suggested that mitochondrial superoxide must be

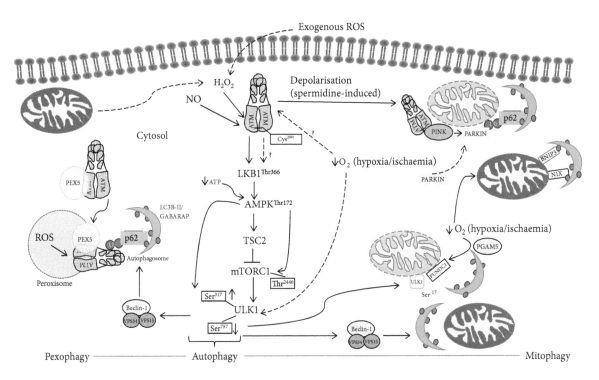

FIGURE 1: ROS can activate cytosolic ATM. ATM is activated in response to both endogenous and exogenous ROS, as well as NO at Cys^{2991}, where it forms a disulphide bond. Once activated, it phosphorylates LKB1 at Thr^{366} which phosphorylates AMPK and drives the inhibition of mTORC1 through TSC2. The inhibition of mTORC1 phosphorylates ULK1 at Ser^{757}, whilst AMPK phosphorylates ULK1 at Ser^{313}. This initiates autophagy and the formation of an autophagosome that targets peroxisomes specifically for degradation through the ATM-mediated ubiquitination of PEX5. It is currently unknown whether ATM is involved in either the activation of AMPK or suppression of mTOR in response to ROS to induce mitophagy. ATM mediates PINK/Parkin mitophagy pathway in response to spermidine treatment, which induces ROS and consequently activate ATM, that is then recruited to the permeabilized mitochondrial membrane where it colocalize with PINK and drives the recruitment of Parkin which is ubiquitinated. The ubiquitin chain binds to LC3 (green balls) on the autophagosome, which then engulfs damaged mitochondria for lysosomal degradation (not shown). Hypoxia or mitochondrial uncoupling can also activate ULK1, driving its translocation to the damaged mitochondrion membrane where it phosphorylates FUNDC1, which enhances its binding to LC3, whereas the dephosphorylation of FUNDC1 by PGAM5 also allows FUNDC1 to directly interact with LC3. BNIP and NIX can act as mitochondrial receptors in response to hypoxia when the mitochondrial membrane is not permeabilized and bind to LC3 on the autophagosome. Damaged mitochondria produce less ATP that activates AMPK, which in turn phosphorylates ULK1 and activates the Beclin1-VSP34-VSP15 complex and drives the formation of an autophagosome. Damaged mitochondria can also produce ROS which inhibits mTOR and leads to the activation of autophagy.

converted to H_2O_2 in order to activate ATM in either the cytosol or nucleus of HeLa cells.

Our group reported that ATM is directly associated with the inner mitochondrial membrane of cardiac mitochondria, and the inhibition thereof decreases oxidative phosphorylation and the ATP synthesis rate in a complex I-mediated manner [120]. Similarly, $ATM^{-/-}$ thymocytes exhibit decreased complex I activity [25], whereas the chemical inhibition of ATM resulted in a posttranslational decrease of COX-IV [121]. This is interesting because the inhibition of COX-IV has been associated with increased ROS production at complex I, albeit in the mitochondrial matrix [122]. Depletion of ATP in neuronal Purkinje cells results in increased ROS production that can activate ATM, consequently leading the phosphorylation of Nrf1 that specifically upregulates the expression of nuclear-encoded mitochondrial genes and improves electron transport chain capacity and restores mitochondrial function [123]. Similarly, Fang et al. [124] reported increased mitochondrial content in ATM-knockdown (ATM-KD) rat neurons

coupled to increased ROS production. The authors suggested that this could reflect decreased ATP production and either inadequate or inefficient mitophagy. Moreover, the study showed that mitophagy is suppressed in ATM-KD HeLa cells and rat neurons but that the phenotype could be rescued by replenishing cellular NAD^+ which significantly improved life-span in $ATM^{-/-}$ mice [124].

Interestingly, Beclin-1 heterozygosity in $ATM^{-/-}$ mice reduces mitochondrial ROS and complex I abnormalities in thymocytes [25]. Beclin-1 forms part of the complex required for the induction of autophagy [125] but is also required for the recruitment of Parkin to the mitochondrial membrane where it induces ubiquitination and proteasomal degradation of proteins on the outer mitochondrial membrane [126]. This leads to the inhibition of fusion and the trafficking of dysfunctional mitochondria [126]. It is still unclear why the allelic loss of Beclin1 would promote improvement of mitochondrial dysfunction in $ATM^{-/-}$ mice, but it has led to the suggestion that Beclin-1 might have additional functions besides its role in autophagy [25].

Terminally differentiated cells such as cardiomyocytes and neuronal cells are dependent on the efficient removal and replacement of dysfunctional mitochondria to ensure cell survival and to maintain cellular homeostasis [111, 127]. A decrease in ATP production and increased ROS production as indicators of mitochondrial dysfunction can result in either the release of apoptotic proteins or the selective clearance of the damaged mitochondria. Mitophagy thus serves as an early cardioprotective response through the removal of damaged mitochondria, and if this fails, apoptosis can be induced in response to excessive oxidative stress [128]. Moreover, reduced autophagy, together with the accumulation of dysfunctional mitochondria, has been associated with heart failure and aging [111].

Pexophagy is the targeted selective degradation of peroxisomes [129] and is another example of selective autophagy [130]. Peroxisomes utilise β-oxidation to reduce long-chain fatty acids into medium length fatty acids that can be shuttled to the mitochondria. These highly metabolic organelles generate ROS during β-oxidation and require homeostatic maintenance to prevent oxidative stress. ATM binds to the peroxisome importer receptor, PEX5, in response to excessive ROS and mediates peroxisome-specific autophagy (pexophagy) by phosphorylating PEX5 at Ser^{141} and promoting mono-ubiquitylation at Lys^{209}, whilst simultaneously inducing autophagy through the activation and phosphorylation of TSC2 and ULK1 [17, 131, 132]. Ubiquitylation of PEX5 is mediated by the complex PEX2-PEX10-PEX12 and is then recognized by the autophagy adapter proteins, p62 and NBR1, which directs the autophagosome to the peroxisomes for pexophagy [129].

Loss of function mutations in ATM, such as the ability to sense oxidative stress, can result in a reduction in mitochondrial antioxidant defences, lead to the accumulation of ROS and oxidative damage to mitochondria and other cellular components [18], as well as protein aggregation [95]. Selective autophagy seems to be mainly mediated by ubiquitination which is essential for conferring selectivity [133], as is the case of ATM-mediated pexophagy. As previously discussed, this also implies a potential role for ATM in aggrephagy (degradation of damaged or misfolded proteins) which is dependent on p62 ubiquitination [92].

6. Conclusion

This broad overview describes the apical protein, ATM protein kinase, at the nexus of oxidative stress-induced autophagy [14, 18] as well as nitrosative stress-induced autophagy [72, 116], mitophagy [113, 114], and pexophagy [17, 132] mainly in the context of nondividing cells such as cardiomyocytes and neurons. Site-specific mutations that renders ATM insensitive to oxidative stress increase protein aggregation [95], whilst loss of function increases perinuclear lysosomal accumulation [80] as well as mitochondrial oxidative stress [25] and dysfunction [24, 25, 120]. Cytoplasmic ATM thus plays a central role in redox homeostasis and ROS-mediated autophagy.

As a master regulator of DNA repair, activation of ATM by exogenous and endogenous oxidative stress, independently of DNA strand breaks, only recently came to light [14, 18]. This finding paved the way to understanding the severe neurodegeneration and associated protein aggregation observed in A-T patients that is largely due to disrupted ATM protein kinase functioning leading to disrupted autophagy, mitophagy, and pexophagy [80, 95]. Additionally, the regulation of ATM levels by autophagy [80] and the role of ATM in oxidative stress-mediated autophagy in an AMPK/mTORC1 dependent manner were discovered [13, 19, 132]. Similarly, ROS-induced pexophagy is modulated by ATM through the TSC2/AMPK/mTORC1 pathway in which the disruption of this signalling pathway leads to interrupted cellular homeostasis causing pathologies linked to neurodegeneration [17, 131, 134].

It has been suggested that the pathogenesis of A-T could be ascribed to excessive ROS and that A-T might therefore be an oxidative stress disease [40]. Several studies have investigated the effect of the absence or inhibition of ATM on mitochondrial function and found that ATM is innately associated with the inner mitochondrial membrane and oxidative phosphorylation of cardiac mitochondria [120]. In addition, the absence of functional ATM in the mitochondria of ATM-null thymocytes and fibroblasts was associated with decreased ATP production, increased ROS production [24, 25], and a decrease in mitophagy [119, 123].

Therefore, activation of ATM by oxidative stress and the consequent maintenance of redox homeostasis through autophagy, pexophagy, aggrephagy, and mitophagy place ATM at the centre of cross-talk between ROS and autophagy signalling.

Authors' Contributions

M.B conceptualized and wrote the manuscript and created Figure 1. SH contributed to the writing of the manuscript. B. H and A. L reviewed and modified the manuscript. All authors approved the final version of the manuscript.

Acknowledgments

This work was supported by the National Research Foundation South Africa (grant numbers CPRR160411161914 (BH), SFP180507326754 (MB)) and a Harry Crossley Foundation project grant (SH).

References

[1] L. Syllaba and K. Henner, "Contribution a l'independance de l'athetose double idiopathique et congenitale," *Revista de Neurologia*, vol. 1, pp. 541–562, 1926.

[2] E. Boder and R. P. Sedgwick, "Ataxia-telangiectasia; a familial syndrome of progressive cerebellar ataxia, oculocutaneous telangiectasia and frequent pulmonary infection," *Pediatrics*, vol. 21, no. 4, pp. 526–554, 1958.

[3] R. A. Gatti, I. Berkel, E. Boder et al., "Localization of an ataxia-telangiectasia gene to chromosome 11q22-23," *Nature*, vol. 336, no. 6199, pp. 577–580, 1988.

[4] K. Savitsky, S. Sfez, D. A. Tagle et al., "The complete sequence of the coding region of the ATM gene reveals similarity to cell cycle regulators in different species," *Human molecular genetics*, vol. 4, pp. 2025–2032, 1995.

[5] Y. Ziv, A. Bar-Shira, I. Pecker et al., "Recombinant ATM protein complements the cellular A-T phenotype," *Oncogene*, vol. 15, no. 2, pp. 159–167, 1997.

[6] R. A. Gatti, S. Becker-Catania, H. H. Chun et al., "The pathogenesis of ataxia-telangiectasia: learning from a Rosetta stone," *Clinical Reviews in Allergy and Immunology*, vol. 20, no. 1, pp. 87–108, 2001.

[7] Y. Shiloh, "The cerebellar degeneration in ataxia-telangiectasia: a case for genome instability," *DNA repair*, vol. 95, p. 102950, 2020.

[8] Y. Su and M. Swift, "Mortality Rates among carriers of ataxia-telangiectasia mutant alleles," *Annals of internal medicine*, vol. 133, no. 10, pp. 770–778, 2000.

[9] P. J. Connelly, N. Smith, R. Chadwick, A. R. Exley, J. M. Shneerson, and E. R. Pearson, "Recessive mutations in the cancer gene Ataxia Telangiectasia Mutated (ATM), at a locus previously associated with metformin response, cause dysglycaemia and insulin resistance," *Diabetic Medicine*, vol. 33, no. 3, pp. 371–375, 2016.

[10] A. Barzilai, G. Rotman, and Y. Shiloh, "ATM deficiency and oxidative stress: a new dimension of defective response to DNA damage," *DNA Repair*, vol. 1, no. 1, pp. 3–25, 2002.

[11] D. J. Watters, "Oxidative stress in ataxia telangiectasia," *Redox report*, vol. 8, pp. 23–29, 2013.

[12] Y. Shiloh, "ATM and related protein kinases: safeguarding genome integrity," *Nature Reviews. Cancer*, vol. 3, no. 3, pp. 155–168, 2003.

[13] A. Alexander and C. L. Walker, "Differential localization of ATM is correlated with activation of distinct downstream signaling pathways," *Cell Cycle*, vol. 9, pp. 3685–3686, 2011.

[14] Z. Guo, S. Kozlov, M. F. Lavin, M. D. Person, and T. T. Paull, "ATM activation by oxidative stress," *Science*, vol. 330, no. 6003, pp. 517–521, 2010.

[15] T. T. Paull, "Mechanisms of ATM activation," *Annual review of biochemistry*, vol. 84, pp. 711–738, 2014.

[16] Y. Shiloh and Y. Ziv, "The ATM protein: the importance of being active," *The Journal of Cell Biology*, vol. 198, no. 3, pp. 273–275, 2012.

[17] J. Zhang, D. N. Tripathi, J. Jing et al., "ATM functions at the peroxisome to induce pexophagy in response to ROS," *Nature cell biology*, vol. 17, pp. 1259–1269, 2015.

[18] Y. Zhang, J. H. Lee, T. T. Paull et al., "Mitochondrial redox sensing by the kinase ATM maintains cellular antioxidant capacity," *Science signaling*, vol. 11, article eaaq0702, 2018.

[19] A. Alexander, S. L. Cai, J. Kim et al., "ATM signals to TSC2 in the cytoplasm to regulate mTORC1 in response to ROS," *Proceedings of the National Academy of Sciences*, vol. 107, no. 9, pp. 4153–4158, 2010.

[20] A. Alexander and C. L. Walker, "The role of LKB1 and AMPK in cellular responses to stress and damage," *FEBS Letters*, vol. 585, no. 7, pp. 952–957, 2011.

[21] C. Cosentino, D. Grieco, and V. Costanzo, "ATM activates the pentose phosphate pathway promoting anti-oxidant defence and DNA repair," *The EMBO Journal*, vol. 30, no. 3, pp. 546–555, 2011.

[22] M. Blignaut, *An investigation into the role of ATM protein in mitochondrial defects associated with cardiovascular pathology resulting from insulin resistance*, PhD Dissertation, Stellenbosch University, 2019.

[23] J. S. Eaton, Z. P. Lin, A. C. Sartorelli, N. D. Bonawitz, and G. S. Shadel, "Ataxia-telangiectasia mutated kinase regulates ribonucleotide reductase and mitochondrial homeostasis," *The Journal of Clinical Investigation*, vol. 117, no. 9, pp. 2723–2734, 2007.

[24] M. Ambrose, J. V. Goldstine, and R. A. Gatti, "Intrinsic mitochondrial dysfunction in ATM-deficient lymphoblastoid cells," *Human Molecular Genetics*, vol. 16, no. 18, pp. 2154–2164, 2007.

[25] Y. A. Valentin-Vega, M. L. KH, J. Tait-Mulder et al., "Mitochondrial dysfunction in ataxia-telangiectasia," *Blood*, vol. 119, no. 6, pp. 1490–1500, 2012.

[26] J. R. Mercer, E. Yu, N. Figg et al., "The mitochondria-targeted antioxidant Mito Q decreases features of the metabolic syndrome in ATM +/-/Apo E -/- mice," *Free Radical Biology and Medicine*, vol. 52, pp. 841–849, 2012.

[27] D. A. D'Souza, I. A. Parish, D. S. Krause, S. M. Kaech, and G. S. Shadel, "Reducing mitochondrial ROS improves disease-related pathology in a mouse model of ataxia-telangiectasia," *Molecular Therapy*, vol. 21, pp. 42–48, 2012.

[28] M. Takagi, H. Uno, R. Nishi et al., "ATM regulates adipocyte differentiation and contributes to glucose homeostasis," *Cell reports*, vol. 10, pp. 957–967, 2015.

[29] J. G. Viniegra, N. Martínez, P. Modirassari et al., "Full activation of PKB/Akt in response to insulin or ionizing radiation is mediated through ATM," *The Journal of Biological Chemistry*, vol. 280, no. 6, pp. 4029–4036, 2005.

[30] M. J. Halaby, J. C. Hibma, J. He, and D. Q. Yang, "ATM protein kinase mediates full activation of Akt and regulates glucose transporter 4 translocation by insulin in muscle cells," *Cellular Signalling*, vol. 20, no. 8, pp. 1555–1563, 2008.

[31] Y. Shiloh and Y. Ziv, "The ATM Protein kinase: regulating the cellular response to genotoxic stress, and more," *Nature reviews Molecular cell biology*, vol. 14, no. 4, pp. 197–210, 2013.

[32] Y. Shi, "Serine/threonine phosphatases: mechanism through structure," *Cell*, vol. 139, no. 3, pp. 468–484, 2009.

[33] K. K. Khanna, M. F. Lavin, S. P. Jackson, and T. D. Mulhern, "ATM, a central controller of cellular responses to DNA damage," *Cell Death and Differentiation*, vol. 8, no. 11, pp. 1052–1065, 2001.

[34] C. J. Bakkenist and M. B. Kastan, "DNA damage activates ATM through intermolecular autophosphorylation and dimer dissociation," *Nature*, vol. 421, no. 6922, pp. 499–506, 2003.

[35] A. Maréchal and L. Zou, "DNA damage sensing by the ATM and," *Cold Spring Harbor Perspectives in Biology*, vol. 5, pp. 1–18, 2013.

[36] R. E. Shackelford, C. L. Innes, S. O. Sieber, A. N. Heinloth, S. A. Leadon, and R. S. Paules, "The ataxia telangiectasia gene product is required for oxidative stress-induced G1 and G2 checkpoint function in human fibroblasts," *Journal of Biological Chemistry*, vol. 276, pp. 21951–21959, 2001.

[37] Z. Bencokova, M. R. Kaufmann, I. M. Pires, P. S. Lecane, A. J. Giaccia, and E. M. Hammond, "ATM activation and signaling under hypoxic conditions," *Molecular and Cellular Biology*, vol. 29, no. 2, pp. 526–537, 2009.

[38] J. Kobayashi, Y. Saito, M. Okui, N. Miwa, and K. Komatsu, "Increased oxidative stress in AOA3 cells disturbs ATM-dependent DNA damage responses," *Mutation Research/Genetic Toxicology and Environmental Mutagenesis*, vol. 782, pp. 42–50, 2015.

[39] S. Ditch and T. T. Paull, "The ATM protein kinase and cellular redox signaling: beyond the DNA damage response," *Trends in biochemical sciences*, vol. 37, no. 1, pp. 15–22, 2012.

[40] M. Ambrose and R. A. Gatti, "Pathogenesis of ataxia-telangiectasia: the next generation of ATM functions," *Blood*, vol. 121, no. 20, pp. 4036–4045, 2013.

[41] K. Bedard and K.-H. Krause, "The NOX family of ROS-generating NADPH oxidases: physiology and pathophysiology," *Physiological reviews*, vol. 87, no. 1, pp. 245–313, 2007.

[42] R. P. Patel, J. McAndrew, H. Sellak et al., "Biological aspects of reactive nitrogen species," *Biochimica et Biophysica Acta (BBA)-Bioenergetics*, vol. 1411, no. 2-3, pp. 385–400, 1999.

[43] E. A. Podrez, D. Schmitt, H. F. Hoff, and S. L. Hazen, "Myeloperoxidase-generated reactive nitrogen species convert LDL into an atherogenic form in vitro," *The Journal of Clinical Investigation*, vol. 103, no. 11, pp. 1547–1560, 1999.

[44] T. Finkel, "Signal transduction by reactive oxygen species," *The Journal of Cell Biology*, vol. 194, no. 1, pp. 7–15, 2011.

[45] I. J. Lodhi and C. F. Semenkovich, "Peroxisomes: a nexus for lipid metabolism and cellular signaling," *Cell metabolism*, vol. 19, no. 3, pp. 380–392, 2014.

[46] S. J. Forrester, D. S. Kikuchi, M. S. Hernandes, Q. Xu, and K. K. Griendling, "Reactive oxygen species in metabolic and inflammatory signaling," *Circulation research*, vol. 122, no. 6, pp. 877–902, 2018.

[47] A. Tarafdar and G. Pula, "The role of NADPH oxidases and oxidative stress in neurodegenerative disorders," *International Journal of Molecular Sciences*, vol. 19, no. 12, p. 3824, 2018.

[48] M. W. Ma, J. Wang, Q. Zhang et al., "NADPH oxidase in brain injury and neurodegenerative disorders," *Molecular neurodegeneration*, vol. 12, pp. 1–28, 2017.

[49] K. M. Holmström and T. Finkel, "Cellular mechanisms and physiological consequences of redox-dependent signalling," *Nature reviews Molecular cell biology*, vol. 15, no. 6, pp. 411–421, 2014.

[50] U. Weyemi, C. E. Redon, T. Aziz et al., "NADPH oxidase 4 is a critical mediator in ataxia telangiectasia disease," *Proceedings of the National Academy of Sciences*, vol. 112, no. 7, pp. 2121–2126, 2015.

[51] N. Mizushima, "Autophagy: process and function," *Genes & Development*, vol. 21, no. 22, pp. 2861–2873, 2007.

[52] G. Filomeni, D. De Zio, and F. Cecconi, "Oxidative stress and autophagy: the clash between damage and metabolic needs," *Cell Death & Differentiation*, vol. 22, no. 3, pp. 377–388, 2015.

[53] G. Kroemer, G. Mariño, and B. Levine, "Autophagy and the integrated stress response," *Molecular Cell*, vol. 40, no. 2, pp. 280–293, 2010.

[54] D. J. Klionsky and P. Codogno, "The mechanism and physiological function of macroautophagy," *Journal of Innate Immunity*, vol. 5, no. 5, pp. 427–433, 2013.

[55] D. Glick, S. Barth, and K. F. Macleod, "Autophagy: cellular and molecular mechanisms," *The Journal of Pathology*, vol. 221, no. 1, pp. 3–12, 2010.

[56] J. Kim, G. Yang, Y. Kim, J. Kim, and J. Ha, "AMPK activators: mechanisms of action and physiological activities," *Experimental & molecular medicine*, vol. 48, no. 4, p. e224, 2016.

[57] S. V. Kozlov, A. J. Waardenberg, K. Engholm-Keller, J. W. Arthur, M. E. Graham, and M. Lavin, "Reactive oxygen species (ROS)-activated ATM-dependent phosphorylation of cytoplasmic substrates identified by large-scale phosphoproteomics screen," *Molecular & Cellular Proteomics*, vol. 15, no. 3, pp. 1032–1047, 2016.

[58] D. M. Gwinn, D. B. Shackelford, D. F. Egan et al., "AMPK phosphorylation of raptor mediates a metabolic checkpoint," *Molecular Cell*, vol. 30, no. 2, pp. 214–226, 2008.

[59] S. W. Y. Cheng, L. G. D. Fryer, D. Carling, and P. R. Shepherd, "Thr2446 is a novel mammalian target of rapamycin (mTOR) phosphorylation site regulated by nutrient status," *Journal of Biological Chemistry*, vol. 279, no. 16, pp. 15719–15722, 2004.

[60] Y. Kim, M. Kundu, B. Viollet, and K.-L. Guan, "AMPK and mTOR regulate autophagy through direct phosphorylation of Ulk1," *Nature Cell Biology*, vol. 13, no. 2, pp. 132–141, 2011.

[61] M. Zachari and I. G. Ganley, "The mammalian ULK1 complex and autophagy initiation," *Essays in Biochemistry*, vol. 61, no. 6, pp. 585–596, 2017.

[62] Z. Yang and D. J. Klionsky, "Mammalian autophagy: core molecular machinery and signaling regulation," *Current opinion in cell biology*, vol. 22, no. 2, pp. 124–131, 2010.

[63] N. T. Ktistakis and S. A. Tooze, "Digesting the expanding mechanisms of autophagy," *Trends in cell biology*, vol. 26, no. 8, pp. 624–635, 2016.

[64] T. Nishimura and S. A. Tooze, "Emerging roles of ATG proteins and membrane lipids in autophagosome formation," *Cell Discovery*, vol. 6, no. 1, 2020.

[65] T. Johansen and T. Lamark, "Selective autophagy: ATG8 family proteins, LIR motifs and cargo receptors," *Journal of molecular biology*, vol. 432, no. 1, pp. 80–103, 2020.

[66] M. B. E. Schaaf, T. G. Keulers, M. A. Vooijs, and K. M. A. Rouschop, "LC3/GABARAP family proteins: autophagy-(un)related functions," *The FASEB Journal*, vol. 30, no. 12, pp. 3961–3978, 2016.

[67] P. Wild, D. G. McEwan, and I. Dikic, "The LC3 interactome at a glance," *Journal of Cell Science*, vol. 127, pp. 3–9, 2013.

[68] J. Dancourt and T. J. Melia, "Lipidation of the autophagy proteins LC3 and GABARAP is a membrane-curvature dependent process," *Autophagy*, vol. 10, no. 8, pp. 1470-1471, 2014.

[69] D. Colacurcio and R. Nixon, "Disorders of lysosomal acidification - the emerging role of v- ATPase in aging and neurodegenerative disease," *Ageing Research Reviews*, vol. 32, pp. 75–88, 2016.

[70] J. Y. Koh, H. N. Kim, J. J. Hwang, Y. H. Kim, and S. E. Park, "Lysosomal dysfunction in proteinopathic neurodegenerative disorders: possible therapeutic roles of cAMP and zinc," *Molecular Brain*, vol. 12, pp. 1–11, 2019.

[71] N. Jimenez-Moreno and J. D. Lane, "Autophagy and redox homeostasis in Parkinson's: a crucial balancing act," *Oxidative Medicine and Cellular Longevity*, vol. 2020, 38 pages, 2020.

[72] D. N. Tripathi, R. Chowdhury, L. J. Trudel et al., "Reactive nitrogen species regulate autophagy through ATM-AMPK-TSC2-mediated suppression of mTORC1," *Proceedings of*

the National Academy of Sciences, vol. 110, no. 32, pp. E2950–E2957, 2013.

[73] G. P. Sapkota, M. Deak, A. Kieloch et al., "Ionizing radiation induces ataxia telangiectasia mutated kinase (ATM)-mediated phosphorylation of LKB1/STK11 at Thr-366," *Biochemical Journal*, vol. 516, pp. 507–516, 2002.

[74] R. J. Shaw, M. Kosmatka, N. Bardeesy et al., "The tumor suppressor LKB1 kinase directly activates AMP-activated kinase and regulates apoptosis in response to energy stress," *Proceedings of the National Academy of Sciences*, vol. 101, no. 10, pp. 3329–3335, 2004.

[75] Y. Ikeda, K. Sato, D. R. Pimentel et al., "Cardiac-specific deletion of LKB1 leads to hypertrophy and dysfunction," *The Journal of Biological Chemistry*, vol. 284, no. 51, pp. 35839–35849, 2009.

[76] B. M. Emerling, F. Weinberg, C. Snyder et al., "Hypoxic activation of AMPK is dependent on mitochondrial ROS but independent of an increase in AMP/ATP ratio," *Free Radical Biology and Medicine*, vol. 46, pp. 1386–1391, 2009.

[77] Y. Chen, M. B. Azad, and S. B. Gibson, "Superoxide is the major reactive oxygen species regulating autophagy," *Cell Death & Differentiation*, vol. 16, no. 7, pp. 1040–1052, 2009.

[78] G. Filomeni, E. Desideri, S. Cardaci, G. Rotilio, and M. R. Ciriolo, "Under the ROS: thiol network is the principal suspect for autophagy commitment commitment," *Autophagy*, vol. 6, pp. 999–1005, 2014.

[79] C. Garza-Lombó, A. Pappa, M. I. Panayiotidis, and R. Franco, "Redox homeostasis, oxidative stress and mitophagy," *Mitochondrion*, vol. 51, pp. 105–117, 2020.

[80] A. Cheng, K. H. Tse, H. M. Chow et al., "ATM loss disrupts the autophagy-lysosomal pathway," *Autophagy*, pp. 1–13, 2020.

[81] J. G. Schneider, B. N. Finck, J. Ren et al., "ATM-dependent suppression of stress signaling reduces vascular disease in metabolic syndrome," *Cell Metabolism*, vol. 4, no. 5, pp. 377–389, 2006.

[82] Y. Espach, A. Lochner, H. Strijdom, and B. Huisamen, "ATM protein kinase signaling, type 2 diabetes and cardiovascular disease," *Cardiovascular Drugs and Therapy*, vol. 29, no. 1, pp. 51–58, 2015.

[83] C. Barlow, C. Ribaut-Barassin, T. A. Zwingman et al., "ATM is a cytoplasmic protein in mouse brain required to prevent lysosomal accumulation," *Proceedings of the National Academy of Sciences*, vol. 97, no. 2, pp. 871–876, 2000.

[84] M. Qian, Z. Liu, L. Peng et al., "Boosting ATM activity alleviates aging and extends lifespan in a mouse model of progeria," *eLife*, vol. 7, pp. 1–25, 2018.

[85] D. Carmona-Gutierrez, A. L. Hughes, F. Madeo, and C. Ruckenstuhl, "The crucial impact of lysosomes in aging and longevity," *Ageing research reviews*, vol. 32, pp. 2–12, 2016.

[86] M. Abdellatif, S. Sedej, D. Carmona-Gutierrez, F. Madeo, and G. Kroemer, "Autophagy in cardiovascular aging," *Circulation Research*, vol. 123, no. 7, pp. 803–824, 2018.

[87] T. Lamark and T. Johansen, "Aggrephagy: selective disposal of protein aggregates by macroautophagy," *International Journal of Cell Biology*, vol. 2012, 21 pages, 2012.

[88] H. Tsutsui, S. Kinugawa, and S. Matsushima, "Oxidative stress and heart failure," *American Journal of Physiology-Heart and Circulatory Physiology*, vol. 301, pp. 2181–2190, 2011.

[89] T. C. Squier, "Oxidative stress and protein aggregation during biological aging," *Experimental gerontology*, vol. 36, pp. 1539–1550, 2001.

[90] A. Monaco and A. Fraldi, "Protein aggregation and dysfunction of autophagy-lysosomal pathway: a vicious cycle in lysosomal storage diseases," *Frontiers in Molecular Neuroscience*, vol. 13, pp. 1–8, 2020.

[91] G. Merlini, V. Bellotti, A. Andreola et al., "Protein aggregation," *Clinical Chemistry and Laboratory Medicine*, vol. 39, pp. 1065–1075, 2001.

[92] T. D. Evans, I. Sergin, X. Zhang, and B. Razani, "Target acquired: selective autophagy in cardiometabolic disease," *Science signaling*, vol. 10, no. 468, p. eaag2298, 2017.

[93] S. Elmore, "Apoptosis: a review of programmed cell death," *Toxicologic Pathology*, vol. 35, pp. 495–516, 2016.

[94] K. D. Sullivan, V. V. Palaniappan, and J. M. Espinosa, "ATM regulates cell fate choice upon p 53 activation by modulating mitochondrial turnover and ROS levels," *Cell Cycle*, vol. 14, no. 1, pp. 56–63, 2015.

[95] J. H. Lee, M. R. Mand, C. H. Kao et al., "ATM directs DNA damage responses and proteostasis via genetically separable pathways," *Science signaling*, vol. 11, no. 512, p. eaan5598, 2018.

[96] C. Barlow, P. A. Dennery, M. K. Shigenaga et al., "Loss of the ataxia–telangiectasia gene product causes oxidative damage in target organs," *Proceedings of the National Academy of Sciences*, vol. 96, no. 17, pp. 9915–9919, 1999.

[97] H. Kato, S. Takashima, Y. Asano et al., "Identification of p 32 as a novel substrate for ATM in heart," *Biochemical and Biophysical Research Communications*, vol. 366, no. 4, pp. 885–891, 2008.

[98] H. Jiao, G. Q. Su, W. Dong et al., "Chaperone-like protein p32 regulates ULK1 stability and autophagy," *Cell Death & Differentiation*, vol. 22, no. 11, pp. 1812–1823, 2015.

[99] W. Tian, W. Li, Y. Chen et al., "Phosphorylation of ULK1 by AMPK regulates translocation of ULK1 to mitochondria and mitophagy," *FEBS letters*, vol. 589, no. 15, pp. 1847–1854, 2015.

[100] A. L. Anding and E. H. Baehrecke, "Cleaning house: selective autophagy of organelles," *Developmental Cell*, vol. 41, no. 1, pp. 10–22, 2017.

[101] W. Wu, W. Tian, Z. Hu et al., "ULK1 translocates to mitochondria and phosphorylates FUNDC1 to regulate mitophagy," *EMBO Reports*, vol. 15, no. 5, pp. 566–575, 2014.

[102] K. Nishida, S. Kyoi, O. Yamaguchi, J. Sadoshima, and K. Otsu, "The role of autophagy in the heart," *Cell Death and Differentiation*, vol. 16, no. 1, pp. 31–38, 2009.

[103] W. X. Ding and X. M. Yin, "Mitophagy: mechanisms, pathophysiological roles, and analysis," *Biological Chemistry*, vol. 393, no. 7, pp. 547–564, 2012.

[104] A. Diot, K. Morten, and J. Poulton, "Mitophagy plays a central role in mitochondrial ageing," *Mammalian Genome*, vol. 27, no. 7-8, pp. 381–395, 2016.

[105] A. Roberta, M. Gottlieb, and A. Thomas, "Mitophagy and mitochondrial quality control mechanisms in the heart," *Current pathobiology reports*, vol. 5, pp. 161–169, 2017.

[106] A. Hamacher-Brady and N. R. Brady, "Mitophagy programs: mechanisms and physiological implications of mitochondrial targeting by autophagy," *Cellular and molecular life sciences*, vol. 73, pp. 775–795, 2016.

[107] T. N. Nguyen, B. S. Padman, and M. Lazarou, "Deciphering the molecular signals of PINK1/Parkin mitophagy," *Trends in cell biology*, vol. 26, no. 10, pp. 733–744, 2016.

[108] S. Sciarretta, Y. Maejima, D. Zablocki, and J. Sadoshima, "The role of autophagy in the heart," *Annual Review of Physiology*, vol. 80, no. 1, pp. 1–26, 2018.

[109] J. Zhang and P. A. Ney, "Role of BNIP3 and NIX in cell death, autophagy, and mitophagy," *Cell Death & Differentiation*, vol. 16, no. 7, pp. 939–946, 2009.

[110] S. Rikka, M. N. Quinsay, R. L. Thomas et al., "Bnip3 impairs mitochondrial bioenergetics and stimulates mitochondrial turnover," *Cell Death & Differentiation*, vol. 18, no. 4, pp. 721–731, 2011.

[111] A. G. Moyzis, J. Sadoshima, and Å. B. Gustafsson, "Mending a broken heart: the role of mitophagy in cardioprotection," *American Journal of Physiology-Heart and Circulatory Physiology*, vol. 308, no. 3, pp. H183–H192, 2015.

[112] H. Wei, L. Liu, and Q. Chen, "Selective removal of mitochondria via mitophagy: distinct pathways for different mitochondrial stresses," *Biochimica et Biophysica Acta (BBA)-Molecular Cell Research*, vol. 1853, pp. 2784–2790, 2015.

[113] X. Gu, Y. Qi, Z. Feng, L. Ma, K. Gao, and Y. Zhang, "Lead (Pb) induced ATM-dependent mitophagy via PINK1/Parkin pathway," *Toxicology letters*, vol. 291, pp. 92–100, 2018.

[114] Y. Qi, Q. Qiu, X. Gu, Y. Tian, and Y. Zhang, "ATM mediates spermidine-induced mitophagy via PINK1 and Parkin regulation in human fibroblasts," *Scientific reports*, vol. 6, p. 24700, 2016.

[115] T. Eisenberg, H. Knauer, A. Schauer et al., "Induction of autophagy by spermidine promotes longevity," *Nature cell biology*, vol. 11, no. 11, pp. 1305–1314, 2009.

[116] C. Cirotti, S. Rizza, P. Giglio et al., "Redox activation of ATM enhances GSNOR translation to sustain mitophagy and tolerance to oxidative stress," *EMBO reports*, vol. 22, article e50500, 2020.

[117] A. Morita, K. Tanimoto, T. Murakami, T. Morinaga, and Y. Hosoi, "Mitochondria are required for ATM activation by extranuclear oxidative stress in cultured human hepatoblastoma cell line Hep G2 cells," *Biochemical and biophysical research communications*, vol. 443, no. 4, pp. 1286–1290, 2014.

[118] D. Watters, P. Kedar, K. Spring et al., "Localization of a portion of extranuclear ATM to peroxisomes," *The Journal of Biological Chemistry*, vol. 274, no. 48, pp. 34277–34282, 1999.

[119] Y. A. Valentin-Vega and M. B. Kastan, "A new role for ATM: regulating mitochondrial function and mitophagy," *Autophagy*, vol. 8, pp. 840–841, 2014.

[120] M. Blignaut, B. Loos, S. W. Botchway, A. W. Parker, and B. Huisamen, "Ataxia-telangiectasia mutated is located in cardiac mitochondria and impacts oxidative phosphorylation," *Scientific Reports*, vol. 9, no. 1, p. 4782, 2019.

[121] A. Y. Patel, T. M. McDonald, L. D. Spears, J. K. Ching, and J. S. Fisher, "Ataxia telangiectasia mutated influences cytochrome _c_ oxidase activity," *Biochemical and biophysical research communications*, vol. 405, no. 4, pp. 599–603, 2011.

[122] Q. Chen, E. J. Vazquez, S. Moghaddas, C. L. Hoppel, and E. J. Lesnefsky, "Production of reactive oxygen species by mitochondria," *The Journal of Biological Chemistry*, vol. 278, no. 38, pp. 36027–36031, 2003.

[123] H. M. Chow, A. Cheng, X. Song, M. R. Swerdel, R. P. Hart, and K. Herrup, "ATM is activated by ATP depletion and

[124] E. F. Fang, H. Kassahun, D. L. Croteau et al., "NAD+ replenishment improves lifespan and healthspan in ataxia telangiectasia models via mitophagy and DNA repair," *Cell Metabolism*, vol. 24, no. 4, pp. 566–581, 2016.

[125] S. Kobayashi and Q. Liang, "Autophagy and mitophagy in diabetic cardiomyopathy," *Biochimica et Biophysica Acta (BBA)-Molecular Basis of Disease*, vol. 1852, no. 2, pp. 252–261, 2015.

[126] V. Choubey, M. Cagalinec, J. Liiv et al., "BECN1 is involved in the initiation of mitophagy: it facilitates PARK2 translocation to mitochondria," *Autophagy*, vol. 10, no. 6, pp. 1105–1119, 2014.

[127] Y. Wang, N. Liu, and B. Lu, "Mechanisms and roles of mitophagy in neurodegenerative diseases," *CNS Neuroscience & Therapeutics*, vol. 25, no. 7, pp. 859–875, 2019.

[128] D. A. Kubli and Å. B. Gustafsson, "Mitochondria and mitophagy: the yin and yang of cell death control," *Circulation Research*, vol. 111, no. 9, pp. 1208–1221, 2012.

[129] K. Germain and P. K. Kim, "Pexophagy : a model for selective autophagy," *International journal of molecular sciences*, vol. ', pp. 1–27, 2020.

[130] C. He and D. J. Klionsky, "Regulation mechanisms and signaling pathways of autophagy," *Annual Review of Genetics*, vol. 43, no. 1, pp. 67–93, 2009.

[131] D. N. Tripathi, J. Zhang, J. Jing, R. Dere, and C. L. Walker, "A new role for ATM in selective autophagy of peroxisomes (pexophagy)," *Autophagy*, vol. 12, no. 4, pp. 711–712, 2016.

[132] J. Zhang, J. Kim, A. Alexander et al., "A tuberous sclerosis complex signalling node at the peroxisome regulates mTORC1 and autophagy in response to ROS," *Nature Cell Biology*, vol. 15, no. 10, pp. 1186–1196, 2013.

[133] C. Kraft, M. Peter, and K. Hofmann, "Selective autophagy: ubiquitin-mediated recognition and beyond," *Nature cell biology*, vol. 12, no. 9, pp. 836–841, 2010.

[134] D. S. Jo and D. H. Cho, "Peroxisomal dysfunction in neurodegenerative diseases," *Archives of pharmacal research*, vol. 42, no. 5, pp. 393–406, 2019.

Anti-Glutamic Acid Decarboxylase Antibody-Associated Ataxia as an Extrahepatic Autoimmune Manifestation of Hepatitis C Infection

Amer Awad,[1] Olaf Stüve,[2,3] Marlyn Mayo,[4] Rafeed Alkawadri,[5] and Bachir Estephan[6]

[1] Baton Rouge Neurology Associates, Baton Rouge General Medical Center, Baton Rouge, LA, USA
[2] Department of Neurology, The University of Texas Southwestern Medical Center, Dallas, TX, USA
[3] Neurology Section, VA North Texas Health Care Systems, Dallas, TX, USA
[4] Department of Internal Medicine-Digestive and Liver Diseases, The University of Texas Southwestern Medical Center, Dallas, TX, USA
[5] Neurological Institute, Cleveland Clinic Foundation, Cleveland, OH, USA
[6] Department of Neurology, University of Kansas Medical Center, Kansas, KS, USA

Correspondence should be addressed to Amer Awad, ameraldo@gmail.com

Academic Editors: A. E. Cavanna, M. Filosto, and J. L. González-Gutiérrez

Extrahepatic immunological manifestations of hepatitis C virus (HCV) are well described. In addition, antiglutamic acid decarboxylase (GAD) antibody-associated cerebellar ataxia is well-established entity. However, there have been no reports in the literature of anti-GAD antibody-associated ataxia as an extrahepatic manifestation of HCV infection. We report the case of a young woman with chronic hepatitis C virus and multiple extrahepatic autoimmune diseases including Sjögren syndrome and pernicious anemia who presented with subacute midline cerebellar syndrome and was found to have positive antiglutamic acid decarboxylase (GAD) antibody in the serum and cerebrospinal fluid. An extensive diagnostic workup to rule out neoplastic growths was negative, suggesting the diagnosis of nonparaneoplastic antiglutamic acid decarboxylase antibody-associated cerebellar ataxia as an additional extrahepatic manifestation of hepatitis C virus infection. The patient failed to respond to high-dose steroids and intravenous immunoglobulin. Treatment with the monoclonal antibody rituximab stabilized the disease. We postulate that anti-GAD associated ataxia could be an extrahepatic manifestation of HCV infection.

1. Introduction

Hepatitis C virus (HCV) is commonly associated with autoimmune diseases as extrahepatic manifestations (EHM) [1] The most important autoimmune diseases associated with HCV are mixed essential cryoglobulinemia (MEC) [2] and Sjögren syndrome (SS) [3]. Other autoimmune diseases have been described in patients with HCV, but the association has not been well documented. These autoimmune diseases include HCV-associated arthritis [4], systemic lupus erythematosus [5], polyarteritis nodosa [6], antiphospholipid antibody syndrome [7], inflammatory myopathies [8], sarcoidosis [9], autoimmune thyroid disease [10], autoimmune glomerulonephritis [11], skin vasculitis [12], and autoimmune thrombocytopenia [13].

The pathogenesis of these EHM is still not fully understood, although most studies suggest that the presence of MEC, particular lymphotropism of the virus, molecular mimicry, and non-MEC autoimmune phenomena constitute the major pathogenic factors [14].

To our knowledge, there have been no previous reports of antiglutamic acid decarboxylase (GAD) antibody-associated cerebellar ataxia as an extrahepatic manifestation of chronic HCV infection. We report here a young woman with chronic HCV infection, who presented with subacute midline (vermis) cerebellar syndrome and tested positive for anti-GAD antibodies in the serum and the cerebrospinal fluid (CSF). We postulate that the patient has a postinfectious or parainfectious autoimmune disease caused by antibodies directed against the neuronal antigen GAD 65.

2. Case Report

The patient is a 48-year-old African American woman with past medical history significant for HCV secondary to blood transfusion, SS, pernicious anemia, and obesity status post-bariatric surgery. She presented to the neurology clinic with history of subacute onset gait ataxia, intermittent vertigo, diplopia, oscillopsia, dysarthria, and dysphagia. The patient was initially treated with high-dose intravenous methylpred-nisolone (IVMP) followed by high-dose oral prednisone with modest response as her ataxia continued to progress. Based on the assumption that her symptoms were secondary to central nervous system (CNS) involvement of SS, she was treated with rituximab with no significant clinical improvement though it stabilized the disease. The patient also did not respond to intravenous immunoglobulin (IVIG) treatment. No history of alcohol use or malnutrition. Her neurological examination revealed hypometric saccades, mild dysarthria, truncal ataxia, and gait ataxia without limb ataxia. A motor exam was unremarkable, and sensory exam was positive for decreased vibratory sensation distally. An extensive workup was initiated. Abnormal results include HCV viral load 193,000 copies per mL, HCV genotype I, liver biopsy (stage I HCV disease), antinuclear antibody (Ab) (ANA) positive, SS-A positive (1 : 230), antiparietal cell Ab positive, anti-intrinsic factor (IF) Ab positive, small M spike on serum protein electrophoresis (SPEP) with normal 24-hour urine protein electrophoresis (UPEP), cerebrospinal fluid (CSF) oligoclonal bands (OCBs) positive with normal cell count and protein, and increased uptake on the right sub-mandibular gland on positron emission tomography (PET). Pertinent negative/normal results include vitamin B12 (on supplements), folic acid (on supplements), vitamin B1 (thiamine on supplements), vitamin B6, vitamin E, lactate, pyruvate, thyroid stimulating hormone (TSH), copper, ceruloplasmin, urine heavy metals, human immunodeficiency virus (HIV), rapid plasma regain (RPR), SS-B, rheumatoid factor (RF), antineutrophilic cytoplasmic Ab (ANCA), antiphospholipid Ab (a PL), angiotensin-converting enzyme (ACE), antiendomysial Ab, erythrocyte sedimentation rate (ESR), C-reactive protein (CRP), C3, C4, cryoglobulins, paraneoplastic panel, anti-amphiphysin antibody, brain and spine magnetic resonance imaging (MRI) with contrast, bone scan, bone marrow biopsy, mammogram, Pap smear, computerized tomography (CT) of the chest, abdomen, and pelvis. The most remarkable finding was a positive anti-GAD 65 Ab in the serum (titer 113.65 units per mL) and in the CSF (titer 29.4 nmole/L with a normal range of <0.02 nmole/L) with positive OCBs despite treatment with steroids, IVIG, and Rituximab. The patient had numerous fasting blood sugars (FBS) done to exclude late onset diabetes. All the FBS values were within normal limits (80–95 mg/dL).

Antiviral therapy with interferon alpha (IFNα) and rib-avirin was discussed with the hepatologist, but the patient was considered a poor candidate due to the possibility of ex-acerbation of a secondary autoimmune disease. Since the pa-tient's cerebellar syndrome was stabilized by rituximab, we continued maintenance therapy with close monitoring of her neurological status.

3. Discussion

The patient presented with symptoms and signs consis-tent with cerebellar vermis syndrome including hypometric saccades, truncal, and gait ataxia without limb ataxia [15, 16]. Thiamine and copper deficiency as potential causes of ataxia, which are common after Bariatric surgery [17, 18], were excluded by normal serum levels. The patient was on vitamin B12 and folic acid supplements. Brain and spine MRI excluded structural causes of ataxia. The thorough workup excluded other potential causes of ataxia including vitamin E deficiency [19], heavy metal toxicity [20, 21], celiac disease-associated ataxia [22]. Finally, numerous fasting blood sugar samples excluded late onset insulin-dependent diabetes mellitus.

The most striking abnormality was the finding of positive anti-GAD 65 Abs in the serum and the CSF. The positivity in the CSF confirms its pathogenic role in the patient's ataxia. Anti-GAD 65 Ab has been associated with a myriad of disor-ders including insulin-dependent diabetes mellitus (IDDM) [23], stiff person syndrome (SPS) [24], limbic encephalitis [25], opsoclonus-myoclonus syndrome [26], epilepsy [27], and ataxia [27, 28]. The positivity for anti-GAD dictated a thorough neoplastic workup because anti-GAD antibody is often associated with neoplastic growth in the context of a paraneoplastic neurological disorder. This is especially true if anti-amphiphysin antibodies are also present [29]. A comprehensive neoplastic workup was negative, and a para-neoplastic antibody panel was negative as well. The clinical picture in parallel with the lab findings suggests the diagnosis of nonparaneoplastic anti-GAD Ab-associated ataxia. Never-theless, the continuous and long-term search for occult neo-plasms is required to confirm the nonparaneoplastic origin since neurological paraneoplastic disorders can precede the diagnosis of occult malignancies by a long period of time.

While ataxia associated with anti-GAD antibodies is a well-described entity, this patient is unusual as her under-lying chronic medical condition is a viral infection of the liver, namely, HCV. A thorough literature review did not uncover previous reports of such an association. We propose that the anti-GAD ataxia in this patient is an extrahepatic autoimmune manifestation of HCV. The association might be incidental, but there are 2 factors that make the association more than just incidental. The first one is the extreme rarity of anti-GAD ataxia making the mathematical possibility of both occurring in the same patient very highly unlikely. The second factor, and the more important reason is the finding of remarkable molecular mimicry between HCV and GAD 65 [30].

With regard to the etiology of this clinical presentation, we hypothesize that this patient is suffering from a para-infectious autoimmune disease caused by of molecular mim-icry. Not unlike in a paraneoplastic syndrome, it is conceiv-able that a neuronal antigen-like determinant is ectopically expressed. Only in this case, it would be expressed not by a malignant cell, but instead either by HCV, or by a host cell infected with HCV. Consequently, this antigen is recognized as "foreign". Initially, the viral neuronal-antigen-like deter-minant is recognized at the site of inoculation by cells of the innate immune system, which then present linear epitopes to T cells. These T cells, once activated, in turn cross-activates antigen-specific B cells. Such activated autoreactive T cells and B cells readily entering the CNS during the course of routine immune surveillance [31]. Incidentally, these cells may encounter a neuronal antigen in the cerebellum that closely resembles the viral neuronal-antigen-like determinant they were originally primed against. Following reactivation by CNS intrinsic antigen presenting cells, these T cells and B cells now initiate and autoimmune disease, which includes the recruitment of nonantigen specific immune cells from the blood that amplify the inflammation.

It would be extremely difficult to test our hypothesis in a human patient. In animal models, the cascade of events described above was successfully demonstrated experimentally by transgenic insertion of a lymphocytic choriomeningitis virus (LCMV) antigen in murine oligodendrocytes. Following intraperitoneal inoculation of these animals with LCMV, the infection was cleared at the entry site. However, 7–14 days later, the inflammation of the CNS was detected, and the experimental animals displayed functional clinical deficits [32].

Treatment of anti-GAD syndrome is not well established yet. However, favorable responses to steroids, IVIG, and plasma exchange were reported in the literature [33–35]. Rituximab was shown to be safe and helpful in treatment of EHM of HCV [36, 37]. More importantly, antiviral treatment of HCV can improve EHM [38] but may worsen the course of autoimmune disorders associated with HCV [39].

4. Conclusion

Our case of HCV-associated anti-GAD ataxia should help alert neurologists and other physicians treating patients with HCV to the presence of this entity. Patients with HCV and neurological symptoms should be evaluated for neuroimmunological disorders by running a comprehensive immune workup including testing for anti-GAD Ab. Early diagnosis is crucial to stabilize the disease and prevent its progression since reversing neuropathology is currently not feasible. Further studies are crucial to study this association and the exact immunopathogenesis behind it.

References

[1] S. Ferri, L. Muratori, M. Lenzi, A. Granito, F. B. Bianchi, and D. Vergani, "HCV and autoimmunity," *Current Pharmaceutical Design*, vol. 14, no. 17, pp. 1678–1685, 2008.

[2] C. Ferri, "Mixed cryoglobulinemia," *Orphanet Journal of Rare Diseases*, vol. 3, no. 1, article 25, 2008.

[3] M. Ramos-Casals, S. Muñoz, F. Medina et al., "Systemic autoimmune diseases in patients with hepatitis C virus infection: characterization of 1020 cases (The HISPAMEC Registry)," *Journal of Rheumatology*, vol. 36, no. 7, pp. 1442–1448, 2009.

[4] C. Lormeau, G. Falgarone, D. Roulot, and M. C. Boissier, "Rheumatologic manifestations of chronic hepatitis C infection," *Joint Bone Spine*, vol. 73, no. 6, pp. 633–638, 2006.

[5] M. M. Ahmed, S. M. Berney, R. E. Wolf et al., "Prevalence of active hepatitis C virus infection in patients with systemic lupus erythematosus," *American Journal of the Medical Sciences*, vol. 331, no. 5, pp. 252–256, 2006.

[6] R. Canada, S. Chaudry, L. Gaber, B. Waters, A. Martinez, and B. Wall, "Polyarteritis nodosa and cryoglobulinemic glomerulonephritis related to chronic hepatitis C," *American Journal of the Medical Sciences*, vol. 331, no. 6, pp. 329–333, 2006.

[7] A. M. Atta, P. Estevam, R. Paraná, C. M. Pereira, B. C. O. Leite, and M. L. B. Sousa-Atta, "Antiphospholipid antibodies in Brazilian hepatitis C virus carriers," *Brazilian Journal of Medical and Biological Research*, vol. 41, no. 6, pp. 489–492, 2008.

[8] A. di Muzio, B. Bonetti, M. Capasso et al., "Hepatitis C virus infection and myositis: a virus localization study," *Neuromuscular Disorders*, vol. 13, no. 1, pp. 68–71, 2003.

[9] M. Ramos-Casals, J. Mañá, N. Nardi et al., "Sarcoidosis in patients with chronic hepatitis C virus infection: analysis of 68 cases," *Medicine (Baltimore)*, vol. 84, no. 2, pp. 69–80, 2005.

[10] A. Antonelli, C. Ferri, S. M. Ferrari, M. Colaci, D. Sansonno, and P. Fallahi, "Endocrine manifestations of hepatitis C virus infection," *Nature Clinical Practice Endocrinology and Metabolism*, vol. 5, no. 1, pp. 26–34, 2009.

[11] P. Martin and F. Fabrizi, "Hepatitis C virus and kidney disease," *Journal of Hepatology*, vol. 49, no. 4, pp. 613–624, 2008.

[12] P. Cacoub and D. Saadoun, "Hepatitis C virus infection induced vasculitis," *Clinical Reviews in Allergy and Immunology*, vol. 35, no. 1-2, pp. 30–39, 2008.

[13] A. J. de Almeida, M. Campos-de-Magalhães, C. L. Antonietti et al., "Autoimmune thrombocytopenia related to chronic hepatitis C virus infection," *Hematology*, vol. 14, no. 1, pp. 49–58, 2009.

[14] C. Ferri, A. Antonelli, M. T. Mascia et al., "B-cells and mixed cryoglobulinemia," *Autoimmunity Reviews*, vol. 7, no. 2, pp. 114–120, 2007.

[15] M. Victor, R. D. Adams, and E. L. Mancall, "A restricted form of cerebellar cortical degeneration occurring in alcoholic patients," *Archives of Neurology*, vol. 1, no. 6, pp. 579–688, 1959.

[16] A. J. Bastian, J. W. Mink, B. A. Kaufman, and W. T. Thach, "Posterior vermal split syndrome," *Annals of Neurology*, vol. 44, no. 4, pp. 601–610, 1998.

[17] G. Sechi, "Prognosis and therapy of Wernicke's encephalopathy after obesity surgery," *American Journal of Gastroenterology*, vol. 103, no. 12, p. 3219, 2008.

[18] A. Von Drygalski and D. A. Andris, "Anemia after bariatric surgery: more than just iron deficiency," *Nutrition in Clinical Practice*, vol. 24, no. 2, pp. 217–226, 2009.

[19] S. Jayaram, A. Soman, S. Tarvade, and V. Londhe, "Cerebellar Ataxia due to isolated Vitamin E deficiency," *Indian Journal of Medical Sciences*, vol. 59, no. 1, pp. 20–23, 2005.

[20] T. W. Clarkson, "The toxicology of mercury," *Critical Reviews in Clinical Laboratory Sciences*, vol. 34, no. 4, pp. 369–403, 1997.

[21] M. F. Gordon, R. I. Abrams, D. B. Rubin, W. B. Barr, and D. D. Correa, "Bismuth toxicity," *Neurology*, vol. 44, no. 12, p. 2418, 1994.

[22] M. Hadjivassiliou, D. S. Sanders, N. Woodroofe, C. Williamson, and R. A. Grünewald, "Gluten ataxia," *Cerebellum*, vol. 7, no. 3, pp. 494–498, 2008.

[23] M. Sue, A. Yoshihara, T. Otani, Y. Tsuchida, M. Higa, and N. Hiroi, "Characteristics of fulminant type 1 diabetes mellitus," *Medical Science Monitor*, vol. 14, no. 10, pp. 97–101, 2008.

[24] M. C. Dalakas, "Advances in the pathogenesis and treatment of patients with stiff person syndrome," *Current Neurology and Neuroscience Reports*, vol. 8, no. 1, pp. 48–55, 2008.

[25] S. Matà, G. C. Muscas, I. Naldi et al., "Non-paraneoplastic limbic encephalitis associated with anti-glutamic acid decarboxylase antibodies," *Journal of Neuroimmunology*, vol. 199, no. 1-2, pp. 155–159, 2008.

[26] I. Markakis, E. Alexiou, M. Xifaras, G. Gekas, and A. Rombos, "Opsoclonus-myoclonus-ataxia syndrome with autoantibodies to glutamic acid decarboxylase," *Clinical Neurology and Neurosurgery*, vol. 110, no. 6, pp. 619–621, 2008.

[27] S. Vulliemoz, G. Vanini, A. Truffert, C. Chizzolini, and M. Seeck, "Epilepsy and cerebellar ataxia associated with anti-glutamic acid decarboxylase antibodies," *Journal of Neurology, Neurosurgery and Psychiatry*, vol. 78, no. 2, pp. 187–189, 2007.

[28] A. Saiz, Y. Blanco, L. Sabater et al., "Spectrum of neurological syndromes associated with glutamic acid decarboxylase antibodies: diagnostic clues for this association," *Brain*, vol. 131, no. 10, pp. 2553–2563, 2008.

[29] B. B. Murinson and J. B. Guarnaccia, "Stiff-person syndrome with amphiphysin antibodies: distinctive features of a rare disease," *Neurology*, vol. 71, no. 24, pp. 1955–1958, 2008.

[30] D. P. Bogdanos and E. I. Rigopoulou, "Viral/self-mimicry and immunological cross-reactivity as a trigger of hepatic C virus associated autoimmune diabetes," *Diabetes Research and Clinical Practice*, vol. 77, no. 1, pp. 155–156, 2007.

[31] W. F. Hickey, "Basic principles of immunological surveillance of the normal central nervous system," *GLIA*, vol. 36, no. 2, pp. 118–124, 2001.

[32] C. F. Evans, M. S. Horwitz, M. V. Hobbs, and M. B. A. Oldstone, "Viral infection of transgenic mice expressing a viral protein in oligodendrocytes leads to chronic central nervous system autoimmune disease," *Journal of Experimental Medicine*, vol. 184, no. 6, pp. 2371–2384, 1996.

[33] G. Lauria, D. Pareyson, M. G. Pitzolu, and E. Bazzigaluppi, "Excellent response to steroid treatment in anti-GAD cerebellar ataxia," *Lancet Neurology*, vol. 2, no. 10, pp. 634–635, 2003.

[34] M. C. Dalakas, "The role of IVIg in the treatment of patients with stiff person syndrome and other neurological diseases associated with anti-GAD antibodies," *Journal of Neurology*, vol. 252, supplement 1, pp. I19–I25, 2005.

[35] L. M. Levy, M. C. Dalakas, and M. K. Floeter, "The stiff-person syndrome: an autoimmune disorder affecting neurotransmission of γ-aminobutyric acid," *Annals of Internal Medicine*, vol. 131, no. 7, pp. 522–530, 1999.

[36] S. de Vita, L. Quartuccio, and M. Fabris, "Rituximab in mixed cryoglobulinemia: increased experience and perspectives," *Digestive and Liver Disease*, vol. 39, supplement 1, pp. S122–S128, 2007.

[37] G. Cervetti, S. Mechelli, R. Riccioni, S. Galimberti, F. Caracciolo, and M. Petrini, "High efficacy of Rituximab in indolent HCV-related lymphoproliferative disorders asociated with systemic autoimmune diseases," *Clinical and Experimental Rheumatology*, vol. 23, no. 6, pp. 877–880, 2005.

[38] J. N. Acharya and V. H. Pacheco, "Neurologic complications of hepatitis C," *Neurologist*, vol. 14, no. 3, pp. 151–156, 2008.

[39] L. E. Wilson, D. Widman, S. H. Dikman, and P. D. Gorevic, "Autoimmune disease complicating antiviral therapy for hepatitis C virus infection," *Seminars in Arthritis and Rheumatism*, vol. 32, no. 3, pp. 163–173, 2002.

A Comparative Study of Conventional Physiotherapy versus Robot-Assisted Gait Training Associated to Physiotherapy in Individuals with Ataxia after Stroke

Marcia Belas dos Santos ⓘ,[1] **Clarissa Barros de Oliveira,**[2] **Arly dos Santos,**[1] **Cristhiane Garabello Pires,**[3] **Viviana Dylewski,**[2] **and Ricardo Mario Arida**[1]

[1]*Physiology Department, Universidade Federal de São Paulo (UNIFESP), São Paulo, SP, Brazil*
[2]*Physiotherapy Department, Associação de Assistência a Criança Deficiente (AACD), São Paulo, SP, Brazil*
[3]*Faculty of Medicine, University of Sao Paulo (USP), São Paulo, SP, Brazil*

Correspondence should be addressed to Marcia Belas dos Santos; mbelassantos@gmail.com

Academic Editor: Tauheed Ishrat

Objectives. To assess the influence of RAGT on balance, coordination, and functional independence in activities of daily living of chronic stroke survivors with ataxia at least one year of injury. *Methods.* It was a randomized controlled trial. The patients were allocated to either therapist-assisted gait training (TAGT) or robotic-assisted gait training (RAGT). Both groups received 3 weekly sessions of physiotherapy with an estimated duration of 60 minutes each and prescribed home exercises. The following outcome measures were evaluated prior to and after the completion of the 5-month protocol treatment: BBS, TUG test, FIM, and SARA. For intragroup comparisons, the Wilcoxon test was used, and the Mann–Whitney test was used for between-group comparison. *Results.* Nineteen stroke survivors with ataxia sequel after one year of injury were recruited. Both groups showed statistically significant improvement ($P < 0.05$) in balance, functional independencein, and general ataxia symptoms. There were no statistically significant differences ($P < 0.05$) for between-group comparisons both at baseline and after completion of the protocol. *Conclusions.* Chronic stroke patients with ataxia had significant improvements in balance and independence in activities of daily living after RAGT along with conventional therapy and home exercises.

1. Introduction

Stroke is the third most common cause of death and the biggest factor for disability in adults of developing nations, just behind cancer and heart diseases [1]. Approximately 795,000 stroke cases occur every year in the USA [2] with 2-3% in the cerebellum area [3]. The loss of motor skills is one of the most common complaints of stroke survivors as approximately 75% of these patients have some walking disability that could result in high risk of falls [4, 5]. In a prospective study, 256 stroke patients were evaluated in the acute phase, with approximately 27% reporting at least one fall in a three-month period [6].

Impairment in the posterior circulation that involves the cerebellum or brainstem region may lead to damages in several important functions, such as balance, movement coordination, speech, hearing, ocular movement, and swallowing [7, 8]. Ataxia is an important sequela observed and recognized for its presentation as a loss of coordination, dysmetria, dysarthria, hypotonia, rebound phenomenon, and nystagmus [9]. Gait ataxia is described by a stumbling walking pattern, an irregular foot placement, an increased step, an enlarged stance, and an abnormal joint torque [10, 11].

When the depletion of balance ability is associated with decreased joint mobility, muscle tone problems, and loss of proprioception, there is an increase in the difficulty to perform activities of daily living for individuals with stroke injury [12]. Consequently, balance training is crucial for rehabilitation treatment. Conventional gait therapy (CGT), such as the Bobath concept, proprioceptive neuromuscular facilitation, therapist-assisted walking, and the use of braces or other devices are common treatment approaches [13]. Furthermore, high severity stroke patients with poor coordination in walking may benefit from treatment with a robotic device that allows task-focused training [14].

Robot-assisted gait training (RAGT) has been used since 1980 to assist patients with dysfunction in movement caused by neurological disorders [15]. This treatment is based on the body weight-supported treadmill (BWSTT) principle and achieves functional motor relearning through the repetitive practice of all different phases of gait [16]. Training the same movement repetitively enables the nervous system to develop circuits for better communication between the motor center and sensory pathways [17].

Treatment by RAGT compared with conventional treatment on the treadmill presents advantages, including training duration, more reproducible symmetrical gait patterns, operation by a single therapist, and a reduction in the energy expenditure imposed upon the therapists [18]. In addition, recent research revealed that robot-assisted treadmill training resulted in a more symmetrical muscle activity pattern in paretic patients compared with conventional treatment [5]. It is important to highlight that there have been very few investigations on RAGT in individuals with ataxia poststroke.

A systematic review on the efficacy of rehabilitation robotics for walking training in neurological disorders showed that patients injured by stroke had statistically significant amelioration in walking speed, functional abilities, and motor functions after treatment [19]. However, a study that compared treadmill training with both partial body weight support and robotic training revealed that therapy with partial body weight support was superior to robotic training for subjects with chronic stroke [20].

One of the possible drawbacks of treatment with RAGT may be the excessive passive guidance of device, which could potentially reduce patient effort and treatment effectiveness [21]. Additionally, another important factor is the patients' limited degree of freedom with the equipment, which could result in abnormal torque [18].

Considering the critical importance of the subject as well as the shortage and inconclusive information about it, this study aimed to assess the influence of robot-assisted gait training on balance and coordination and to verify the functional independence in activities of daily living of chronic stroke survivors with ataxia after at least one year of injury.

2. Methods

2.1. Subjects. This was a randomized controlled trial approved by the Universidade Federal do Estado de São Paulo (UNIFESP) ethics committee (number 933.112). All the patients who participated or their legal representatives gave written informed consent voluntarily without financial gains.

The inclusion criteria were stroke survivors with ataxia, minimum time of injury over 1 year (in the chronic phase of rehabilitation), cerebellar stroke verified by an initial MRI, clinical stability, presence of hemiplegia or quadriplegia motor impairment, and admission to the Associação de Assistência a Criança Deficiente (AACD) Rehabilitation Center from September 23, 2014, to December 20, 2015. Patients from both genders who were at least 18 years of age were accepted. A physician examined all the patients and described their diagnosis in medical records.

The exclusion criteria were physical disability that made training with the robotic device unsafe such as cognitive impairment, dementia, aphasia, presence of other orthopedic or neurosurgical problems in the lower extremities, pressure ulcers on the hips or lower extremities, weight higher than 120 kg, ataxia originated by progressive disease, and not accomplishing the proposed treatment.

The participants were allocated to each arm of this study using a weekly timetable, which illustrated a list of sessions available for the proposed treatment. This specific schedule was formulated given ten different schedule options per week. Depending on their preferable time session chosen, they were allocated to one of the two arms of this study: therapist-assisted gait training (TAGT) or RAGT. Each participant completed three sessions per week. Furthermore, their timeline was organized with the availability and capacity of the institution for both proposed interventions.

2.2. Evaluation Protocol. All participants were examined by a blinded evaluator at two-time points: before and after the protocol treatment was completed. The Berg Balance Scale (BBS), the Functional Independence Measure (FIM), the Timed Up and Go Test (TUG), and the Scale for the Assessment and Rating of Ataxia (SARA) were the tools used for baseline and outcome evaluation.

The BBS test is used to evaluate balance and risk of fall. The BBS focuses on static and dynamic balance, which includes 14 tasks with a maximum score of 56 [22, 23].

The TUG test evaluates sitting balance, transfers from sitting to standing, stability in ambulation, and gait course changes [24].

The FIM is used to assess neuropsychological and motor disability. This functional scale includes 18 items allocated into 6 domains: 2 cognitive and 4 motors. Each item has an increasing score from 1 to 7 (1 = maximum of functional dependence and 7 = maximum of functional independence). The minimum value of the entire range is 18, and the total score is 126 [22].

The SARA is used to assess the severity and treatment effectiveness of cerebellar ataxia. Some studies have shown its usefulness in stroke individuals [25, 26]. The total score ranges from 0 (no ataxia) to 40 (severe ataxia), and it is composed of the following 8 items [27]: 1 gait (0–8); 2 stance (0–6); 3 sitting (0–4); 4 speech disturbance (0–6); 5 finger chase (0–4); 6 nose finger test (0–4); 7 fast alternating hand movement (0–4); and 8 heel-shin slide (0–4); the four extremities are evaluated bilaterally, and the mean values are used to calculate the total score [26].

TABLE 1: Summary of demographic and baseline characteristics by intervention therapy.

Demographic and baseline characteristics	Therapist-assisted ($n = 8$) X (SD)	Robot-assisted ($n = 7$) X (SD)	P value
Mean age (year)	56.4 (11.8)	44.4 (12.7)	0.064
Gender, number (M/F)	6/2	5/2	0.876
Diagnosis, number (I/H)	2/6	2/5	0.876
Right side motor impairment, number	2	2	0.876
Left side motor impairment, number	2	2	0.876
Both side motor impairment, number	4	3	0.782
Onset (year)	10.5 (5.4)	4.8 (0.92)	0.021*

P value represents between-group differences. *Requirement for a statistically significant difference: $P < 0.05$. SD: standard deviation; M: male; F: female; I: ischemic; H: hemorrhagic.

2.3. Training Protocol. The patients were allocated into two groups according to the treatment received for gait training: therapist-assisted gait training (TAGT) and robot-assisted gait training (RAGT). Both groups were submitted to 3 intensive sessions of physiotherapy per week and were prescribed home exercises. Each group had 2 sessions of conventional physiotherapy and 1 session of gait training with an estimated duration of 60 minutes each. The TAGT was delivered over ground with the use of a walker device, if necessary. The RAGT was performed with a robot-driven exoskeleton orthosis equipment Lokomat® 5.0. In an automated electromechanical gait rehabilitation, the Lokomat device consists of a robotic gait orthosis combined with a harness-supported body weight system used in combination with a treadmill. The estimated protocol time was 5 months.

For both groups, the rehabilitation program consisted of muscle stretching and strengthening, balance training, postural stability control, sensory techniques, and functional daily activities. Furthermore, the patients were encouraged to continue practicing exercises at home. The professional in charge of the physiotherapy treatment was very knowledgeable and experienced in treating neurological disorders.

The main aim of RAGT was to improve the quality of movement and the coordination of both legs. The parameters were performed at a low speed (between 0.8 kph and 1.5 kph) and were adjusted gradually according to the patients' evolution. The body weight support was 50% of the patient weight at the beginning of the protocol treatment, which was gradually reduced until a minimum of 10% at the end the protocol training.

2.4. Statistical Analysis. All parametric results are illustrated as the mean ± standard deviation for each group in the tables and text. A level of significance of $P < 0.05$ was accepted for this study. The data were analyzed using change scores from pre- to posttraining with intragroup and between-group comparisons. Only data from subjects who completed the protocol training were used. The demographic characteristics (age and median onset time) were analyzed using the Mann–Whitney U test. Gender, the distribution of diagnosis, and side motor impairment were analyzed using the two-ratio test. The Wilcoxon test was used for intragroup comparisons, and the Mann–Whitney U test for between-group comparison. The data were analyzed using SPSS software V17, Minitab 16, and Excel Office 2010.

3. Results

A total of 19 patients were enrolled in this study from September 23, 2014, to December 20, 2015. The TAGT group contained 8 subjects. The RAGT group contained 11 subjects, of whom 4 were excluded for not complying with the protocol treatment criteria, leaving 7 subjects. The median age of all patients was 50.8 ± 13.3 years. The median onset time of all patients was 7.8 ± 4.8 years. The population studied was predominantly composed of hemorrhagic stroke patients ($P = 0.017$) (two-ratio test). The distribution of motor impairment side was homogeneous for both groups. The demographic distribution and baseline characteristics for each group are reported separately in Table 1.

After protocol treatment, both groups showed statistically significant improvement ($P < 0.05$) in balance, functional independence in daily living activities, and general ataxia sequela symptoms. Such betterment was evidenced by the intragroup comparison of all functional scales scores from pre- and posttreatment, which are described in Table 2.

Figure 1 shows the difference in the means of the SARA score for both TAGT and RAGT at baseline and after the conclusion of the protocol treatment. There was a significant improvement in the SARA score at the completion of the protocol training for both groups.

Although the two groups had different mean values for the functional scale scores (Table 2), there was no statistically significant difference for the between-group comparison at both baseline and after completion of the protocol treatment (BBS pre $P = 0.816$, post $P = 0.862$; TUG pre $P = 0.807$, post $P = 0.684$; FIM pre $P = 0.318$, post $P = 0.343$; and SARA pre $P = 0.817$, post: $P = 0.643$).

4. Discussion

In general, the major goal of a rehabilitation program is to improve gait capacity, which has been directly connected to the quality of life in poststroke patients [28]. Moreover, other frequently addressed complaints are postural instability and balance impairments, which are related to a loss in independence to perform activities of daily living [29].

Balance involves a range of motor skills that are directly connected to sensory-motor processes, functional contexts, and the environment [30]. Stroke is frequently associated with the impairment of these abilities. However, there are

TABLE 2: Outcome measures at baseline and after protocol treatment by intervention therapy.

Functional scale	Therapist-assisted		P value	Robot-assisted		P value
	Pre	Post		Pre	Post	
BBS	27.3 ± 10.8	35.5 ± 14.1	0.012^*	26.6 ± 18.0	32.4 ± 18.8	0.018^*
TUG	$0:28 \pm 0:11$	$0:22 \pm 0:10$	0.017^*	$0:46 \pm 0.40$	$0:27 \pm 0:17$	0.011^*
FIM	80.9 ± 9.6	85.4 ± 8.2	0.016^*	73.9 ± 14.6	78.5 ± 12.9	0.042^*
SARA	18.9 ± 6.8	15.4 ± 5.6	0.012^*	18.7 ± 7.6	15.2 ± 6.8	0.018^*

All values are shown as the mean $\pm$ SD. P value represents intragroup differences. *Requirement for a statistically significant difference: $P < 0.05$. The nonparametric Wilcoxon test was used to compare pre- and posttreatment measurements. BBS: Berg Balance Scale; TUG: Timed Up and Go Test reported in seconds; FIM: Functional Independence Measure; SARA: Scale Assessment and Rating of Ataxia.

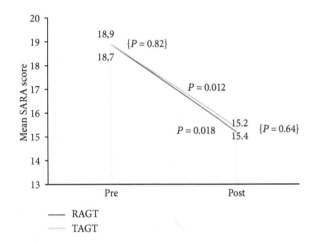

FIGURE 1: Changes in assessment and rating of ataxia. P value represents intragroup differences. Requirement for a statistically significant difference: $P < 0.05$. P value for between-group comparison: $\{P = 0.82; P = 0.64\}$. Requirement for a statistically significant difference: $P < 0.05$.

few studies that have reported the effect of RAGT on balance [18]. This research aimed to assess the influence of robot-assisted gait training on balance and to verify the functional independence in daily living activities of chronic stroke survivors with ataxia after at least one year of injury.

In the present study, we used the BBS and TUG tests to assess balance control. The results indicated a significant improvement in balance for both RAGT and TAGT groups. These findings agree with previous reports [18, 31, 32]. Furthermore, when the balance outcomes were compared between groups, that is, RAGT versus TAGT, no significant difference was demonstrated, which is also supported by several studies [18, 32–35]. In contrast, Dundar et al. showed greater improvement in balance for the group that received RAGT; their treatment protocol included patients with a stroke onset ranging from 28 days to 365 days, which differs from the current study that included only subjects with chronic stroke [22].

After the protocol treatment was completed, both RAGT and TAGT groups revealed a significant improvement in mean FIM scale results, which indicates that both strategies could be effective in improving independence in activities of daily living. Moreover, no significant difference was encountered when these outcomes were compared between

groups. Tong et al. also compared the therapeutic effects of TAGT and RAGT interventions [32]. Our findings agree with regard to the improvement in general independence and the absence of significant differences for the intergroup comparison. On the contrary, other studies presented statistically superior improvement in general activities for the group that received RAGT [22, 28]. This discrepancy in the findings is still relatively unexplained and should be investigated further.

In the present study, an improvement in the SARA outcome measure after protocol treatment was observed in stroke patients with ataxia sequela, showing a better control in postural disorders. When the total SARA scores were compared between groups, there was no statistically significant difference. Only a few studies have focused on the assessment and rehabilitation treatment of ataxia disorders and have demonstrated the beneficial effects of rehabilitation programs [36, 37]. Although there are published investigations of different techniques, such as virtual reality, biofeedback, and treadmill exercise with or without body weight support [36–39], none have evaluated the effect of RAGT on chronic stroke patients with ataxia.

Gait ability is closely associated with balance control [40]. A systematic review concluded that RAGT may increase the chance of recovering independent walking ability in poststroke patients [22]. The greatest improvement in independent walking and walking speed was observed during the early months after stroke [22, 41].

A multicenter randomized clinical trial that compared RAGT with TAGT interventions in subjects affected by subacute stroke showed that TAGT rendered better outcomes for gait improvement [33]. Similarly, another comparative study showed greater improvements in overground walking speed in chronic stroke survivors who received TAGT [20].

In the last two decades, several studies have demonstrated different results regarding the effects of RAGT treatment for gait rehabilitation on poststroke individuals [14, 31, 33, 42, 43]. Robotic assistance is a valuable resource for recovering gait ability. Notwithstanding, only a few studies have investigated its effectiveness for balance recovery in chronic stroke survivors. Additionally, there is no published study that has specifically focused on treating ataxia with RAGT. This study has addressed this gap in knowledge and has contributed to the evidence that robotic therapy may also be an additional asset for the balance treatment of ataxic patients.

This study has some limitations. In particular, some limitations are related to the small sample size. Moreover, future studies should evaluate a longer follow-up time and patients in acute and subacute stroke phases. Additionally, we recommend that future studies should address the analysis of RAGT in larger samples with a comparative measurement and include patients in all stages of stroke. Furthermore, we also suggest the investigation of supplementary interventional methods to gain a comprehensive understanding of the balance control mechanism in ataxic patients.

5. Conclusions

This study concluded that chronic stroke patients with ataxia sequela had a significant improvement in balance and independence in activities of daily living after treatment with RAGT along with conventional therapy and home exercises. For this sample size, the outcomes were similar regardless of the applied treatment strategy, that is, RAGT or TAGT. Both treatment approaches should be included as options in balance rehabilitation programs for ataxic patients.

References

[1] A. Pennycott, D. Wyss, H. Vallery, V. Klamroth-Marganska, and R. Riener, "Towards more effective robotic gait training for stroke rehabilitation: a review," *Journal of NeuroEngineering and Rehabilitation*, vol. 9, no. 1, pp. 65–13, 2012.

[2] D. Lloyd-Jones, R. J. Adams, T. M. Brown et al., "Executive summary: heart disease and stroke statistics-2010 update: a report from the American heart association," *Circulation*, vol. 121, no. 7, pp. 948–954, 2010.

[3] U. Bultmann, D. Pierscianek, E. R. Gizewski et al., "Functional recovery and rehabilitation of postural impairment and gait ataxia in patients with acute cerebellar stroke," *Gait & Posture*, vol. 39, no. 1, pp. 563–569, 2014.

[4] B. Husemann, F. Müller, C. Krewer, S. Heller, and E. Koenig, "Effects of locomotion training with assistance of a robot-driven gait orthosis in hemiparetic patients after stroke: a randomized controlled pilot study," *Stroke*, vol. 38, no. 2, pp. 349–354, 2007.

[5] C. Krishnan, D. Kotsapouikis, Y. Y. Dhaher, and W. Z. Rymer, "Reducing robotic guidance during robot-assisted gait training improves gait function: a case report on a stroke survivor," *Archives of Physical Medicine and Rehabilitation*, vol. 94, no. 6, pp. 1202–1206, 2013.

[6] B. Indredavik, G. Rohweder, E. Naalsund, and S. Lydersen, "Medical complications in a comprehensive stroke unit and an early supported discharge service," *Stroke*, vol. 39, no. 2, pp. 414–420, 2008.

[7] S. Bonnì, V. Ponzo, C. Caltagirone, and G. Koch, "Cerebellar theta burst stimulation in stroke patients with ataxia," *Functional Neurology*, vol. 29, no. 1, pp. 41–45, 2014.

[8] S. Maeshima, A. Osawa, Y. Miyazaki, H. Takeda, and N. Tanahashi, "Functional outcome in patients with pontine infarction after acute rehabilitation," *Neurological Sciences*, vol. 33, no. 4, pp. 759–764, 2012.

[9] S. Datar and A. A. Rabinstein, "Cerebellar hemorrhage," *Neurologic Clinics*, vol. 32, no. 4, pp. 993–1007, 2014.

[10] W. Ilg, H. Golla, P. Thier, and M. A. Giese, "Specific influences of cerebellar dysfunctions on gait," *Brain*, vol. 130, no. 3, pp. 786–798, 2007.

[11] S. M. Morton, Y.-W. Tseng, K. M. Zackowski, J. R. Daline, and A. J. Bastian, "Longitudinal tracking of gait and balance impairments in cerebellar disease," *Movement Disorders*, vol. 25, no. 12, pp. 1944–1952, 2010.

[12] Z. Sawacha, E. Carraro, P. Contessa, A. Guiotto, S. Masiero, and C. Cobelli, "Relationship between clinical and instrumental balance assessments in chronic post-stroke hemiparesis subjects," *Journal of NeuroEngineering and Rehabilitation*, vol. 10, no. 1, p. 95, 2013.

[13] S. Hesse, "Treadmill training with partial body weight support after stroke: a review," *NeuroRehabilitation*, vol. 23, no. 1, pp. 55–65, 2008.

[14] D. Y. Cho, S.-W. Park, M. J. Lee, D. S. Park, and E. J. Kim, "Effects of robot-assisted gait training on the balance and gait of chronic stroke patients: focus on dependent ambulators," *Journal of Physical Therapy Science*, vol. 27, no. 10, pp. 3053–3057, 2015.

[15] S. Kubota, Y. Nakata, K. Eguchi et al., "Feasibility of rehabilitation training with a newly developed wearable robot for patients with limited mobility," *Archives of Physical Medicine and Rehabilitation*, vol. 94, no. 6, pp. 1080–1087, 2013.

[16] S. Jezernik, G. Colombo, T. Keller, H. Frueh, and M. Morari, "Robotic orthosis lokomat: a rehabilitation and research tool," *Neuromodulation: Technology at the Neural Interface*, vol. 6, no. 2, pp. 108–115, 2003.

[17] L. Wallard, G. Dietrich, Y. Kerlirzin, and J. Bredin, "Effects of robotic gait rehabilitation on biomechanical parameters in the chronic hemiplegic patients," *Neurophysiologie Clinique/Clinical Neurophysiology*, vol. 45, no. 3, pp. 215–219, 2015.

[18] E. Swinnen, D. Beckwée, R. Meeusen, J.-P. Baeyens, and E. Kerckhofs, "Does robot-assisted gait rehabilitation improve balance in stroke patients? A systematic review," *Topics in Stroke Rehabilitation*, vol. 21, no. 2, pp. 87–100, 2014.

[19] C. Tefertiller, B. Pharo, N. Evans, and P. Winchester, "Efficacy of rehabilitation robotics for walking training in neurological disorders: a review," *Journal of Rehabilitation Research & Development*, vol. 48, no. 4, pp. 387–416, 2011.

[20] T. G. Hornby, D. D. Campbell, J. H. Kahn, T. Demott, J. L. Moore, and H. R. Roth, "Enhanced gait-related improvements after therapist-versus robotic-assisted locomotor training in subjects with chronic stroke: a randomized controlled study," *Stroke*, vol. 39, no. 6, pp. 1786–1792, 2008.

[21] J. F. Israel, D. D. Campbell, J. H. Kahn, and T. G. Hornby, "Metabolic costs and muscle activity patterns during robotic- and therapist-assisted treadmill walking in individuals with incomplete spinal cord injury," *Physical Therapy*, vol. 86, no. 11, pp. 1466–1478, 2006.

[22] U. Dundar, H. Toktas, O. Solak, A. M. Ulasli, and S. Eroglu, "A comparative study of conventional physiotherapy versus robotic training combined with physiotherapy in patients with stroke," *Topics in Stoke Rehabilitation*, vol. 21, no. 6, pp. 453–461, 2014.

[23] S. T. Miyamoto, I. Lombardi Junior, K. O. Berg, L. R. Ramos, and J. Natour, "Brazilian version of the Berg balance scale," *Brazilian Journal of Medical and Biological Research*, vol. 37, no. 9, pp. 1411–1421, 2004.

[24] T. B. Hafsteinsdóttir, M. Rensink, and M. Schuurmans, "Clinimetric properties of the timed up and go test for patients with stroke: a systematic review," *Topics in Stroke Rehabilitation*, vol. 21, no. 3, pp. 197–210, 2014.

[25] B.-R. Kim, J.-Y. Lee, M. J. Kim, H. Jung, and J. Lee, "Korean version of the scale for the assessment and rating of ataxia in ataxic stroke patients," *Annals of Rehabilitation Medicine*, vol. 38, no. 6, pp. 742–751, 2014.

[26] B.-R. Kim, J.-H. Lim, S. A. Lee et al., "Usefulness of the scale for the assessment and rating of ataxia (SARA) in ataxic stroke patients," *Annals of Rehabilitation Medicine*, vol. 35, no. 6, pp. 772–780, 2011.

[27] P. Braga-Neto, C. Godeiro-Junior, L. A. Dutra, J. L. Pedroso, and O. G. P. Barsottini, "Translation and validation into Brazilian version of the scale of the assessment and rating of ataxia (SARA)," *Arquivos de Neuro-Psiquiatria*, vol. 68, no. 2, pp. 228–230, 2010.

[28] G. Taveggia, A. Borboni, C. Mulé, J. H. Villafañe, and S. Negrini, "Conflicting results of robot-assisted versus usual gait training during postacute rehabilitation of stroke patients: a randomized clinical trial," *International Journal of Rehabilitation Research*, vol. 39, no. 1, pp. 29–35, 2016.

[29] P. G. Lopes, J. A. F. Lopes, C. M. Brito, F. M. Alfieri, and L. Rizzo Battistella, "Relationships of balance, gait performance, and functional outcome in chronic stroke patients: a comparison of left and right lesions," *BioMed Research International*, vol. 2015, Article ID 716042, 8 pages, 2015.

[30] C. B. de Oliveira, I. R. de Medeiros, N. A. Frota, M. E. Greters, and A. B. Conforto, "Balance control in hemiparetic stroke patients: main tools for evaluation," *Journal of Rehabilitation Research & Development*, vol. 45, no. 8, pp. 1215–1226, 2008.

[31] L. Conesa, Ú. Costa, E. Morales et al., "An observational report of intensive robotic and manual gait training in sub-acute stroke," *Journal of NeuroEngineering and Rehabilitation*, vol. 9, no. 1, p. 13, 2012.

[32] R. K. Tong, M. F. Ng, and L. S. Li, "Effectiveness of gait training using an electromechanical gait trainer, with and without functional electric stimulation, in subacute stroke: a randomized controlled trial," *Archives of Physical Medicine and Rehabilitation*, vol. 87, no. 10, pp. 1298–1304, 2006.

[33] J. Hidler, D. Nichols, M. Pelliccio et al., "Multicenter randomized clinical trial evaluating the effectiveness of the lokomat in subacute stroke," *Neurorehabilitation and Neural Repair*, vol. 23, no. 1, pp. 5–13, 2009.

[34] D. Dias, J. Laíns, A. Pereira et al., "Can we improve gait skills in chronic hemiplegics? A randomised control trial with gait trainer," *Europa Medicophysica*, vol. 43, no. 4, pp. 499–504, 2007.

[35] M. F. W. Ng, R. K. Y. Tong, and L. S. W. Li, "A pilot study of randomized clinical controlled trial of gait training in subacute stroke patients with partial body-weight support electromechanical gait trainer and functional electrical stimulation: six-month follow-up," *Stroke*, vol. 39, no. 1, pp. 154–160, 2008.

[36] A. Marquer, G. Barbieri, and D. Pérennou, "The assessment and treatment of postural disorders in cerebellar ataxia: a systematic review," *Annals of Physical and Rehabilitation Medicine*, vol. 57, no. 2, pp. 67–78, 2014.

[37] K. Cernak, V. Stevens, R. Price, and A. Shumway-Cook, "Locomotor training using body-weight support on a treadmill in conjunction with ongoing physical therapy in a child with severe cerebellar ataxia," *Physical Therapy*, vol. 88, no. 1, pp. 88–97, 2007.

[38] J. E. Freund and D. M. Stetts, "Use of trunk stabilization and locomotor training in an adult with cerebellar ataxia: a single system design," *Physiotherapy Theory and Practice*, vol. 26, no. 7, pp. 447–458, 2010.

[39] D. V. Vaz, C. Schettino R de, T. R. Rolla de Castro, V. R. Teixeira, S. R. Cavalcanti Furtado, and E. de Mello Figueiredo, "Treadmill training for ataxic patients: a single-subject experimental design," *Clinical Rehabilitation*, vol. 22, no. 3, pp. 234–241, 2008.

[40] T. J. Kim, K. M. Seo, D.-K. Kim, and S. H. Kang, "The relationship between initial trunk performances and functional prognosis in patients with stroke," *Annals of Rehabilitation Medicine*, vol. 39, no. 1, pp. 66–73, 2015.

[41] J. Mehrholz, C. Werner, J. Kugler, and M. Pohl, "Electromechanical-assisted training for walking after stroke-review," *The Cochrane Collaboration*, no. 9, 2010.

[42] D. E. Uçar, N. Paker, and D. Buğdaycı, "Lokomat: a therapeutic chance for patients with chronic hemiplegia," *NeuroRehabilitation*, vol. 34, no. 3, pp. 447–453, 2014.

[43] B. H. Dobkin, "Progressive staging of pilot studies to improve phase III trials for motor interventions," *Neurorehabilitation and Neural Repair*, vol. 23, no. 3, pp. 197–206, 2009.

11

Intensive Outpatient Treatment of Depression in a Spinocerebellar Ataxia Type 1 Patient

Eric Black ⓘ

Assistant Professor of Psychiatry, Southern Illinois University, USA

Correspondence should be addressed to Eric Black; ericblack@gmx.net

Academic Editor: Toshiya Inada

Objective. Spinocerebellar ataxia type 1 (SCA1) is but one subtype of spinocerebellar ataxia (SCA), each of which can possibly be considered a separate neurological condition (N. Whaley, S. Fujioka, Z. K. Wszolek, 2011). SCA is hereditary, progressive, and degenerative. SCA1 symptoms initially include coordination problems and ataxia. SCA1 can also include speech and swallowing difficulties, spasticity, ophthalmoplegia, cognitive difficulties, and even sensory neuropathy, dystonia, atrophy, and fasciculations. Literature has established that depressive symptoms can be exhibited with spinocerebellar ataxia patients regardless of type (T. Schmitz-Hübsch, 2011). While a higher risk for depression occurs with more severe SCA disease, successful treatment to mitigate symptoms has been documented (N. Okamoto, M. Ogawa, Y. Murata, et al., 2010). In this case a SCA1 patient with advanced neurological disease was enrolled in a psychiatric intensive outpatient (IOP) treatment program in the midwestern United States to address his comorbid depressive symptoms. This treatment option allowed a less restrictive environment while providing a more structured therapeutic setting and social support for the patient, much more so than that which is typically offered in a traditional outpatient setting. *Case Report*. A patient with relatively advanced SCA1 successfully participated in a psychiatric IOP program or depressive symptoms and benefitted from the program's structure and additional psychosocial support. *Conclusion*. Awareness among physicians, particularly psychiatrists and neurologists, regarding IOP programs as a treatment option for comorbid depression in the clinical setting of progressive SCA or other neurological conditions can be beneficial to patients requiring an increased level of psychiatric treatment.

1. Introduction

Patients with various subtypes of SCA can exhibit depressive symptoms. The pathology of such depressive symptoms in the setting of SCA is not fully explained [1, 2]. Either the symptoms clinically arise due to stress resulting from progressively decreased neurological motor function, or there possibly exists a neurodegenerative process manifesting in depression. The treatment of major depressive disorder (MDD) complicated by SCA has been reported in the literature [2–4]. The benefits of pharmacotherapy, specifically utilizing selective serotonin reuptake inhibitors (SSRIs) which have proven effective even when depression occurs with advanced SCA, points to reversible abnormalities of serotonin transmission as a depression etiology [3]. This successful treatment, however, does not completely exclude the possibility that the depressive symptoms were, at least in part, reactive to the stress from decreased motor function in SCA. Numerous SCA analyses have been done, producing data ranging from basic quantitative SCA survival data [5], to patient-reported outcome measures (PROMs) as a complement to neurological scales [6]. PROMs including depressive symptoms within the Patient Health Questionnaire (PHQ-9) have been tracked, underlying the importance of PROMs as additional outcome measures for SCA patients [6]. To this end, the specific management and treatment of depression arising from the patient's progressive SCA functional limitations need even further attention in the literature. This unique aspect of depression treatment is addressed in this report, describing a SCA1 patient with advanced neurological disease enrolled in a psychiatric IOP program to provide social support in a structured therapeutic setting. The utilization and effectiveness of this type of psychosocial intervention for depression in the setting of SCA is not mentioned in the literature as part of a treatment plan for a patient. However, IOPs in general have been utilized successfully for a variety of psychiatric conditions [7]. The additional longitudinal emotional and psychological support along with monitored pharmacotherapy with SSRIs improved the quality of life for a SCA1 patient despite the progression of his neurological symptoms. The objective is to highlight that this more comprehensive treatment option, when available to SCA patients suffering from depression, may warrant more consideration from neurologists and psychiatrists in the management of this chronic condition.

2. Case Report

A 49-year-old Caucasian male was evaluated at the Department of Adult Psychiatry Intensive Outpatient (IOP) Treatment Program for initial intake after having been referred from the Department of Neurology Outpatient Clinic. He had complaints of depressed mood, lack of enjoyment of pleasurable activities, sleep disturbances, poor concentration, and occasional passive suicidal thoughts. These symptoms were in association with ongoing progression of symptoms related to his diagnosis of SCA1. His neurologic symptoms included coordination problems and ataxia initially at diagnosis, but in recent years speech impairment, swallowing difficulties, some spasticity, and eventually muscle atrophy were presented. He had to utilize a motorized wheelchair as a result of his progressive disability. His current house was not fully wheelchair accessible. He lived alone but had siblings who visited at least several times per week. He also seemed to lack insight into the relationship between his thoughts, feelings, and physical limitations.

At the psychiatric evaluation, he expressed that his self-esteem was strongly affected by his limited physical mobility due to his SCA1, and he seemed extremely unhappy. He reported passive death wishes at least once a week, usually without a suicidal plan or intent. Laboratory evaluations including hemogram, liver function tests, total protein, vitamin B12, folic acid, T3, T4, and TSH were within normal limits. Baseline psychiatric evaluation with the Beck Depression Inventory (BDI-II) [8] revealed scores of 23 (moderate depression). According to clinical evaluation as well as DSM-V [9] criteria, the patient was diagnosed with major depressive disorder and he was started on sertraline 50 milligrams (mg) by mouth per day. He had never taken medications for depression before. Group cognitive behavioral therapy focusing on negative cognitions as well as aspects of dialectical behavioral therapy were initiated as part of the IOP protocol [10]. These group sessions occurred three times a week for several hours a session totaling approximately 12 hours per week. Individual cognitive behavioral therapy with a psychologist also occurred weekly for the first several weeks of the IOP program. He also met with a psychiatrist weekly, then every two weeks, and finally monthly for medication management. His sertraline was increased over this time period to 100 mg per day. He reported compliance with medications and reported no side effects. He also participated in 3 family sessions whereby his family members were also engaged in psychoeducation and therapy. Partial response to treatment was observed at the 12th week with reduction of BDI-II [8] score to 12 (mild mood disturbance). He participated in the IOP program for approximately 6 months in total, becoming increasingly more engaged, and eventually reported a subjective significant reduction in depressed mood, anhedonia, and suicidal thoughts. His sleep and concentration also improved. He reported improved insight into the mind-body connection between his physical and emotional conditions. He acquired new coping skills to limit counterproductive behaviors and irrational emotional responses to his occasional negative thoughts. With help of IOP staff and social workers, he found an assisted living accepting of his limited ambulation, moving to a better housing situation. He then was eventually scheduled for medication management and monitoring follow-up appointments in the Department of Adult Psychiatry Outpatient clinic once discharged from the IOP treatment program.

3. Limitations

While this case report fills a niche in the literature regarding the role of an IOP in treating comorbid depression in the setting of a chronically deteriorating condition such as SCA1, there are some limitations involved. Firstly, there are numerous varieties of SCA, and this case focuses on a patient with SCA1. It may serve as an area of future research when other depressive symptoms are studied in other subtypes of SCA. Also, pharmacotherapy (an SSRI) was used in this case to treat MDD, and this modality is not exclusive to an IOP program's offerings. Reversible abnormalities of serotonin transmission as a depression etiology in SCA patients have been noted [3], and this aspect of treatment can be addressed in any psychiatric setting, not just an IOP. PROMs in past research have included PHQ-9 as a measure of depression in SCA patients [6], and here the BDI-II [8] was utilized as an outcome measure. While both are valid instruments in clinical practice, future research may lead to more standardization in this specific patient population. The length of time the patient participating in the IOP program was about 6 months, which can vary among different countries and regions. The availability, strength of services offered, and the experience of the IOP program staff compared to traditional clinics can all vary as well. This unfortunately may be the greatest limitation, speaking to the need for more promotion and development of such valuable psychosocial programs for patients.

4. Discussion

In clinical psychiatric practice, treating patients with comorbid physical impairments can be challenging as the scope of their overall impairment may be better addressed through a broader variety of approaches [11, 12]. Standard psychiatric outpatient medication management clinics are typically challenged for resources. They may lack extensive social and psychological services that patients with physical disabilities need to more globally assess their overall condition as it affects their mental health, representing a significant disparity for those patients [12]. IOP treatment programs, particularly those in the United States where this case occurred, offer unique resources and longitudinal structure providing intensive, goal-oriented, group-based programming to foster increased self-awareness, and behavioral change. Target areas for intervention in a robust IOP program with a full array of social workers and psychologists include symptom management, self-esteem and emotional regulation, interpersonal effectiveness, distress tolerance, and adaptive coping [7]. Addressing substance use has traditionally been part of United States IOP programs as well [13]. Programs also include routine monitoring of the patients by a psychiatrist. As was noted earlier, such an extensive IOP program unfortunately may not always be available, pointing to a glaring need in certain mental health communities.

In the present case, although response was achieved through psychological and pharmacological treatment with respect to the patient's MDD, the report of success through an IOP treatment program specifically in a comorbid SCA1 patient is notable. This favorable outcome points to a possibly better alternative than a traditional psychiatric outpatient clinic for patients with significant psychosocial stress due to progressive physical limitations. It should be noted that the level of care provided in traditional psychiatric clinics and services offered can vary greatly, so some may compare more favorably to IOP programs. This case also illustrates that the IOP program availability and promotion in the community must be robust, and here the initial referral came from a Neurology outpatient clinic as staff there were aware of the program, believing it to be a good fit for the patient's needs. It is noted again here too that such resources may not be available in all countries or regions.

In conclusion, physicians, especially psychiatrists and neurologists, should remain mindful of the utility of IOP programs as treatment options for mental health conditions. The more intensive psychosocial treatment can be particularly beneficial for those patients with chronic physical conditions, especially those with significant psychiatric comorbidities, such as SCA. Pharmacological targets for therapy and the stress of living with a chronic progressive physical disease are optimally addressed in such a program. Healthcare professionals owe this holistic approach to their patients as part of a comprehensive model of caring for them.

Authors' Contributions

Eric Black contributed to the patient's treatment and follow-up and was responsible for case conception and design, review of the literature drafting of the manuscript. Eric Black was also responsible for the critical revision of the manuscript.

References

[1] N. Whaley, S. Fujioka, and Z. K. Wszolek, "Autosomal dominant cerebellar ataxia type I: A review of the phenotypic and genotypic characteristics," *Orphanet Journal of Rare Diseases*, vol. 6, article no 33, 2011.

[2] T. Schmitz-Hübsch, "Depression comorbidity in spinocerebellar ataxia," *Movement Disorders Journal*, vol. 26, no. 5, pp. 870–876, 2011.

[3] N. Okamoto, M. Ogawa, Y. Murata et al., "Major depressive disorder complicated with spinocerebellar ataxia: Report of 2 cases," *Case Reports in Neurology*, vol. 2, no. 2, pp. 52–56, 2010.

[4] F. Mario and M. D. Mendez, "Depressive and memory symptoms as presenting features of spinocerebellar ataxia," *Journal of Neuropsychiatry and Clinical Neurosciences*, vol. 18, no. 3, pp. 420–422, 2006.

[5] A. Diallo, H. Jacobi, A. Cook et al., "Survival in patients with spinocerebellar ataxia types 1, 2, 3, and 6 (EUROSCA): A longitudinal cohort study," *The Lancet Neurology*, vol. 17, no. 4, pp. 327–334, 2018.

[6] H. Jacobi, S. T. du Montcel, P. Bauer et al., "Long-term evolution of patient-reported outcome measures in spinocerebellar ataxias," *Journal of Neurology*, vol. 265, no. 9, pp. 2040–2051, 2018.

[7] G. W. Smith, A. Ruiz-Sancho, and J. G. Gunderson, "An intensive outpatient program for patients with borderline personality disorder," *American Psychiatric Association*, vol. 52, no. 4, pp. 532-533, 2001.

[8] A. T. Beck, R. A. Steer, and G. K. Brown, *Manual for the Beck Depression Inventory-II*, Psychological Corporation, San Antonio,Tex, USA, 1996.

[9] American Psychiatric Association, *Diagnostic and Statistical Manual of Mental Disorders: DSM-V*, vol. 28, American Psychiatric Association, Washington, DC, 5th edition, 2013.

[10] L. A. Ritschel, J. S. Cheavens, and J. Nelson, "Dialectical behavior therapy in an intensive outpatient program with a mixed-diagnostic sample," *Journal of Clinical Psychology*, vol. 68, no. 3, pp. 221–235, 2012.

[11] N. Sartorious, "Comorbidity of mental and physical diseases: A main challenge for medicine of the 21st century," *Shanghai Archives of Psychiatry*, vol. 25, no. 2, pp. 68-69, 2013.

[12] M. de Hert, C. U. Correll, J. Bobes et al., "Physical illness in patients with severe mental disorders. I. Prevalence, impact of medications and disparities in health care," *World Psychiatry*, vol. 10, no. 1, pp. 52–77, 2011.

[13] "Substance abuse: Clinical issues in intensive outpatient treatment," Treatment Improvement Protocol (TIP) Series, No. 4 (SMA) 06-4182, Center for Substance Abuse Treatment, Substance Abuse and Mental Health Services Administration (US), Rockville (MD), 2006.

12

Drosophila melanogaster Models of Friedreich's Ataxia

P. Calap-Quintana,[1] **J. A. Navarro,**[2] **J. González-Fernández,**[1,3] **M. J. Martínez-Sebastián,**[1] **M. D. Moltó ⓘ,**[1,3,4] **and J. V. Llorens**[1]

[1]*Department of Genetics, University of Valencia, Campus of Burjassot, Valencia, Spain*
[2]*Institute of Zoology, University of Regensburg, Regensburg, Germany*
[3]*Biomedical Research Institute INCLIVA, Valencia, Spain*
[4]*Centro de Investigación Biomédica en Red de Salud Mental (CIBERSAM), Madrid, Spain*

Correspondence should be addressed to M. D. Moltó; dmolto@uv.es

Academic Editor: Antonio Baonza

Friedreich's ataxia (FRDA) is a rare inherited recessive disorder affecting the central and peripheral nervous systems and other extraneural organs such as the heart and pancreas. This incapacitating condition usually manifests in childhood or adolescence, exhibits an irreversible progression that confines the patient to a wheelchair, and leads to early death. FRDA is caused by a reduced level of the nuclear-encoded mitochondrial protein frataxin due to an abnormal GAA triplet repeat expansion in the first intron of the human *FXN* gene. *FXN* is evolutionarily conserved, with orthologs in essentially all eukaryotes and some prokaryotes, leading to the development of experimental models of this disease in different organisms. These FRDA models have contributed substantially to our current knowledge of frataxin function and the pathogenesis of the disease, as well as to explorations of suitable treatments. *Drosophila melanogaster*, an organism that is easy to manipulate genetically, has also become important in FRDA research. This review describes the substantial contribution of *Drosophila* to FRDA research since the characterization of the fly frataxin ortholog more than 15 years ago. Fly models have provided a comprehensive characterization of the defects associated with frataxin deficiency and have revealed genetic modifiers of disease phenotypes. In addition, these models are now being used in the search for potential therapeutic compounds for the treatment of this severe and still incurable disease.

1. Introduction

Friedreich's ataxia (FRDA) is an autosomal recessive neurodegenerative disorder and the most common form of hereditary ataxia among populations of European origin (2–4/100,000) [1]. This disabling condition typically manifests before age 25, with progressive neurodegeneration of the dorsal root ganglia, sensory peripheral nerves, corticospinal tracts, and dentate nuclei of the cerebellum. A large proportion of patients develop hypertrophic cardiomyopathy, which is the major cause of reduced life expectancy in this disease. Diabetes mellitus and impaired glucose tolerance are also seen in a significant number of FRDA patients (reviewed in [2]).

FRDA is caused by loss-of-function mutations in the *FXN* gene, which encodes the frataxin protein [3]. Frataxin is a small protein encoded in the nucleus, expressed as

a precursor polypeptide in the cytoplasm and imported into mitochondria [4–6]. The majority of FRDA patients are homozygous for an abnormally expanded GAA repeat in intron 1 of *FXN*, resulting in strongly reduced frataxin protein expression (from 5% to 30% of the normal level) [7]. The remaining FRDA patients are compound heterozygotes, carrying the GAA repeat expansion on one *FXN* allele and another pathogenic mutation on the other allele, including point mutations and insertion and/or deletion mutations [8].

A lack of available patients and the inherent limitations of cellular models often hinder the discovery and detailed analyses of genes and pathways relevant to the pathology of rare human disorders such as FRDA. Fortunately, the high evolutionary conservation of frataxin (Figure 1) has enabled the development of disease models in several organisms, from bacteria to mice, that have significantly contributed to the

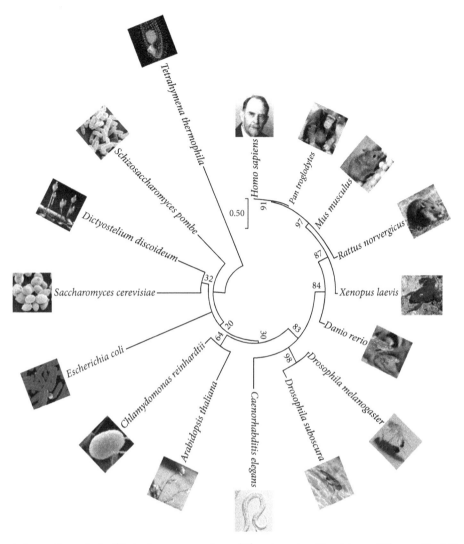

FIGURE 1: Molecular phylogenetic analysis of frataxin sequences from different species. The picture of Thomas Hunt Morgan was chosen to represent *Homo sapiens* because, as a result of his work, *D. melanogaster* became a major model organism in genetics. Methods: evolutionary history was inferred with the maximum likelihood method based on Le and Gascuel model [9]. The tree with the highest log likelihood (−2026.7976) is shown. Initial trees for the heuristic search were obtained automatically by applying the Neighbor-Joining and BioNJ algorithms to a matrix of pairwise distances estimated using a JTT model and then selecting the topology with the superior log likelihood value. A discrete gamma distribution was used to model evolutionary rate differences among sites (5 categories (+G, parameter = 2.4842)). The tree is drawn to scale, with branch lengths representing the number of substitutions per site. The analysis involved 16 amino acid sequences. All positions containing gaps and missing data were eliminated. A total of 90 positions were present in the final dataset. Evolutionary analyses were conducted in MEGA7 [10].

understanding of frataxin function. The development of these disease models is an essential step in elucidating underlying pathological mechanisms and identifying efficient treatments in FRDA.

Seminal findings reported by key studies in model organisms (reviewed in [14–23]) have suggested potential roles for frataxin in iron homeostasis and cellular defense against reactive oxygen species (ROS), as an activator of the mitochondrial respiratory chain, as a mitochondrial chaperone, and as a regulator of Fe-S cluster (ISC) assembly. Although frataxin function is not yet fully characterized, its role in ISC biogenesis is generally accepted [24–26]. Major alterations associated with frataxin deficiency include mitochondrial

iron accumulation, oxidative stress hypersensitivity, impaired ISC biogenesis, and aconitase and respiratory chain dysfunction (reviewed in [27–29]).

Although the arthropod lineage diverged from the vertebrate lineage more than 600 MYA, genome sequencing projects have revealed a large number of biological processes that are conserved between flies and vertebrates. Most of the genes implicated in familial forms of disease have at least one *Drosophila* ortholog [30, 31]. This species offers many different genetic tools that can be applied to investigate basic biological questions in a multicellular organism, with the advantages of easy manipulation and culture.

2. The *Drosophila* Ortholog of the *FXN* Gene

The *D. melanogaster* frataxin ortholog was cloned and characterized in our laboratory in the early 2000s. It was named *dfh* (*Drosophila frataxin homolog*) [32]. This gene is referred to as *fh* (*frataxin homolog*) in FlyBase (CG8971, FBgn0030092), and this name will be used throughout this review. We isolated *fh* by screening a genomic library from *D. subobscura* using human *FXN* probes. Database searches employing the sequence of *D. subobscura* positive clones led to the identification of the *D. melanogaster* STS 125a12, mapped to the 8CD region on the X chromosome and cloned in cosmid 125a12. Further characterization of this cosmid showed an open reading frame (ORF) encoding a frataxin-like protein. Screening of an adult cDNA library from *D. melanogaster*, using the genomic frataxin ORF, revealed two transcripts with two different polyadenylation signals. We confirmed that this gene is located in the 8CD region by in situ hybridization analysis of polytene chromosomes of *D. melanogaster* using *fh* cDNA as a probe.

The genomic organization of *fh* is much simpler than that of the human gene (Figure 2(a)) [32]. *fh* is approximately 1 kb and is composed of two exons of 340 bp and 282 bp, separated by an intron of 69 bp. RNA in situ hybridization in whole embryos showed ubiquitous expression of *fh* in all developmental stages examined (from 2 to 16 h). ~1 kb major transcript was identified by Northern blot analysis, in agreement with the predicted size of one of the two mRNA sequences detected by cDNA library screening. This transcript was found in embryonic, larval, pupal, and adult stages [32]. Accordingly, the protein was present in all developmental stages at varying levels, reaching its highest level in late embryos [33].

The encoded fly protein was predicted to have 190 amino acids, with a molecular weight of ~21 kDa. A sequence comparison of frataxin proteins from different species showed better alignment in the central and the C-terminal regions (Figure 2(b)), whereas no alignment was found in the N-terminal region of the protein. Importantly, this region of fly frataxin (FH) also showed typical frataxin features, such as a mitochondrial signal peptide and a putative α-helix with abundant positively charged amino acids and few negatively charged residues [32]. Colocalization experiments using an FH-enhanced green fluorescent fusion protein (EGFP) and a mitochondrial marker confirmed the localization of FH in mitochondria [34]. The mature form of FH has a molecular weight of ~15 kDa [33]. The secondary structure of FH matches the α-β sandwich motif characteristic of other frataxin proteins encoded by orthologous genes [32]. Predictions of the 3D structure generated using the Phyre 2 [11] and Chimera 1.12 [12] software show that FH has an organization similar to that of the human protein (Figure 2(c)). The biophysical properties of FH indicate that its thermal and chemical stabilities closely resemble those of human frataxin [35]. Unlike other eukaryotic frataxin proteins, FH shows enhanced stability *in vitro*, making it a more attractive candidate for evaluation of metal binding and delivery properties. In these experimental conditions, FH can bind and deliver Fe(II), which is required for ISC biosynthesis [35], and, as previously described for human frataxin [36], it interacts with Isu (the Fe cofactor assembly platform for ISC cellular production) in an iron-dependent manner [35]. Recently, some authors have provided experimental evidence that the initial complex of the mitochondrial ISC biosynthetic machinery is conserved in *Drosophila* [37, 38]. These results, along with those reported in mouse (reviewed in [39]), suggest an evolutionarily conserved role for frataxin in ISC biosynthesis.

3. Modeling FRDA in Flies

Several models of FRDA have been developed in *D. melanogaster*, mainly taking advantage of GAL4/UAS transgene-based RNA interference (RNAi) methodology. RNAi allows the posttranscriptional silencing of a gene via the expression of transgenic double-stranded RNAs [40]. The GAL4/UAS system [13] has been incredibly successful in *D. melanogaster* and can induce the expression of a transgene under the control of UAS (Upstream Activating Sequences) and the transcriptional activator protein GAL4 (Figure 3). This experimental strategy has been used to induce tissue-specific and ubiquitous knockdown of *fh* (Table 1). Therefore, this strategy allows the phenotypes of FRDA patients to be mimicked by reducing rather than completely eliminating FH.

The first UAS-transgene construct for RNAi-mediated silencing of *fh* expression was reported by Anderson et al. [33]. This construct consisted of inverted repeats containing the first 391 nucleotides of the *fh* coding region, which were subcloned into the pUAST vector. Fly transformants were crossed to the da^{G32} GAL4-driver line (which exhibits widespread GAL4 protein expression throughout development and in most tissues under the control of regulatory sequences of *daughterless*) to examine *fh* silencing. Three transgenic lines (UDIR1, UDIR2, and UDIR3) were selected in which the GAL4-regulated transgene substantially reduced the FH protein level [33, 41]. Similarly, Llorens et al. [34] generated another UAS-transgene construct (named UAS-*fh*IR) containing two copies of the *fh* coding region in opposite orientations, separated by a GFP fragment as a spacer. A transgenic line (*fh*RNAi line) was selected showing milder effect than the GAL4-regulated transgene in UDIR1/2/3 when crossed with the da^{G32} GAL4 line (Table 1).

The RNAi lines from John Phillips's laboratory [33] have also been combined with a ligand-inducible GAL4/UAS system to deplete frataxin in the *Drosophila* heart [42]. This system is based on a steroid-activated chimeric GAL4 protein, specifically the GAL4-progesterone-receptor fusion protein that is activated by RU486 (mifepristone) [43, 44]. Transgene expression is induced by supplementing the fly food with RU486, and the level of expression is controlled by changing the dosage of the steroid ligand [43].

More recently, Chen et al. [45] identified the first mutant allele of *fh* (*fh*^1) in an unbiased genetic screen of the X chromosome designed to isolate mutations that cause neurodegenerative phenotypes. The mutant allele consisted of an ethyl-methanesulfonate-induced missense mutation (S136R) located in a highly conserved region (S157 in the human protein) required for the binding of human frataxin to the

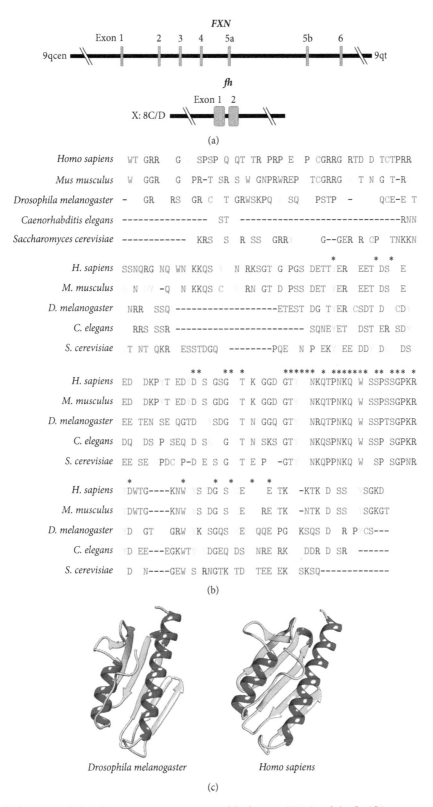

FIGURE 2: The *Drosophila* frataxin ortholog. (a) Genomic organization of the human *(FXN)* and the fly *(fh)* genes encoding frataxin. *FXN* is located in 9q21.11 and contains seven exons. *fh* is located in chromosome X: 8C14 and has two exons. (b) Multiple alignment of the frataxin protein sequences of *Homo sapiens, Mus musculus, D. melanogaster, Caenorhabditis elegans*, and *Saccharomyces cerevisiae*. The letters indicate the amino acid in each position, and the colors classify the amino acids according to their biochemical properties, as described in the MEGA7 program [10]. Invariant amino acids are marked with an asterisk. (c) The 3D structure prediction of the frataxin protein using the Phyre 2 [11] and Chimera 1.12 software [12]; α-helixes appear in blue and β-sheets in green.

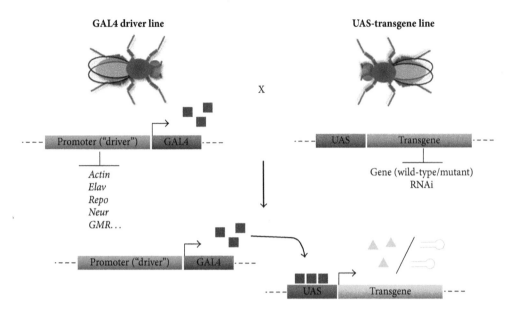

FIGURE 3: The GAL4/UAS system, adapted from yeast, involves the use of two transgenic lines in *Drosophila* [13]. One line carries the GAL4 transcription factor under the control of a promoter of known expression pattern (the driver line), and the other line contains the transgene of interest downstream of UAS (the responder line). Many GAL4 driver lines are available, carrying the promoters of genes such as *actin* (ubiquitous), *elav* (pan-neuronal), *repo* (glial cells), *neur* (sensory organs), and *GMR* (eye). This system is very versatile and allows the expression of specific genes or gene constructs to be induced or suppressed. Triangles indicate a wild-type or mutant protein; the hairpins represent double-stranded RNA molecules that mediate RNAi.

ISC assembly complex [45, 46]. The authors also generated mosaic *fh* mutant mitotic clones of adult photoreceptor neurons using the eyeless-FLP/FRT system to bypass the lethality associated with the fh^1 mutation [45].

These *Drosophila* models of FRDA have been employed to study frataxin function, analyze conserved pathological mechanisms, and search for genetic modifiers and potential therapies. The main results of such studies are described in the following sections.

4. Phenotypes of Frataxin Deficiency in *Drosophila*

The loss of *fh* function in *Drosophila* recapitulates important biochemical, cellular, and physiological phenotypes of FRDA. In addition, some phenotypes have been described for the first time in this organism, revealing new key players in FRDA pathogenesis. All these phenotypes have been obtained using the *fh* constructs and alleles that were described above. Table 1 details these features as well as the temperature of the crosses when available, because the GAL4/UAS system is sensitive to this parameter.

Near-complete frataxin depletion in *Drosophila* seriously affects viability, similar to observations in the FRDA mouse model [47] and most likely in humans, since no patients carrying a pathogenic point mutation or deletion or insertion mutations in both *FXN* alleles have been reported. Ubiquitous *fh* suppression affects larva and pupa development, and individuals do not reach the adult phase [33, 34]. In agreement with these results, individuals that are hemizygous for the fh^1 mutant, carrying the missense S136R mutation, show lethality from the instar 3 larva to pupa stages [45]. Silencing

of *fh* in developing muscle and heart tissue (using the *24B* and *Dot* driver lines) is also lethal in pupal stages, while reduction of *fh* expression in subsets of neurons (C96, *Ddc*, *D42*, *c698a*, and *neur*) allows the development of viable adults. Importantly, when *fh* expression is specifically reduced in the peripheral nervous system (PNS), using the *C96* and *neur* GAL4 lines, the adult flies show a shortened lifespan and reduced climbing ability [33, 34]. These results indicated that, in *Drosophila*, as in humans, frataxin is an essential protein and that different tissues have distinct sensitivity to frataxin deficiency.

Tricoire et al. [42] obtained the first fly *in vivo* heart images after heart-specific depletion of frataxin using the UDIR2 line and the RU486-inducible Geneswitch driver HandGS. They observed major cardiac dysfunction including impaired systolic function and substantial heart dilatation, resembling the phenotypes observed in FRDA patients. The cellular neuropathology of frataxin deficiency was examined in larval motor neurons using the UDIR1 line [48]. Loss of mitochondrial membrane potential was detected in the cell bodies, axons, and neuromuscular junction of segmental nerves from second to late third instar larvae. These effects were followed by defects in mitochondrial retrograde transport in the distal axons, leading to a concomitant dying-back neuropathy. A dying-back mechanism has also been described in sensory neurons and the spinocerebellar and corticospinal motor tract in patients (reviewed in [29]).

To more closely mimic the patient situation, viable adults with ubiquitous reduction of FH were obtained by Llorens et al. [34] by crossing the *fh*RNAi line with the actin-GAL4 driver at 25°C. Under these experimental conditions, the *fh* mRNA level was reduced to one-third compared with

TABLE 1: *Drosophila* models of frataxin deficiency. The *fh* construct or allele and the GAL4 driver used to obtain the different phenotypes of frataxin reduction are specified.

RNAi/mutant allele	GAL4 driver line	Phenotypes
UDIR1–3 [33] frataxin reduction to undetectable levels (25°C)*	*da*^{G32} Ubiquitous	(i) Prolonged larval stages, reduced larvae viability, and inability to pupate [33, 88] (ii) When raised at 18°C, survivor adults exhibit high initial mortality, with some escapers that survive up to 40 days [33, 83] (iii) Reduction of activity of aconitase and respiratory complexes II, III, and IV in larvae and adults [33] (iv) Increase in free fatty acid content in larvae [83]
	C96 Adult peripheral nervous system	(i) Viable adults with a shortened lifespan and increased sensitivity to H_2O_2 [33, 41]
	D42 Motor neurons and interneurons in L3. Adult motor neurons	(i) Normal development and longevity [33] (ii) Loss of mitochondrial membrane potential and reduced mitochondrial transport in the distal axons. Distal axonal degeneration and cell body loss in the ventral ganglion in late L3 [48] (iii) Normal ROS levels [48]
	Repo Pan-glial	(i) Viable adults accompanied by some preadult lethality [83] (ii) Reduction of lifespan, increased sensitivity to hyperoxia (99.5% O_2), and impaired climbing capability [66, 83] (iii) Lipid droplet accumulation in glial cells and brain vacuolization [66, 83]
	HandGS Heart-specific RU486-inducible Geneswitch driver	(i) Induction starting at L3. Viable adults that display heart dilatation and impaired systolic function [42, 88]
	GMR Developing eye	(i) Mild rough eye phenotype [82]

TABLE 1: Continued.

RNAi/mutant allele	GAL4 driver line	Phenotypes
UAS-fhIR [34]: Up to 70% frataxin reduction (25°C)*	actin and da^G32 Ubiquitous	(i) Lethal at the mature pupa stage at 29°C [34] (ii) Viable adults that exhibit shortened lifespan, sensitivity to oxidative stress, and reduced climbing ability [34, 49, 66, 81, 82] (iii) Exposure to hyperoxia causes a substantial reduction in aconitase activity and oxygen consumption [34, 81, 83] (iv) Increased levels of lipid peroxides [81–83] (v) Increased mitochondrial iron content [49] (vi) Sensitive to increased iron content in diet [66] (vii) Complete ablation of iron-dependent ferritin accumulation, reduction of IRP-1A expression, and enhanced expression levels of *mfrn (mitoferrin)* [66] (viii) Increased levels of Fe, Zn, Cu, Mn, and Al [82]
	neur Sensory organs and their precursors	(i) Viable adults at 29°C [34] (ii) Reduced lifespan and climbing capability at 25 and 29°C [34, 49]
	Nervous system: D42, motor neurons Ddc, aminergic neurons and c698a, brain	(i) Viable adults at 29°C [34] (ii) Lifespan and climbing capability unaffected at 29°C [34]
	Repo Pan-glial	(i) Viable adults [83] (ii) Reduction of lifespan, increased sensitivity to hyperoxia (99.5% O_2), and impaired climbing capability [66, 83]
	Other tissues: Dot, heart and 24B, mesoderm	(i) Lethal at the mature pupa stage at 29°C [34]
fh^1 [45]: Ethyl-methanesulfonate-induced missense mutation (S136R). Severe loss of *fh* function Mosaic *fh* mutant clones of adult photoreceptor neurons by the eyeless-FLP/FRT system		(i) Hemizygous fh^1 mutants are lethal from L3 to pupa stage [45] (ii) Removal of maternal *fh* mRNA or protein in the egg causes embryonic lethality [45] (iii) Age-dependent degeneration of photoreceptors [45] (iv) Abnormal mitochondrial cristae morphology, reduced ETC CI activity, and impaired ATP production [45] (v) No increase in ROS [45] (vi) Accumulation of Fe^{2+} and/or Fe^{3+} and iron-dependent stimulation of sphingolipid synthesis and activation of the Pdk1/Mef2 pathway [45]

*The most used temperature in the different experiments.

the normal level. As in humans [7], the remaining frataxin (approximately 30% of the normal level) allowed normal embryonic development but resulted in decreased lifespan and impaired motor performance in adulthood. Specifically, survival analysis showed a decrease of 60% and 32% in the mean and maximum lifespan, respectively, compared with controls. The FRDA flies showed limited climbing ability in negative geotaxis assays, with 5-day-old adults exhibiting a 45% decline compared with control flies.

Frataxin deficiency in flies also triggers iron accumulation [45, 49] restricted to mitochondria [49], consistent with findings in other model organisms and FRDA patients. Importantly, the role of iron in the pathophysiology of FRDA has not yet been completely established and is still a matter of debate. The discovery of iron deposits in the hearts of FRDA patients in the late seventies [50, 51] was the first indication of an association between frataxin and this transition metal. This relationship became more important after the discovery that the loss-of-function of the yeast frataxin ortholog results in mitochondrial iron accumulation [52]. Since then, iron-enriched granules have been further confirmed in patient hearts [53–55] and in several other patient tissues [56, 57]. Surprisingly, analyses of iron levels in neuronal tissues have shown inconsistent results, even in tissues with high frataxin expression. On the one hand, histological and imaging approaches have detected alterations in the expression of iron-related proteins that support the hypothesis that iron redistribution rather than iron accumulation is the key defect underlying frataxin deficiency in the nervous system [58, 59]. On the other hand, increased iron content has been reported in critical brain areas of FRDA patients [60, 61]. In Drosophila, Chen et al. showed that iron accumulates in the nervous system in fh^1 mutants [45]. These authors also found increased levels of iron in the nervous system in an FRDA mouse model that exhibits less than 40% of the normal level of frataxin mRNA in this tissue [62]. By contrast, no iron deposits have been reported in the nervous system in other mouse models of FRDA [47, 63–65]. In line with the proposed iron toxicity in FRDA, all Drosophila models share an enhanced sensitivity to increased iron content in food [33, 45, 66].

The analysis of the iron-frataxin relationship in several FRDA models has provided experimental evidence supporting a role for frataxin in iron homeostasis (storage, redistribution, chaperone, and ISC biosynthesis, reviewed in [23, 24]). Supporting a role for frataxin in ISC assembly, loss of FH expression is associated with impaired activity of Fe-S containing enzymes, including proteins involved in the mitochondrial electron transport chain (ETC) and aconitase [33, 34]. This effect causes problems in ATP production, which is reduced in Drosophila models independently of the levels of functional frataxin [33, 34, 45], as well as in FRDA patients [67, 68]. In addition, the biochemical and biophysical characterization of FH is consistent with its expected role as an iron chaperone acting as a regulator during ISC biosynthesis [35]. In line with this role for frataxin, its suppression in the prothoracic gland impairs the ability of larvae to initiate pupariation [69]. This organ produces ecdysteroid hormones, such as 20-hydroxyecdysone, that mediate developmental transitions. Interestingly, some Fe-S-containing enzymes such as Neverland (converts cholesterol into 7-dehydrocholesterol) and the fly ferredoxins Fdxh and Fdxh2 participate in the metabolism of ecdysone, and their activities are likely impaired in frataxin-deficient larvae. In agreement with this hypothesis, 20-hydroxyecdysone supplementation improves the defective transitions associated with frataxin deficiency in the prothoracic gland [69]. An ecdysone deficiency would explain the giant, long-lived larvae phenotype reported by Anderson et al. in their fly model using the UDIR2 line and da^{G32} GAL4 driver [33]. Interestingly, Drosophila models have also revealed that iron deregulation occurs before the decrease in the activity of mitochondrial enzymes [49, 66]. This is in agreement with results from an inducible yeast model in which the iron regulon was activated long before decreased aconitase activity was observed [70].

It has been suggested that ROS are generated by iron accumulation through Fenton's reaction, damaging the mitochondrial ETC and mediating the pathophysiology of FRDA (reviewed in [20, 71]). However, the role of oxidative stress in the disease is still questioned, and controversial results have also been reported in Drosophila. Overexpression of ROS-scavenging enzymes such as catalase (CAT), superoxide dismutase 1 (SOD1), or SOD2 could not rescue the pupae lethality caused by ubiquitous UDIR1 and UDIR2 expression [33] or the photoreceptor neurodegeneration in fh^1 mutant clones [45]. CAT overexpression and treatment with EUK8 (a synthetic superoxide dismutase and catalase mimetic) also failed to improve cardiac function in frataxin-depleted hearts [42]. Shidara and Hollenbeck [48] did not detect increased ROS levels in frataxin-deficient motor neurons, but these neurons responded to the complex III inhibitor antimycin A with a larger increase in ROS than control neurons.

However, increasing evidence from different FRDA models and patient samples suggests that oxidative stress is a major player in FRDA [34, 41, 65, 72–80]. In Drosophila, increased levels of malondialdehyde (MDA, a lipoperoxidation product) have been reported in flies with ubiquitous FH suppression using the fhRNAi line and the actin GAL4-driver line [81, 82]. These flies and flies with tissue-specific frataxin deficiency in the PNS (C96) or glial cells (repo) showed increased sensitivity to external oxidative insults (see Table 1) such as hyperoxia or H_2O_2 treatment [41, 81, 83]. Hyperoxia induces enhanced aconitase inactivation in the frataxin knockdown flies [34, 83], which compromises the entire respiratory process. In fact, hyperoxia leads to reduced oxygen consumption rates in mitochondrial extracts of the frataxin-depleted flies [34]. Overexpression of the H_2O_2-scavenging enzymes CAT, mitoCAT (using a synthetic transgene that targets CAT to the mitochondria), or mitochondrial peroxiredoxin (mTPx) rescues the shortened lifespan and increased sensitivity to H_2O_2 in flies with reduced frataxin expression in the PNS (C96) [41]. These scavengers also restore aconitase activity in flies with systemic reduction of FH using the UDIR1 line and the da^{G32} GAL4 driver [41], supporting the role of oxidative stress in aconitase inactivation. In addition, scavengers of lipid peroxides have been shown to improve frataxin-deficient phenotypes [83, 84].

Recently, Hugo Bellen's laboratory identified a new mechanism for neuronal degeneration in FRDA, in which iron toxicity is not associated with ROS damage [45]. These authors showed in their *fh* mutant that iron accumulation induces sphingolipid synthesis and activates the expression of the genes *3-phosphoinositide dependent protein kinase-1 (Pdk1)* and *myocyte enhancer factor-2 (Mef2)* and their downstream targets, causing loss of photoreceptors in fly ommatidia. In agreement with these results, inhibition of sphingolipid synthesis by downregulating the expression of the rate-limiting enzyme lace (the fly ortholog of serine palmitoyltransferase) or feeding the mutant flies Myriocin (a compound that inhibits serine palmitoyltransferase) was sufficient to partially revert the cellular degeneration [45]. Similarly, silencing *Pdk1* or *Mef2* expression also suppressed the neurodegenerative phenotype. Remarkably, the authors found that loss of frataxin in the nervous system in mice and in heart tissue from patients also activates the same pathway, suggesting a conserved mechanism [62]. These results highlight, once more, the relevance of *Drosophila* in the study of human disorders such as FRDA. In addition, they strongly suggest that iron plays an instrumental role in *Drosophila* frataxin biology.

Similarly, *Drosophila* has also been a pioneer model organism in highlighting the role of frataxin in lipid homeostasis [83]. Ubiquitous frataxin knockdown or targeted frataxin downregulation in glia cells triggered lipid accumulation. Increased amounts of myristic acid (C14:0), palmitic acid (C16:0), palmitoleic acid (C16:1), oleic acid (C18:1), and linoleic acid (C18:2) were found. These results suggested that loss of mitochondrial function also affects fatty acid beta-oxidation, leading to the accumulation of the most abundant lipid species [83]. The presence of lipid droplets had already been characterized in mouse models [63], and the fly findings indicated the content of these droplets and their likely association with the disease pathophysiology. These findings were followed by assessments of lipid deregulation in other models [85] and in patient samples [86]. The association between frataxin and lipid metabolism has been extensively reviewed elsewhere [87].

5. Frataxin Overexpression Phenotypes

Although frataxin overexpression does not model the disease, it is an excellent complementary tool to further describe the cellular roles of frataxin. In this regard, *Drosophila* models have shown that some increase in frataxin expression is beneficial, whereas its excess beyond certain thresholds is clearly detrimental. Table 2 summarizes the phenotypes reported for frataxin overexpression in flies using several GAL4 lines that drive ubiquitous or tissue-specific *fh* expression.

Flies with ubiquitous *fh* expression at a level approximately fourfold higher than the physiological level show increased longevity, antioxidant defense responses, and resistance to treatment with paraquat (a chemical known to specifically affect mitochondrial complex I and to generate free radicals), H_2O_2, and dietary iron [89]. Similarly, it has

been reported that frataxin overexpression in mice [90, 91] or in cultured cells [92–94] is innocuous or has a positive effect, stimulating ATP production or inducing antioxidant defense responses.

A systemic 9-fold increase in *fh* mRNA expression impairs muscle, heart, and PNS development in fly embryos, leading to lethality from larva to pupa stages [34]. Frataxin overexpression restricted to developing heart and muscle tissue (*Dot, 24B*; Table 2) also has deleterious effects [34]. In contrast, overexpressing FH pan-neuronally (*Appl, elav*), in sensory organs (*neur*), motor neurons (*D42*), and glial cells (*repo*) produces viable adults, but they show a reduced lifespan and decreased locomotor performance [34, 95]. The effect of human frataxin expression has also been tested in *Drosophila*. FXN is correctly expressed and targeted to mitochondria in flies and can rescue the aconitase activity of UDIR2-knockdown flies [95]. These results provide *in vivo* evidence that human and fly frataxins have conserved functions, which was further confirmed by Tricoire et al. [42] and Chen et al. [45]. As expected, FXN overexpression in flies produces similar but slightly stronger phenotypes at biochemical, physiological, and developmental levels than those observed in flies overexpressing FH [95]. Initially, it was proposed that frataxin overexpression might act as a dominant negative mutation and that its toxic effect might be mediated by oxidative stress [95]. The mechanism underlying frataxin overexpression has recently been further investigated [96]. In this study, the authors reported that frataxin overexpression increases oxidative phosphorylation and modifies iron homeostasis. Such an increase of mitochondrial activity alters mitochondrial morphology and sensitizes cells to oxidative damage leading to neurodegeneration and cell death. Importantly, authors found that iron was a pivotal factor in the neurodegeneration [96].

These results in *Drosophila* show that frataxin requires an optimal balance in expression to function properly and that control of its expression is important in treatments that aim to increase its protein level.

6. Genetic Modifiers of FRDA

Drosophila models are important because they offer the ability to carry out genetic screens for mutations that affect a particular biological process. This powerful tool provides a way to identify genetic modifiers of human diseases (Figures 4(a) and 4(c)). Our group has collaborated with Juan Botas's laboratory in two studies using this methodology in *Drosophila* models of FRDA. These studies followed a biased candidate approach, selecting genes related to disease pathophysiology [81, 82]. We set out to test whether genetic modification of key pathways would improve FRDA phenotypes in flies. Candidate genes were selected from pathways involved in metal homeostasis, the response to oxidative stress, apoptosis, and autophagy. Approximately 300 lines were analyzed, including RNAi lines from the Vienna *Drosophila* Resource Center and loss-of-function and overexpression lines from the Bloomington Stock Center (Indiana University). The external eye morphology and motor performance of adult flies were used

TABLE 2: Frataxin overexpression in *Drosophila*. The *fh* construct and the GAL4 driver used to obtain the different phenotypes are indicated.

Overexpression line	GAL4 driver line	Phenotypes
UAS-dfh¹ and *UAS-dfh²* [89]: fourfold increase in *fh* mRNA expression (25°C)*	*Actin* Ubiquitous	(i) Viable adults [89] (ii) Increased lifespan [89] (iii) Significant increase in tolerance to iron-induced stress ($FeCl_3$), paraquat, and H_2O_2 (measuring survival) [89] (iv) Significant increase in total antioxidant activity (bathocuproine dye) [89]
	Actin and *da*^G32 Ubiquitous	(i) Lethal at early pupae or 3rd instar larvae at 29°C [34] (ii) Defects in developing muscles, axonal tracks, and axonal pathfinding (1D4 staining) and an increase in the number of sensory ventral neurons. No abnormalities detected in the CNS [34] (iii) At 25°C, viable adults that are sensitive to oxidative stress and iron [34, 96]. Young individuals have higher catalase and aconitase activities and ATP production than controls but are hypersensitive to hyperoxia [96]
	Appl and *elav* Pan-neural	(i) Viable at 29°C and 25°C (ii) Reduced lifespan and climbing capability [95, 96]. Locomotor defects are rescued by mitochondrial catalase expression and *mfrn* silencing [96]. (iii) Reduced ferritin and mitoferrin levels [96] (iv) Brain vacuolization [96]
UAS-fh [34]: 9-fold increase in *fh* mRNA expression and a strong increase in protein levels (29°C)*	*Other neuronal drivers* *neur* Sensory organs and their precursors *D42* Motor neurons *Ddc* Aminergic neurons *TH* Dopaminergic neurons *c698a* Brain	(i) Viable adults at 29°C and 25°C [34] (ii) Reduced climbing capability and lifespan at both temperatures (*neur/D42*) [34, 95]. (iii) Lifespan is recovered by mitochondrial catalase (*neur*) [95] (iv) *Ddc, TH*, and *c698a*: lifespan and climbing capability unaffected at 29°C or 25°C [34, 96] (v) Strong promotion of mitochondrial fusion and ROS-mediated cell death of dopaminergic neurons (*TH*) [96]
	Repo Pan-glial	(i) Reduced lifespan and climbing capability [95] (ii) Expression of mitochondrial catalase increases lifespan and climbing capability [95]
	Other tissues: *Dot*, heart and *24B*, mesoderm	(i) Lethal from the early pupa stage to adult eclosion from the puparium at 29°C and 25°C [34, 95] (ii) Lack of some pericardial cells along the tubular structure of the developing heart (ECII staining) in embryos at 29°C [34]

TABLE 2: Continued.

Overexpression line	GAL4 driver line	Phenotypes
	Actin and da^{G32} Ubiquitous	(i) Lethal in pupae [95] (ii) Reduced aconitase activity in larvae [95] (iii) Reduced NDUFS3 protein levels in larvae [95]
UAS-FXN[#] [95]: Expression of human frataxin. Stronger phenotypes than UAS-fh (25°C)*	Appl Pan-neural	(i) Viable adults, lethal at 29°C [95]
	neur Sensory organs and their precursors	(i) Reduced lifespan and climbing capability and increased sensitivity to oxidative insult [95] (ii) Expression of mitochondrial catalase increases lifespan [95]
	Repo Pan-glial	(i) Morphological disruption of glial cells and formation of lipid droplets [95] (ii) Expression of mitochondrial catalase increases lifespan and improves climbing capability [95]
	24B Mesoderm	(i) Lethal during pupariation [95]

*The most used temperature in the experiments. [#] UAS-FXN triggers the same defects as UAS-fh. To avoid repetition, only new phenotypes have been included; CNS: Central Nervous System.

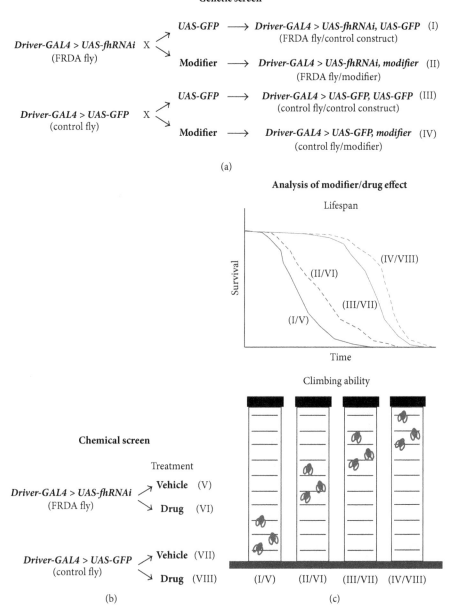

FIGURE 4: Schematic design of a genetic (a) or chemical (b) screen to identify genetic modifiers or potential therapeutic compounds in FRDA using *Drosophila* as a model organism. The effect of a genetic modifier or drug is evaluated by monitoring the lifespan and climbing ability of FRDA flies. (c) A UAS-GFP construct is included in this strategy as an internal control to determine whether the drug can interfere with the GAL4/UAS system and the potential dilution of the GAL4 protein due to the presence of two UAS construct. In parallel, the effect of the modifier or drug treatment is analyzed in control flies to identify frataxin interactors. GFP: green fluorescent protein. Vehicle: DMSO/H_2O depending on the drug solubility.

as screening phenotypes. The UDIR2 line [33] (with a 90% reduction in FH expression when expressed ubiquitously) produces a mild rough eye phenotype when expressed in the developing eye [82]. The *fh*RNAi line [34] (with a 70% reduction in FH expression that is compatible with normal development) impairs motor performance when expressed ubiquitously. We applied a tiered strategy to examine the effect of metal-related genes on eye morphology, followed by the effect of eye modifiers on motor performance [82]. In Calap-Quintana et al. [81], we reported the effect of the remaining candidate genes on the motor performance of the *fh*RNAi line.

Five suppressors of both the eye and motor performance phenotypes were identified: the iron regulatory proteins encoded by the genes *Irp-1A* and *Irp-1B*, their target Transferrin (*Tsf1* and *Tsf3*), and *Malvolio (Mvl)*, the *Drosophila* ortholog of the mammalian gene *Divalent metal transporter-1 (DMT1)*. The suppression of these FRDA phenotypes was mediated by reducing the iron abundance associated with frataxin deficiency [82]. On the one hand, reduced expression of *Mvl*, *Tsf1*, and *Tsf3* decreases cellular iron uptake, which in turn reduces mitochondrial iron accumulation. On the other hand, downregulation of *Irp-1A* and *Irp-1B* reduces IRP activity, as suggested in [33, 66], and thus recovers ferritin expression and normal cellular iron distribution. In agreement with these findings, *Irp1* knockout reduces mitochondrial iron accumulation in frataxin-depleted mouse livers [97].

Another iron player that can suppress FRDA phenotypes in flies was identified by Navarro et al. [66]. It is a member of the mitochondrial solute carrier family named mitoferrin (Mfrn), which is located in the inner mitochondrial membrane, and its function is to translocate iron into mitochondria [98–100]. Downregulation of *mfrn* was sufficient to improve iron metabolism in frataxin-deficient flies and to ameliorate neurodegeneration triggered by targeted frataxin silencing in glia cells [66]. In this study, overexpression of ferritin subunits was unable to counteract neurodegeneration, whereas another study reported that ferritin overexpression had a positive effect in *fh* mutant clones of fly photoreceptors [45]. It is likely that the different metabolic requirements of each cell type might be reflected in the factors that can exert protective roles.

Knockdown of zinc transporters and copper chaperones also ameliorates FRDA phenotypes in flies [82]. Members of the two conserved gene families of zinc transporters (the ZnT and Zip families) improve the eye and motor performance phenotypes by normalizing iron levels in some cases. It has been previously reported that several members of the Zip family can also transport iron in addition to zinc [101–103]. Genetic reduction of *Atox1*, which encodes a chaperone that delivers copper to ATP7 transporters located in the trans-Golgi network [104], and *dCutC*, encoding a protein involved in the uptake, storage, delivery, and efflux of copper [105], suppressed both FRDA phenotypes. We also found that the *Metal-Responsive Transcription Factor-1 Gene (MTF-1)* is a modifier of the motor impairment phenotype, acting as a suppressor when overexpressed and as an enhancer when downregulated. Overexpression of *MTF-1* in *Drosophila* also reduces the toxicity associated with oxidative stress [106], human Aβ42 peptide expression [107], and a parkin null mutation [108]. Under stress conditions, such as metal overload and oxidative stress, MTF-1 is translocated to the nucleus and binds to metal response elements (MREs) in the regulatory regions of its target genes, such as metal-sequestering metallothioneins (Mtns). Mtns are small cysteine-rich proteins that maintain low levels of intracellular free metal due to their ability to bind metals with high affinity. Contrary to what was expected, Mtn knockdown suppressed FRDA phenotypes [82], which could be explained by the role of Mtns as prooxidants under oxidative stress conditions [109–111]. Therefore, the beneficial effect of *MTF-1* overexpression may not be mediated by Mtns but rather by reduced iron accumulation, because the iron level is normalized in *fh*RNAi flies with *MTF-1* overexpression [82]. These results demonstrate that metal dysregulation in FRDA affects other metals in addition to iron. Importantly, zinc and copper redistribution have been reported in the dentate nucleus of the cerebellum in FRDA patients [112].

The genetic screen conducted in Calap-Quintana et al. [81] revealed four modifiers of the motor performance phenotype in FRDA flies. These genes encode tuberous sclerosis complex protein 1 *(Tsc1)*, ribosomal protein S6 kinase *(S6k)*, eukaryotic translation initiation factor 4E *(eIF-4F)*, and leucine-rich repeat kinase *(Lrrk)*. These proteins are involved in the TORC1 signaling pathway, which regulates many major cellular functions such as protein synthesis, lipid biogenesis, and autophagy. We found that genetic reduction in TORC1 signaling activity is beneficial, while its genetic activation produces a detrimental effect in frataxin knockdown flies by inducing semilethality. Table 3 shows these genetic mediators of frataxin deficiency as well as other modifiers individually identified in other studies.

7. Potential Therapeutic Compounds for FRDA Treatment

Currently, there is no effective treatment for FRDA, although different therapeutic strategies are being developed or tested in clinical trials (http://www.curefa.org/pipeline). These strategies include lowering oxidative damage, reducing iron-mediated toxicity, increasing antioxidant defense, and increasing frataxin expression and gene therapy [83, 113, 114]. *Drosophila* models are also gaining increasing significance in biomedical and pharmaceutical research as a valuable tool for testing potential treatments (Figures 4(b) and 4(c)).

Table 4 lists the compounds that have been found to improve some FRDA phenotypes in *Drosophila*. Our group has validated the utility of frataxin-depleted flies for drug screening [49]. We separately tested the effect of two compounds, the iron chelator deferiprone (DFP) and the antioxidant idebenone (IDE), that were already in use in clinical trials for this disease. DFP is a small-molecule, blood-brain-barrier-permeable drug that preferentially binds iron and prevents its reaction with ROS. IDE is a synthetic analog of coenzyme Q10 and can undergo reversible redox reactions, improving electron flux along the ETC. Each drug was administered in the fly food at two starting points: early treatment (from larva to adult stage) and adult treatment (in adult phase). Both drugs improved the lifespan and motor ability of flies expressing the *fh*-RNAi allele in a ubiquitous pattern or in the PNS *(neur)*, especially when given at the early treatment timepoint. DFP improved the FRDA phenotypes by sequestering mitochondrial iron and preventing toxicity induced by iron accumulation. IDE rescued aconitase activity in flies subjected to external oxidative stress [49].

Another compound with electron carrier properties, methylene blue (MB), has been described as a potent therapeutic drug for heart dysfunction in FRDA [42]. Cardiac defects were decreased in a dose-dependent manner in flies with heart-specific frataxin depletion treated with different concentrations of MB. The authors demonstrated that this drug was also able to reduce heart dilatation associated with deficiencies in several components of complexes I and III in mutant flies. These results indicate that respiratory chain impairment is involved in the cardiac defects associated with frataxin deficiency and that compounds showing electron

---

TABLE 3: Genetic modifiers of FRDA phenotypes in *Drosophila*.

Modifier	Pathway	Effect
Fer1HCH/Fer2LCH (Co-expression)	Iron storage	Suppressor of reduced life span [66], ERG, and photoreceptor neurodegeneration [45]
Fer3HCH (OE)	Iron storage and oxidative stress protection	Suppressor of reduced life span [66] ERG, and photoreceptor neurodegeneration [45]
Irp-1A (RNAi) *Irp-1B* (RNAi) *Irp-1B* (LOF)	Iron sensor	Suppressor of mild rough eye and impaired motor performance [82]
mfrn (RNAi)	Mitochondrial iron importer	Suppressor of reduced aconitase activity and IRP-1A and ferritin levels, impaired motor performance, and increased brain vacuolization [66]
mfrn (OE)		Enhancer of locomotor defects and brain vacuolization [66]
Mvl (RNAi)	Iron absorption	Suppressor of mild rough eye and impaired motor performance [82]
Tsf1 (LOF) *Tsf3* (RNAi)	Serum iron binding transport proteins	Suppressor of mild rough eye and impaired motor performance [82]
dZip42C.1 (RNAi) *dZip42C.2* (RNAi) *dZip88E* (RNAi)	Zinc importer	Suppressor of mild rough eye and impaired motor performance [82]
dZnT35C (RNAi)	Zinc transporter to vesicles	Suppressor of mild rough eye and impaired motor performance [82]
dZnT41F (RNAi)	Zinc homeostasis	Suppressor of mild rough eye and impaired motor performance [82]
dZnT63C (RNAi)	Zinc exporter	Suppressor of mild rough eye and impaired motor performance [82]
foi (LOF)	Zinc importer	Suppressor of impaired motor performance [82]
Atox1 (RNAi)	Copper chaperone donor	Suppressor of mild rough eye and impaired motor performance [82]
dCutC (RNAi)	Copper uptake and storage	Suppressor of mild rough eye and impaired motor performance [82]
MTF-1 (OE)	Metal responsive Transcription Factor	Suppressor of impaired motor performance [82]
MTF-1 (LOF)		Enhancer of impaired motor performance [82]
MtnA (RNAi)	Heavy metal detoxification	Suppressor of mild rough eye and impaired motor performance [82]
MtnB (RNAi) *MtnC* (RNAi)	Heavy metal detoxification	Suppressor of mild rough eye [82]
Tsc1 (RNAi)	TORC1 pathway	Enhancer of reduced survival [81]
S6K (DN)	TORC1 pathway	Suppressor of impaired motor performance [81]
S6K (CA)		Enhancer of reduced survival [81]
eIF-4E (LOF)	TORC1 pathway	Suppressor of impaired motor performance [81]
Lrrk (RNAi)	TORC1 pathway	Suppressor of impaired motor performance [81]
Cat (OE) *mCat* (OE) *mTPx* (OE)	Antioxidant (hydrogen peroxide scavengers)	Suppressor of reduced lifespan when overexpressed in the PNS [41]

TABLE 3: Continued.

Modifier	Pathway	Effect
dGLaz (OE)	Antioxidant defense	Suppressor of reduced life span, impaired motor performance, aconitase inactivation, and lipid peroxidation [83]
Pdk1 (RNAi)	Embryonic development (insulin receptor transduction pathway and apoptotic pathway)	Suppressor of photoreceptor neurodegeneration [45]
Mef2 (RNAi)	Muscle differentiation	Suppressor of photoreceptor neurodegeneration [45]
lace (RNAi)	Sphingosine biosynthesis pathway	Suppressor of photoreceptor neurodegeneration [45]

CA: constitutively active mutation; DN: dominant negative mutation; ERG: electroretinograms; LOF: loss-of-function mutation; OE: overexpression; RNAi: RNA interference.

TABLE 4: Compounds that showed beneficial effects in *Drosophila* models of FRDA.

Compound	Mechanism of action	Improved phenotype
Idebenone	Antioxidant	Motor performance and lifespan in adults [42, 49]
Methylene blue	Electron carrier	Adult heart function [42]
Toluidine blue	Electron carrier	Adult heart function [42]
Deferiprone	Iron chelator	Motor performance and lifespan in adults [49]
Deferoxamine	Iron chelator	Pupa development [88]
LPS 01-03-L-F03	Possible iron chelator	Pupa development [88]
LPS 02-25-L-E10	Possible iron chelator	Pupa development [88]
LPS 02-13-L-E04	Possible iron chelator	Pupa development [88]
LPS 01-04-L-G10	n.d.	Pupa development [88] Adult heart function [88]
LPS 02-14-L-B11	n.d.	Pupa development [88]
Rapamycin	TORC1 inhibitor	Motor performance and oxidative stress in adults [81]
Myriocin	Serine palmitoyltransferase inhibitor	Photoreceptor function [45]

n.d.: not described.

transfer properties could prevent heart dysfunction in FRDA patients.

A yeast/*Drosophila* screen to identify new compounds for FRDA treatment was carried out by Seguin et al. [88]. The authors showed the utility of using a strategy based on two complementary models, a unicellular and a multicellular organism. Accordingly, a frataxin-deleted yeast strain was used in a primary screen, and positive hits were tested in flies ubiquitously expressing the UDIR2 allele (secondary screen). Approximately 6380 compounds were evaluated from two chemical libraries (the French National Chemical Library and the Prestwick Collection) to test the ability of the drugs to improve the fitness of yeast mutants using raffinose as the main carbon source. Yeast cells with frataxin deficiency grew slowly when raffinose was provided as the carbon source [115]. A total of 12 compounds, representative of the different chemical families, were selected from the yeast-based screen and their effect was analyzed on the FRDA fly model. Six of them improved the pupariation impairment of flies, with

LPS 01-04-LG10 and Deferoxamine B (DFOB) being the most promising compounds. DFOB, an iron chelator, was suggested to increase the pools of bioavailable iron and to reduce iron accumulation in mitochondria. LPS 01-04-L-G10, a cinnamic derivative, partially rescued heart dilatation in flies with heart-specific frataxin depletion [88].

The efficacy of iron chelators as potential treatments has already been assessed in FRDA patients, but unfortunately the results were not conclusive. Studies have reported improvement of the cardiac and/or neurological conditions [61, 116, 117], no significant effect [118], or even worsening of some conditions [119]. However, the *Drosophila* models of FRDA indicate that iron is an important factor in FRDA pathophysiology. Genetic or pharmacological interventions through pathways regulating iron homeostasis and the sphingolipid/Pdk1/Mef-2 pathway are new approaches that might be explored in preclinical studies. In addition, *Drosophila* has shown for the first time that alteration of genes involved in metal detoxification and metal homeostasis (copper and zinc in addition to iron) is also a potential therapeutic strategy.

Finally, the results obtained from the genetic screen in *Drosophila* [81] also suggest that rapamycin and its analogs (rapalogs) are promising molecules for FRDA treatment. Inhibition of TORC1 signaling by rapamycin increases climbing speed, survival, and ATP levels in flies [81]. This compound enhances antioxidant defenses in both control and FRDA flies by increasing the nuclear translocation of the transcription factor encoded by the gene *cap-n-collar*, the *Drosophila* ortholog of *Nrf2*. As a result, it induces the expression of a battery of antioxidant genes. In addition, rapamycin protects against external oxidative stress by inducing autophagy. Rapamycin is a well-described drug approved for human uses. There is a large amount of data regarding the safety, tolerability, and side effects of this drug and rapalogs, which could facilitate their potential use in FRDA.

8. Conclusions

D. melanogaster is one of the most studied organisms in biological research. The conservation of many cellular and organismal processes between humans and flies and the constant increase in the number of genetic tools for *Drosophila* have made this organism one of the best choices for studying human genetic diseases. Following the identification of Friedreich's ataxia gene by positional cloning, model organisms have played a decisive role in the investigation of the function of frataxin and consequently the underlying pathophysiological mechanisms of FRDA. Here, we have presented the main contributions of *Drosophila* in this area of research. Frataxin-depleted flies recapitulate important biochemical, cellular, and physiological hallmarks of FRDA. In addition, the model flies exhibit new phenotypes that reveal, for the first time, other key players in FRDA pathogenesis. These models have allowed the identification of genetic and pharmacological factors capable of modifying some FRDA phenotypes, revealing new and promising ways to find effective treatments. Nevertheless, there are still many other questions that can be addressed by taking advantage of *Drosophila* models. Additional models of FRDA in flies are expected to help us understand the transcriptional silencing of *FXN* mediated by the GAA repeat expansion. These new models will advance our knowledge of the molecular bases of this disease and facilitate the development of new drugs for FRDA.

Acknowledgments

This study was supported by a grant from Generalitat Valenciana, Spain (PROMETEOII/2014/067). Pablo Calap-Quintana was a recipient of a fellowship from Generalitat Valenciana, Spain, and José Vicente Llorens is supported by a research contract from FARA and FARA Ireland.

References

[1] A. Harding, "Clinical features and classification of inherited ataxias," *Advances in Neurology*, vol. 61, pp. 1–14, 1993.

[2] S. I. Bidichandani and M. B. Delatycki, "Friedreich Ataxia," GeneReviews®. 2017.

[3] V. Campuzano, L. Montermini, M. D. Moltò et al., "Friedreich's ataxia: autosomal recessive disease caused by an intronic GAA triplet repeat expansion," *Science*, vol. 271, no. 5254, pp. 1423–1427, 1996.

[4] H. Koutnikova, V. Campuzano, F. Foury, P. Dollé, O. Cazzalini, and M. Koenig, "Studies of human, mouse and yeast homologues indicate a mitochondrial function for frataxin," *Nature Genetics*, vol. 16, no. 4, pp. 345–351, 1997.

[5] H. Koutnikova, V. Campuzano, and M. Koenig, "Maturation of wild-type and mutated frataxin by the mitochondrial processing peptidase," *Human Molecular Genetics*, vol. 7, no. 9, pp. 1485–1489, 1998.

[6] I. Condò, N. Ventura, F. Malisan, A. Rufini, B. Tomassini, and R. Testi, "In vivo maturation of human frataxin," *Human Molecular Genetics*, vol. 16, no. 13, pp. 1534–1540, 2007.

[7] V. Campuzano, L. Montermini, Y. Lutz et al., "Frataxin is reduced in Friedreich ataxia patients and is associated with mitochondrial membranes," *Human Molecular Genetics*, vol. 6, no. 11, pp. 1771–1780, 1997.

[8] C. A. Galea, A. Huq, P. J. Lockhart et al., "Compound heterozygous FXN mutations and clinical outcome in friedreich ataxia," *Annals of Neurology*, vol. 79, no. 3, pp. 485–495, 2016.

[9] S. Q. Le and O. Gascuel, "Accounting for solvent accessibility and secondary structure in protein phylogenetics is clearly beneficial," *Systematic Biology*, vol. 59, no. 3, pp. 277–287, 2010.

[10] S. Kumar, G. Stecher, and K. Tamura, "MEGA7: Molecular Evolutionary Genetics Analysis version 7.0 for bigger datasets," *Molecular Biology and Evolution*, vol. 33, no. 7, pp. 1870–1874, 2016.

[11] L. A. Kelley, S. Mezulis, C. M. Yates, M. N. Wass, and M. J. E. Sternberg, "The Phyre2 web portal for protein modeling, prediction and analysis," *Nature Protocols*, vol. 10, no. 6, pp. 845–858, 2015.

[12] E. F. Pettersen, T. D. Goddard, C. C. Huang et al., "UCSF Chimera—a visualization system for exploratory research and analysis," *Journal of Computational Chemistry*, vol. 25, no. 13, pp. 1605–1612, 2004.

[13] A. H. Brand and N. Perrimon, "Targeted gene expression as a means of altering cell fates and generating dominant phenotypes," *Development*, vol. 118, no. 2, pp. 401–415, 1993.

[14] P. González-Cabo, J. Vicente Llorens, F. Palau, and M. Dolores Moltó, "Friedreich ataxia: An update on animal models, frataxin function and therapies," *Advances in Experimental Medicine and Biology*, vol. 652, pp. 247–261, 2009.

[15] M. Pandolfo and A. Pastore, "The pathogenesis of Friedreich ataxia and the structure and function of frataxin," *Journal of Neurology*, vol. 256, supplement 1, pp. 9–17, 2009.

[16] T. L. Stemmler, E. Lesuisse, D. Pain, and A. Dancis, "Frataxin and mitochondrial FeS cluster biogenesis," *The Journal of Biological Chemistry*, vol. 285, no. 35, pp. 26737–26743, 2010.

[17] D. Marmolino, "Friedreich's ataxia: Past, present and future," *Brain Research Reviews*, vol. 67, no. 1-2, pp. 311–330, 2011.

[18] M. V. Busi and D. F. Gomez-Casati, "Exploring frataxin function," *IUBMB Life*, vol. 64, no. 1, pp. 56–63, 2012.

[19] C. M. Gomes and R. Santos, "Neurodegeneration in Friedreich's ataxia: From defective frataxin to oxidative stress," *Oxidative Medicine and Cellular Longevity*, Article ID 487534, 2013.

[20] R. A. Vaubel and G. Isaya, "Iron-sulfur cluster synthesis, iron homeostasis and oxidative stress in Friedreich ataxia," *Molecular and Cellular Neuroscience*, vol. 55, pp. 50–61, 2013.

[21] A. Pastore and H. Puccio, "Frataxin: A protein in search for a function," *Journal of Neurochemistry*, vol. 126, no. 1, pp. 43–52, 2013.

[22] A. Anzovino, D. J. R. Lane, M. L.-H. Huang, and D. R. Richardson, "Fixing frataxin: 'Ironing out' the metabolic defect in Friedreich's ataxia," *British Journal of Pharmacology*, vol. 171, no. 8, pp. 2174–2190, 2014.

[23] S. Chiang, Z. Kovacevic, S. Sahni et al., "Frataxin and the molecular mechanism of mitochondrial iron-loading in Friedreich's ataxia," *Clinical Science*, vol. 130, no. 11, pp. 853–870, 2016.

[24] A. Martelli and H. Puccio, "Dysregulation of cellular iron metabolism in Friedreich ataxia: from primary iron-sulfur cluster deficit to mitochondrial iron accumulation," *Frontiers in Pharmacology*, vol. 5, article 130, 2014.

[25] N. Maio and T. A. Rouault, "Iron-sulfur cluster biogenesis in mammalian cells: new insights into the molecular mechanisms of cluster delivery," *Biochimica et Biophysica Acta (BBA)—Molecular Cell Research*, vol. 1853, no. 6, pp. 1493–1512, 2015.

[26] A. Parent, X. Elduque, D. Cornu et al., "Mammalian frataxin directly enhances sulfur transfer of NFS1 persulfide to both ISCU and free thiols," *Nature Communications*, vol. 6, article no. 5686, 2015.

[27] R. Santos, S. Lefevre, D. Sliwa, A. Seguin, J.-M. Camadro, and E. Lesuisse, "Friedreich ataxia: molecular mechanisms, redox considerations, and therapeutic opportunities," *Antioxidants & Redox Signaling*, vol. 13, no. 5, pp. 651–690, 2010.

[28] A. Bayot and P. Rustin, "Friedreich's ataxia, frataxin, PIP5K1B: Echo of a distant fracas," *Oxidative Medicine and Cellular Longevity*, Article ID 725635, 2013.

[29] P. González-Cabo and F. Palau, "Mitochondrial pathophysiology in Friedreich's ataxia," *Journal of Neurochemistry*, vol. 126, no. 1, pp. 53–64, 2013.

[30] L. T. Reiter, L. Potocki, S. Chien, M. Gribskov, and E. Bier, "A systematic analysis of human disease-associated gene sequences in *Drosophila melanogaster*," *Genome Research*, vol. 11, no. 6, pp. 1114–1125, 2001.

[31] M. E. Fortini, M. P. Skupski, M. S. Boguski, and I. K. Hariharan, "A survey of human disease gene counterparts in the *Drosophila* genome," *The Journal of Cell Biology*, vol. 150, no. 2, pp. F23–F30, 2000.

[32] J. Cañizares, J. M. Blanca, J. A. Navarro, E. Monrós, F. Palau, and M. D. Moltó, "dfh is a Drosophila homolog of the Friedreich's ataxia disease gene," *Gene*, vol. 256, no. 1-2, pp. 35–42, 2000.

[33] P. R. Anderson, K. Kirby, A. J. Hilliker, and J. P. Phillips, "RNAi-mediated suppression of the mitochondrial iron chaperone, frataxin, in *Drosophila*," *Human Molecular Genetics*, vol. 14, no. 22, pp. 3397–3405, 2005.

[34] J. V. Llorens, J. A. Navarro, M. J. Martínez-Sebastían et al., "Causative role of oxidative stress in a *Drosophila* model of Friedreich ataxia," *The FASEB Journal*, vol. 21, no. 2, pp. 333–344, 2007.

[35] K. C. Kondapalli, N. M. Kok, A. Dancis, and T. L. Stemmler, "Drosophila frataxin: An iron chaperone during cellular Fe-S cluster bioassembly," *Biochemistry*, vol. 47, no. 26, pp. 6917–6927, 2008.

[36] T. Yoon and J. A. Cowan, "Frataxin-mediated iron delivery to ferrochelatase in the final step of heme biosynthesis," *The Journal of Biological Chemistry*, vol. 279, no. 25, pp. 25943–25946, 2004.

[37] S. P. Dzul, A. G. Rocha, S. Rawat et al., "In vitro characterization of a novel Isu homologue from Drosophila melanogaster for de novo FeS-cluster formation," *Metallomics*, vol. 9, no. 1, pp. 48–60, 2017.

[38] Z. Marelja, S. Leimkühler, and F. Missirlis, "Iron Sulfur and Molybdenum Cofactor Enzymes Regulate the Drosophila Life Cycle by Controlling Cell Metabolism," *Frontiers in Physiology*, vol. 9, 2018.

[39] M. Perdomini, A. Hick, H. Puccio, and M. A. Pook, "Animal and cellular models of Friedreich ataxia," *Journal of Neurochemistry*, vol. 126, no. 1, pp. 65–79, 2013.

[40] J. R. Kennerdell and R. W. Carthew, "Heritable gene silencing in Drosophila using double-stranded RNA," *Nature Biotechnology*, vol. 18, no. 8, pp. 896–898, 2000.

[41] P. R. Anderson, K. Kirby, W. C. Orr, A. J. Hilliker, and J. P. Phillips, "Hydrogen peroxide scavenging rescues frataxin deficiency in a *Drosophila* model of Friedreich's ataxia," *Proceedings of the National Acadamy of Sciences of the United States of America*, vol. 105, no. 2, pp. 611–616, 2008.

[42] H. Tricoire, A. Palandri, A. Bourdais, J.-M. Camadro, and V. Monnier, "Methylene blue rescues heart defects in a *Drosophila* model of Friedreich's ataxia," *Human Molecular Genetics*, vol. 23, no. 4, pp. 968–979, 2014.

[43] T. Osterwalder, K. S. Yoon, B. H. White, and H. Keshishian, "A conditional tissue-specific transgene expression system using inducible GAL4," *Proceedings of the National Acadamy of Sciences of the United States of America*, vol. 98, no. 22, pp. 12596–12601, 2001.

[44] G. Roman, K. Endo, L. Zong, and R. L. Davis, "Pswitch, a system for spatial and temporal control of gene expression in drosophila melanogaster," *Proceedings of the National Acadamy of Sciences of the United States of America*, vol. 98, no. 22, pp. 12602–12607, 2001.

[45] K. Chen, G. Lin, N. A. Haelterman et al., "Loss of frataxin induces iron toxicity, sphingolipid synthesis, and Pdk1/Mef2 activation, leading to neurodegeneration," *eLife*, vol. 5, no. 2016, Article ID e16043, 2016.

[46] J. Bridwell-Rabb, N. G. Fox, C.-L. Tsai, A. M. Winn, and D. P. Barondeau, "Human frataxin activates Fe-S cluster biosynthesis by facilitating sulfur transfer chemistry," *Biochemistry*, vol. 53, no. 30, pp. 4904–4913, 2014.

[47] M. Cossée, H. Puccio, A. Gansmuller et al., "Inactivation of the Friedreich ataxia mouse gene leads to early embryonic lethality without iron accumulation," *Human Molecular Genetics*, vol. 9, no. 8, pp. 1219–1226, 2000.

[48] Y. Shidara and P. J. Hollenbeck, "Defects in mitochondrial axonal transport and membrane potential without increased reactive oxygen species production in a Drosophila mdel of Friedreich aaxia," *The Journal of Neuroscience*, vol. 30, no. 34, pp. 11369–11378, 2010.

[49] S. Soriano, J. V. Llorens, L. Blanco-Sobero et al., "Deferiprone and idebenone rescue frataxin depletion phenotypes in a Drosophila model of Friedreich's ataxia," *Gene*, vol. 521, no. 2, pp. 274–281, 2013.

[50] G. Sanchez-Casis, M. Cote, and A. Barbeau, "Pathology of the Heart in Friedreich's Ataxia: Review of the Literature and Report of One Case," *Canadian Journal of Neurological Sciences /*

Journal Canadien des Sciences Neurologiques, vol. 3, no. 4, pp. 349–354, 1976.

[51] J. B. Lamarche, M. Côté, and B. Lemieux, "The Cardiomyopathy of Friedreich's Ataxia Morphological Observations in 3 Cases," *Canadian Journal of Neurological Sciences / Journal Canadien des Sciences Neurologiques*, vol. 7, no. 4, pp. 389–396, 1980.

[52] F. Foury and O. Cazzalini, "Deletion of the yeast homologue of the human gene associated with Friedreich's ataxia elicits iron accumulation in mitochondria," *FEBS Letters*, vol. 411, no. 2-3, pp. 373–377, 1997.

[53] S. Michael, S. V. Petrocine, J. Qian et al., "Iron and iron-responsive proteins in the cardiomyopathy of Friedreich's ataxia," *The Cerebellum*, vol. 5, no. 4, pp. 257–267, 2006.

[54] R. L. Ramirez, J. Qian, P. Santambrogio, S. Levi, and A. H. Koeppen, "Relation of cytosolic iron excess to cardiomyopathy of friedreich's ataxia," *American Journal of Cardiology*, vol. 110, no. 12, pp. 1820–1827, 2012.

[55] A. H. Koeppen, R. L. Ramirez, A. B. Becker et al., "The pathogenesis of cardiomyopathy in Friedreich ataxia," *PLoS ONE*, vol. 10, no. 3, Article ID e0116396, 2015.

[56] D. Waldvogel, P. Van Gelderen, and M. Hallett, "Increased iron in the dentate nucleus of patients with Friedreich's ataxia," *Annals of Neurology*, vol. 46, no. 1, pp. 123–125, 1999.

[57] J. L. Bradley, J. C. Blake, S. Chamberlain, P. K. Thomas, J. M. Cooper, and A. H. V. Schapira, "Clinical, biochemical and molecular genetic correlations in Friedreich's ataxia," *Human Molecular Genetics*, vol. 9, no. 2, pp. 275–282, 2000.

[58] A. H. Koeppen, S. C. Michael, M. D. Knutson et al., "The dentate nucleus in Friedreich's ataxia: The role of iron-responsive proteins," *Acta Neuropathologica*, vol. 114, no. 2, pp. 163–173, 2007.

[59] A. H. Koeppen, J. A. Morral, A. N. Davis et al., "The dorsal root ganglion in Friedreich's ataxia," *Acta Neuropathologica*, vol. 118, no. 6, pp. 763–776, 2009.

[60] I. H. Harding, P. Raniga, M. B. Delatycki et al., "Tissue atrophy and elevated iron concentration in the extrapyramidal motor system in Friedreich ataxia: The IMAGE-FRDA study," *Journal of Neurology, Neurosurgery & Psychiatry*, vol. 87, no. 11, pp. 1260–1263, 2016.

[61] N. Boddaert, K. H. L. Q. Sang, A. Rötig et al., "Selective iron chelation in Friedreich ataxia: Biologic and clinical implications," *Blood*, vol. 110, no. 1, pp. 401–408, 2007.

[62] K. Chen, T. S.-Y. Ho, G. Lin, K. L. Tan, M. N. Rasband, and H. J. Bellen, "Loss of frataxin activates the iron/sphingolipid/PDK1/Mef2 pathway in mammals," *eLife*, vol. 5, no. 2016, Article ID e20732, 2016.

[63] H. Puccio, D. Simon, M. Cossée et al., "Mouse models for Friedreich ataxia exhibit cardiomyopathy, sensory nerve defect and Fe-S enzyme deficiency followed by intramitochondrial iron deposits," *Nature Genetics*, vol. 27, no. 2, pp. 181–186, 2001.

[64] D. Simon, H. Seznec, A. Gansmuller et al., "Friedreich Ataxia Mouse Models with Progressive Cerebellar and Sensory Ataxia Reveal Autophagic Neurodegeneration in Dorsal Root Ganglia," *The Journal of Neuroscience*, vol. 24, no. 8, pp. 1987–1995, 2004.

[65] S. Al-Mahdawi, R. M. Pinto, D. Varshney et al., "GAA repeat expansion mutation mouse models of Friedreich ataxia exhibit oxidative stress leading to progressive neuronal and cardiac pathology," *Genomics*, vol. 88, no. 5, pp. 580–590, 2006.

[66] J. A. Navarro, J. A. Botella, C. Metzendorf, M. I. Lind, and S. Schneuwly, "Mitoferrin modulates iron toxicity in a *Drosophila* model of Friedreich's ataxia," *Free Radical Biology & Medicine*, vol. 85, pp. 71–82, 2015.

[67] A. Rotig, P. de Lonlay, D. Chretien et al., "Aconitase and mitochondrial iron-sulphur protein deficiency in friedreich ataxia," *Nature Genetics*, vol. 17, no. 2, pp. 215–217, 1997.

[68] D. R. Lynch Gwen Lech, J. M. Farmer, L. J. Balcer, W. Bank, B. Chance, and R. B. Wilson, "Near infrared muscle spectroscopy in patients with Friedreich's ataxia," *Muscle & Nerve*, vol. 25, no. 5, pp. 664–673, 2002.

[69] A. Palandri, D. L'hôte, J. Cohen-Tannoudji, H. Tricoire, and V. Monnier, "Frataxin inactivation leads to steroid deficiency in flies and human ovarian cells," *Human Molecular Genetics*, vol. 24, no. 9, pp. 2615–2626, 2015.

[70] A. Moreno-Cermeño, È. Obis, G. Bellí, E. Cabiscol, J. Ros, and J. Tamarit, "Frataxin depletion in yeast triggers up-regulation of iron transport systems before affecting iron-sulfur enzyme activities," *The Journal of Biological Chemistry*, vol. 285, no. 53, pp. 41653–41664, 2010.

[71] J. S. Armstrong, O. Khdour, and S. M. Hecht, "Does oxidative stress contribute to the pathology of Friedreich's ataxia? A radical question," *The FASEB Journal*, vol. 24, no. 7, pp. 2152–2163, 2010.

[72] A.-L. Bulteau, A. Dancis, M. Gareil, J.-J. Montagne, J.-M. Camadro, and E. Lesuisse, "Oxidative stress and protease dysfunction in the yeast model of Friedreich ataxia," *Free Radical Biology & Medicine*, vol. 42, no. 10, pp. 1561–1570, 2007.

[73] R. P. Vázquez-Manrique, P. González-Cabo, S. Ros, H. Aziz, H. A. Baylis, and F. Palau, "Reduction of Caenorhabditis elegans frataxin increases sensitivity to oxidative stress, reduces lifespan, and causes lethality in a mitochondrial complex II mutant," *The FASEB Journal*, vol. 20, no. 1, pp. 172–174, 2006.

[74] A. Wong, J. Yang, P. Cavadini et al., "The Friedreich's ataxia mutation confers cellular sensitivity to oxidant stress which is rescued by chelators of iron and calcium and inhibitors of apoptosis," *Human Molecular Genetics*, vol. 8, no. 3, pp. 425–430, 1999.

[75] R. Santos, N. Buisson, S. A. B. Knight, A. Dancis, J.-M. Camadro, and E. Lesuisse, "Candida albicans lacking the frataxin homologue: A relevant yeast model for studying the role of frataxin," *Molecular Microbiology*, vol. 54, no. 2, pp. 507–519, 2004.

[76] M. V. Busi, M. V. Maliandi, H. Valdez et al., "Deficiency of Arabidopsis thaliana frataxin alters activity of mitochondrial Fe-S proteins and induces oxidative stress," *The Plant Journal*, vol. 48, no. 6, pp. 873–882, 2006.

[77] I. Condo, N. Ventura, F. Malisan, B. Tomassini, and R. Testi, "A pool of extramitochondrial frataxin that promotes cell survival," *The Journal of Biological Chemistry*, vol. 281, no. 24, pp. 16750–16756, 2006.

[78] E. Napoli, F. Taroni, and G. A. Cortopassi, "Frataxin, iron-sulfur clusters, heme, ROS, and aging," *Antioxidants & Redox Signaling*, vol. 8, no. 3-4, pp. 506–516, 2006.

[79] V. Irazusta, A. Moreno-Cermeño, E. Cabiscol, J. Ros, and J. Tamarit, "Major targets of iron-induced protein oxidative damage in frataxin-deficient yeasts are magnesium-binding proteins," *Free Radical Biology & Medicine*, vol. 44, no. 9, pp. 1712–1723, 2008.

[80] P. Rustin, J.-C. Von Kleist-Retzow, K. Chantrel-Groussard, D. Sidi, A. Munnich, and A. Rötig, "Effect of idebenone on cardiomyopathy in Friedreich's ataxia: A preliminary study," *The Lancet*, vol. 354, no. 9177, pp. 477–479, 1999.

[81] P. Calap-Quintana, S. Soriano, J. V. Llorens et al., "TORC1 inhibition by rapamycin promotes antioxidant defences in a drosophila model of friedreich's ataxia," *PLoS ONE*, vol. 10, no. 7, Article ID e0132376, 2015.

[82] S. Soriano, P. Calap-Quintana, J. V. Llorens et al., "Metal homeostasis regulators suppress FRDA phenotypes in a drosophila model of the disease," *PLoS ONE*, vol. 11, no. 7, Article ID e0159209, 2016.

[83] J. A. Navarro, E. Ohmann, D. Sanchez et al., "Altered lipid metabolism in a *Drosophila* model of Friedreich's ataxia," *Human Molecular Genetics*, vol. 19, no. 14, Article ID ddq183, pp. 2828–2840, 2010.

[84] R. Abeti, E. Uzun, I. Renganathan, T. Honda, M. A. Pook, and P. Giunti, "Targeting lipid peroxidation and mitochondrial imbalance in Friedreich's ataxia," *Pharmacological Research*, vol. 99, article no. 2842, pp. 344–350, 2015.

[85] A. Martelli, L. S. Friedman, L. Reutenauer et al., "Clinical data and characterization of the liver conditional mouse model exclude neoplasia as a non-neurological manifestation associated with Friedreich's ataxia," *Disease Models & Mechanisms*, vol. 5, no. 6, pp. 860–869, 2012.

[86] A. J. Worth, S. S. Basu, E. C. Deutsch et al., "Stable isotopes and LC-MS for monitoring metabolic disturbances in Friedreich's ataxia platelets," *Bioanalysis*, vol. 7, no. 15, pp. 1843–1855, 2015.

[87] J. Tamarit, È. Obis, and J. Ros, "Oxidative stress and altered lipid metabolism in Friedreich ataxia," *Free Radical Biology & Medicine*, vol. 100, pp. 138–146, 2016.

[88] A. Seguin, V. Monnier, A. Palandri et al., "A Yeast/Drosophila Screen to Identify New Compounds Overcoming Frataxin Deficiency," *Oxidative Medicine and Cellular Longevity*, vol. 2015, Article ID 565140, 2015.

[89] A. P. Runko, A. J. Griswold, and K.-T. Min, "Overexpression of frataxin in the mitochondria increases resistance to oxidative stress and extends lifespan in Drosophila," *FEBS Letters*, vol. 582, no. 5, pp. 715–719, 2008.

[90] T. J. Schulz, D. Westermann, F. Isken et al., "Activation of mitochondrial energy metabolism protects against cardiac failure," *AGING*, vol. 2, no. 11, pp. 843–853, 2010.

[91] C. J. Miranda, M. M. Santos, K. Ohshima, M. Tessaro, J. Sequeiros, and M. Pandolfo, "Frataxin overexpressing mice," *FEBS Letters*, vol. 572, no. 1-3, pp. 281–288, 2004.

[92] M. Ristow, M. F. Pfister, A. J. Yee et al., "Frataxin activates mitochondrial energy conversion and oxidative phosphorylation," *Proceedings of the National Acadamy of Sciences of the United States of America*, vol. 97, no. 22, pp. 12239–12243, 2000.

[93] S. A. Shoichet, A. T. Bäumer, D. Stamenkovic et al., "Frataxin promotes antioxidant defense in a thiol-dependent manner resulting in diminished malignant transformation in vitro," *Human Molecular Genetics*, vol. 11, no. 7, pp. 815–821, 2002.

[94] T. J. Schulz, R. Thierbach, A. Voigt et al., "Induction of oxidative metabolism by mitochondrial frataxin inhibits cancer growth: Otto Warburg revisited," *The Journal of Biological Chemistry*, vol. 281, no. 2, pp. 977–981, 2006.

[95] J. A. Navarro, J. V. Llorens, S. Soriano et al., "Overexpression of human and fly frataxins in drosophila provokes deleterious effects at biochemical, physiological and developmental levels," *PLoS ONE*, vol. 6, no. 7, Article ID e21017, 2011.

[96] O. Edenharter, J. Clement, S. Schneuwly, and J. A. Navarro, "Overexpression of Drosophila frataxin triggers cell death in an iron-dependent manner," *Journal of Neurogenetics*, pp. 1–14, 2017.

[97] A. Martelli, S. Schmucker, L. Reutenauer et al., "Iron Regulatory Protein 1 Sustains Mitochondrial Iron Loading and Function in Frataxin Deficiency," *Cell Metabolism*, vol. 21, no. 2, pp. 311–322, 2015.

[98] U. Mühlenhoff, J. Gerber, N. Richhardt, and R. Lill, "Components involved in assembly and dislocation of iron-sulfur clusters on the scaffold protein Isu1p," *EMBO Journal*, vol. 22, no. 18, pp. 4815–4825, 2003.

[99] E. M. Froschauer, R. J. Schweyen, and G. Wiesenberger, "The yeast mitochondrial carrier proteins Mrs3p/Mrs4p mediate iron transport across the inner mitochondrial membrane," *Biochimica et Biophysica Acta (BBA) - Biomembranes*, vol. 1788, no. 5, pp. 1044–1050, 2009.

[100] X. Brazzolotto, F. Pierrel, and L. Pelosi, "Three conserved histidine residues contribute to mitochondrial iron transport through mitoferrins," *Biochemical Journal*, vol. 460, no. 1, pp. 79–89, 2014.

[101] J. P. Liuzzi, F. Aydemir, H. Nam, M. D. Knutson, and R. J. Cousins, "Zip14 (Slc39a14) mediates non-transferrin-bound iron uptake into cells," *Proceedings of the National Acadamy of Sciences of the United States of America*, vol. 103, no. 37, pp. 13612–13617, 2006.

[102] C.-Y. Wang, S. Jenkitkasemwong, S. Duarte et al., "ZIP8 is an iron and zinc transporter whose cell-surface expression is up-regulated by cellular iron loading," *The Journal of Biological Chemistry*, vol. 287, no. 41, pp. 34032–34043, 2012.

[103] G. Xiao, Z. Wan, Q. Fan, X. Tang, and B. Zhou, "The metal transporter ZIP13 supplies iron into the secretory pathway in Drosophila melanogaster," *eLife*, vol. 3, p. e03191, 2014.

[104] J. M. Walker, R. Tsivkovskii, and S. Lutsenko, "Metallochaperone Atox1 transfers copper to the NH2-terminal domain of the Wilson's disease protein and regulates its catalytic activity," *The Journal of Biological Chemistry*, vol. 277, no. 31, pp. 27953–27959, 2002.

[105] Y. Li, J. Du, P. Zhang, and J. Ding, "Crystal structure of human copper homeostasis protein CutC reveals a potential copper-binding site," *Journal of Structural Biology*, vol. 169, no. 3, pp. 399–405, 2010.

[106] S. Bahadorani, S. Mukai, D. Egli, and A. J. Hilliker, "Overexpression of metal-responsive transcription factor (MTF-1) in Drosophila melanogaster ameliorates life-span reductions associated with oxidative stress and metal toxicity," *Neurobiology of Aging*, vol. 31, no. 7, pp. 1215–1226, 2010.

[107] H. Hua, L. Münter, A. Harmeier, O. Georgiev, G. Multhaup, and W. Schaffner, "Toxicity of Alzheimer's disease-associated Aβ peptide is ameliorated in a Drosophila model by tight control of zinc and copper availability," *biological chemistry*, vol. 392, no. 10, pp. 919–926, 2011.

[108] N. Saini, O. Georgiev, and W. Schaffner, "The parkin mutant phenotype in the fly is largely rescued by metal-responsive transcription factor (MTF-1)," *Molecular and Cellular Biology*, vol. 31, no. 10, pp. 2151–2161, 2011.

[109] J. P. Fabisiak, L. L. Pearce, G. G. Borisenko et al., "Bifunctional Anti-/Prooxidant Potential of Metallothionein: Redox Signaling of Copper Binding and Release," *Antioxidants & Redox Signaling*, vol. 1, no. 3, pp. 349–364, 1999.

[110] Z. E. Suntres and E. M. K. Lui, "Prooxidative effect of copper-metallothionein in the acute cytotoxicity of hydrogen peroxide in Ehrlich ascites tumour cells," *Toxicology*, vol. 217, no. 2-3, pp. 155–168, 2006.

[111] K. T. Suzuki, M. Rui, J.-I. Ueda, and T. Ozawa, "Production of hydroxyl radicals by copper-containing metallothionein: Roles as prooxidant," *Toxicology and Applied Pharmacology*, vol. 141, no. 1, pp. 231–237, 1996.

[112] A. H. Koeppen, R. L. Ramirez, D. Yu et al., "Friedreich's ataxia causes redistribution of iron, copper, and zinc in the dentate nucleus," *The Cerebellum*, vol. 11, no. 4, pp. 845–860, 2012.

[113] R. B. Wilson, "Therapeutic developments in Friedreich ataxia," *Journal of Child Neurology*, vol. 27, no. 9, pp. 1212–1216, 2012.

[114] T. E. Richardson, H. N. Kelly, A. E. Yu, and J. W. Simpkins, "Therapeutic strategies in Friedreich's ataxia," *Brain Research*, vol. 1514, pp. 91–97, 2013.

[115] E. Lesuisse, R. Santos, B. F. Matzanke, S. A. B. Knight, J.-M. Camadro, and A. Dancis, "Iron use for haeme synthesis is under control of the yeast frataxin homologue (Yfh1)," *Human Molecular Genetics*, vol. 12, no. 8, pp. 879–889, 2003.

[116] D. Velasco-Sánchez, A. Aracil, R. Montero et al., "Combined therapy with idebenone and deferiprone in patients with Friedreich's ataxia," *The Cerebellum*, vol. 10, no. 1, pp. 1–8, 2011.

[117] S. Elincx-Benizri, A. Glik, D. Merkel et al., "Clinical Experience with Deferiprone Treatment for Friedreich Ataxia," *Journal of Child Neurology*, vol. 31, no. 8, pp. 1036–1040, 2016.

[118] J. Arpa, I. Sanz-Gallego, F. J. Rodríguez-de-Rivera et al., "Triple therapy with deferiprone, idebenone and riboflavin in Friedreich's ataxia - open-label trial," *Acta Neurologica Scandinavica*, vol. 129, no. 1, pp. 32–40, 2014.

[119] M. Pandolfo, J. Arpa, M. B. Delatycki et al., "Deferiprone in Friedreich ataxia: A 6-month randomized controlled trial," *Annals of Neurology*, vol. 76, no. 4, pp. 509–521, 2014.

13

Atypical Features in a Large Turkish Family Affected with Friedreich Ataxia

Semiha Kurt,[1] **Betul Cevik,**[1] **Durdane Aksoy,**[1] **E. Irmak Sahbaz,**[2] **Aslı Gundogdu Eken,**[2] **and A. Nazli Basak**[2]

[1]*Department of Neurology, Gaziosmanpasa University Faculty of Medicine, 60100 Tokat, Turkey*
[2]*Suna and Inan Kıraç Foundation Neurodegeneration Research Laboratory, Molecular Biology and Genetics Department, Bogazici University, 34342 Istanbul, Turkey*

Correspondence should be addressed to Semiha Kurt; gsemihakurt@hotmail.com

Academic Editor: Dominic B. Fee

Here, we describe the clinical features of several members of the same family diagnosed with Friedreich ataxia (FRDA) and cerebral lesions, demyelinating neuropathy, and late-age onset without a significant cardiac involvement and presenting with similar symptoms, although genetic testing was negative for the GAA repeat expansion in one patient of the family. The GAA repeat expansion in the frataxin gene was shown in all of the family members except in a young female patient. MRI revealed arachnoid cysts in two patients; MRI was consistent with both cavum septum pellucidum-cavum vergae and nodular signal intensity increase in one patient. EMG showed demyelinating sensorimotor polyneuropathy in another patient. The GAA expansion-negative 11-year-old female patient had mental-motor retardation, epilepsy, and ataxia. None of the patients had significant cardiac symptoms. Description of FRDA families with different ethnic backgrounds may assist in identifying possible phenotypic and genetic features of the disease. Furthermore, the genetic heterogeneity observed in this family draws attention to the difficulty of genetic counseling in an inbred population and to the need for genotyping all affected members before delivering comprehensive genetic counseling.

1. Introduction

Friedreich ataxia (FRDA) is an autosomal recessive neurodegenerative disorder and the most common hereditary ataxia. The FRDA locus was detected on chromosome 9 in 1988 [1]. The frataxin gene, which encodes a protein that probably acts as a mitochondrial iron transporter, was detected in 1996 [1]. Most mutations appear to be unstable expansions of a GAA repeat in the first intron of the gene [1].

Harding described the essential clinical features as (1) autosomal recessive inheritance, (2) onset before 25 years of age, (3) progressive limb and gait ataxia, (4) absent tendon reflexes in the lower extremities, (5) electrophysiological signs of axonal sensory neuropathy (within 5 years of onset), (6) dysarthria, (7) areflexia at all four extremities, (8) distal loss of position and vibration sense, (9) extensor plantar reflex, and (10) muscle weakness in the lower extremities [2].

The "typical" or "classic" form of the disease is defined as a disease form exhibiting all the clinical features listed by Harding [2, 3]. Disease forms which do not meet these criteria are referred to as atypical Friedreich ataxia. Skeletal deformities, cardiomyopathy, and diabetes are the most common systemic conditions associated with FRDA [4]. The disease is characterized by clinical variability regarding the age at onset, the rate of progression, and presence/absence of areflexia, muscle weakness, or cardiomyopathy. However, the clinical manifestations tend to be similar in affected siblings in the same family [4], indicating the crucial role of genetic factors for phenotypic expression of the disease.

In FRDA patients, magnetic resonance imaging scans reveal spinal cord atrophy along with normal brainstem, cerebellum, and cerebrum [2]. Demyelinating neuropathy and late disease onset after the age of 25 years are the manifestations excluding the classical form of FRDA [1, 3]. Cardiac involvement occurs in most of the patients with FRDA [2]. Similar symptoms related to multiple diseases are also rare in the same family [5].

Here, we describe the atypical clinical features of several members of the same family diagnosed with Friedreich ataxia (FRDA) and cerebral lesions, demyelinating neuropathy, and late-age onset without a significant cardiac involvement and presenting with similar symptoms, although genetic testing was negative for the GAA repeat expansion in one patient of the family.

2. Patients and Methods

Our index case was a 37-year-old man admitted to our outpatient clinic following a history of ataxia. Family members with similar symptoms were identified in Tokat, a city in the Middle Black Sea region of Turkey. This study was performed in accordance with the Helsinki Declaration. All adult participants provided written informed consent. Parents of participating minors provided written informed consent; literate minors who could write also provided signed assent. All subjects received a detailed explanation of the study and genetic counseling as appropriate. A pedigree was prepared in the field. A detailed history was obtained from each subject, and each subject received a detailed neurological examination. All available previous tests and imaging studies of the patients were recorded in detail.

Five stages of disease disability were distinguished: stage 0: patients at risk with normal examination results; stage 1: clinical signs of FRDA found at clinical exam; stage 2: functional signs but able to walk unaided; stage 3: clinical and functional signs, unable to walk without help; stage 4: confined to wheelchair, able to stand but not to walk; stage 5: bedridden: unable to stand [1].

Electrophysiological Examination. Electrophysiological studies were performed using standard nerve conduction techniques with Medelec-Oxford EMG equipment. Sensory nerve conduction studies were performed orthodromically on median and ulnar nerves and antidromically on the sural and superficial peroneal nerves. Motor nerve conduction studies were conducted on the median, ulnar, tibial, and peroneal nerves. Electromyography was performed on at least two proximal and distal muscles from the upper and lower extremities.

DNA Sample Collection and Genetic Analysis. Blood samples were taken from the cubital vein into EDTA-containing tubes during field work. DNA was isolated using the Magna Pure Compact System from Roche, followed by PCR analysis.

3. Results

Figure 1 shows the pedigree structure of the family. Blood samples were obtained from five symptomatic and 15 asymptomatic family members during family screening. Neurological examination of 15 asymptomatic family members did not reveal any abnormal finding. Ten out of these fifteen family members were carriers of GAA repeat expansion.

Clinical, electrophysiological, and neuroradiological data were obtained from two male and two female family members suffering from ataxia (Table 1). One male patient was evaluated clinically and genetically. Patients I.1 (the index patient) and II.5 were brothers, and Patient III.5 was their niece. Patients II.10 and II.11 were siblings and first cousins of Patients II.1 and II.5.

4. Clinical Presentation of the Family

4.1. Patient II.5 (Index Case). The 37-year-old male patient presented with a history of imbalance and numbness in hands and feet starting from the age of 18 without any other previous complaints. Although numbness in the hands and feet has improved in time, the imbalance had worsened. Following the increasing deterioration of the writing hand, muscle weakness in the hands and feet increased. Speech disturbance started about 6-7 years ago. 2-3 years ago, he started to require unilateral aid to walk due to the increased risk of fall. The patient defined similar complaints in his brother, in a female and male cousins, and in his niece. His neurological examination revealed dysarthric speech and a mild effacement of the left nasolabial fold, diffuse weakness and atrophy in the legs, and a mild distal atrophy in the hands. Deep tendon reflexes were absent in the upper and lower extremities. He had a moderate dysmetria and dysdiadochokinesia. His gait was ataxic in spite of unilateral walking aid. Joint-position sense was impaired in the toes. Plantar reflexes were absent on both sides. A mild thoracic scoliosis, pes cavus, and hammer toes were detected in his examination. The results of routine hematological and biochemical investigations were normal. He had no clinical symptoms of a cardiac disease and ECG was normal. In the electrophysiological studies, sensory action potentials were absent in the sural, superficial peroneal, median, and ulnar nerves. Median nerve conduction velocity (NCV) was 38.7 m/s, terminal latency (TL) was 4.3 ms, and F latency was 36.5 ms. Ulnar NCV was 33.45 m/s, TL was 4 ms, and F latency was 37.3 ms. Peroneal NCV was 27.3 m/s, TL was 6.2 ms, and F latency was 68.5 ms. Tibial NCV was 25.4 m/s, TL was 6.55 ms, and F latency was 64.4 ms. Conduction abnormalities matched demyelinating neuropathy criteria [6]. Brain MRI scans revealed an image of arachnoid cyst approximately 25 mm in diameter in posterior vermian area (Figure 2(a)).

4.2. Patient II.1. The 47-year-old male patient stated imbalance that started at the age of 27. Later on, speech disturbance was added to his complaints. Both imbalance and speech disturbance have gradually worsened and he was barely able to take a few steps with bilateral walking aid for the last 5-6 years, usually using a wheelchair. His neurological examination revealed dysarthric speech and bilateral horizontal nystagmus, a mild loss of muscle strength in the lower extremities in spite of normal muscle strength in the upper extremities, a normal superficial sensation and loss of vibration sense in the distal foot, absent deep tendon reflexes, and extensor plantar responses on both sides. Dysmetria

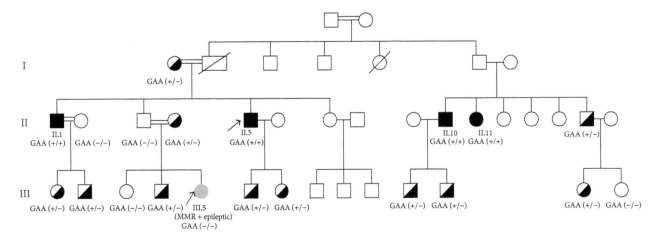

FIGURE 1: Pedigree of a family with FRDA. Black boxes indicate affected FRDA patients. The index case is indicated by an arrow. Semiblack boxes indicate FRDA carriers. The FRDA(−) case is indicated by grey box and the number III.5.

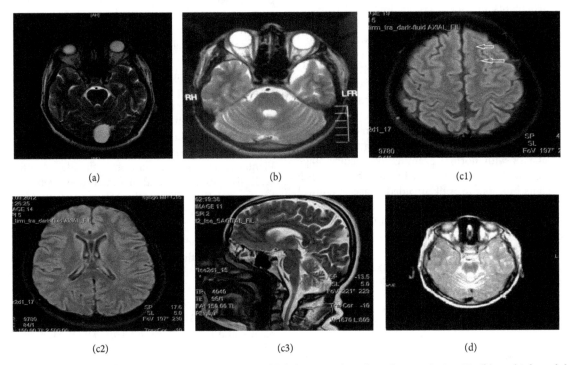

FIGURE 2: Arachnoid cyst in posterior vermian area in Patient II.5 (a); left temporal arachnoid cyst in Patient II.1 (b); multiple nodular (white arrows) lesions (c1), cavum septum pellucidum-cavum vergae variation (c2), and cerebellar atrophy in Patient II.11 (c3); cerebellar atrophy in Patient III.5 (d).

and dysdiadochokinesia were detected in the upper limbs. He was barely able to stand and take a few steps. The results of routine hematological and biochemical investigations were normal. He had no clinical symptoms of cardiac disease and ECG was normal. Echocardiography revealed a mild diastolic dysfunction. On electrophysiological examination, sensory action potentials were absent in the sural nerve and moderately reduced in amplitude and velocity in the median and ulnar nerves. The median, ulnar, peroneal, and tibial motor conduction studies were normal.

Patient's previous MRI scans of the brain revealed a left temporal CSF-isointense lesion consistent with arachnoid cyst (Figure 2(b)) and previous MRI and X-ray of the thoracolumbar spine showed S-shaped scoliosis.

4.3. Patient II.10. The 52-year-old male patient stated gait imbalance and speech disturbance first started when he was sixteen. He became wheelchair-bound in 1997 due to gradually increased ataxia. His neurological examination revealed severe dysarthria, bilateral horizontal nystagmus, a normal superficial sensation, and reduced sense of vibration and position in the distal foot. There was no significant loss of muscle strength. Triceps and biceps reflexes were

TABLE 1: Clinical and laboratory characteristics of the patients.

Feature	Patient II.5	Patient II.1	Patient II.10	Patient II.11	Patient III.5
Age at evaluation	37	47	52	40	11
Age at onset	18	27	16	16	Infant
Duration of the disease	19	20	36	24	11
Sex	M	M	M	F	F
First symptom	Ataxia, paresthesia	Ataxia	Ataxia	Ataxia	MMR
Ataxia	++	+++	+++	+++	+++
Dysarthria	+	++	++	++	++
Muscle weakness					
Upper limbs	+	−	−	+	++
Lower limbs	+	+	−	+++	+++
Deep tendon reflexes					
Upper limbs	Absent	Absent	Diminished	Absent	Absent
Lower limbs	Absent	Absent	Absent	Absent	Absent
Joint position/vibration sense abnormalities					
Upper limbs	−	−	−	+	NP
Lower limbs	+	+	+	+	NP
Babinski sign	Absent	Extensor	Flexor	Extensor	Extensor
Extraneurological findings	Scoliosis, hammer toes	Scoliosis	Scoliosis	Scoliosis	Scoliosis
Cardiomyopathy	−	−	−	−	−
Cranial MRI	Arachnoid cyst	Arachnoid cyst	NP	CV, CSP, NL, and C-Ce atrophy	Ce-atrophy
NCS	Demyelinating neuropathy	Sensorial neuropathy	NP	Sensorial neuropathy	Sensorial neuropathy
Functional score	Unable to walk without help	Confined to wheelchair	Confined to wheelchair	Confined to wheelchair	Confined to wheelchair

M: male, F: female, MMR: mental motor retardation, NP: not performed, NL: nodular lesions, CV: cavum vergae, CSP: cavum septum pellucidum, C: cerebral, and Ce: cerebellar. +++: severe; ++: moderate; +: mild; −: no.

diminished while other deep tendon reflexes were absent too. Flexor plantar responses were obtained on both sides and severe bilateral dysmetria and dysdiadochokinesia were detected predominantly on the left side and he was unable to stand. Scoliosis was noted by visual inspection. The patient had no cardiac complaints and did not accept to undergo investigations other than genetic analysis.

4.4. Patient II.11. The 40-year-old female patient first started to have difficulty in walking when she was sixteen. The gait disorder was followed by a speech disturbance and loss of muscle strength particularly in the lower limbs, and she became wheelchair-bound at the age of 25. Her neurological examination revealed dysarthria, bilateral horizontal nystagmus, and muscle strength of 4/5 in the upper extremities and 0/5 in the lower limbs apart from muscle strength of 2/5 in the dorsiflexion and plantar flexion of the toes, on both sides. Muscle tone was reduced in the lower extremities. Vibration sense was reduced in the distal parts of the hands and foot, in addition to the glove-stocking hypoesthesia. Deep tendon reflexes were absent and an extensor plantar response

was obtained on both sides. Severe bilateral dysmetria and dysdiadochokinesia were detected predominantly on the left side and she was unable to stand even with bilateral assistance. Moderate thoracic scoliosis was evident. The results of routine hematological and biochemical investigations were normal. She had no clinical symptoms of a heart disease and ECG was normal. On electrophysiological examination, sensory action potentials were absent in the sural, superficial peroneal, median, and ulnar nerves. The median, ulnar, peroneal, and tibial motor conduction studies were normal. MRI scan of the brain of the patient revealed signal changes of the white matter indicating multiple nodular lesions in the cerebral parenchyma at the level of corona radiata, centrum semiovale, a congenital cavum septum pellucidum, cavum vergae variation in the interventricular space, and cerebral and cerebellar atrophy (Figures 2(c1), 2(c2), and 2(c3)).

4.5. Patient III.5. The 11-year-old female patient with motor and mental retardation was born by Cesarean section for breech presentation at term. She kept her head steady at 8 months of age and sat without support at the age of three, crawled at the age of four and started to walk at the age of five. Subsequently, she has gradually developed a gait ataxia and required the assistance of a walker and then she became unable to walk. She had her first seizure when she was 6 months old. First valproic acid was started and then it was switched to lamotrigine. The seizures were taken under control by lamotrigine and the treatment was discontinued following two years of seizure-free period of time. It was reported that she was unable to talk in sentences but she could speak a few words and she was partly able to understand. In the neurological examination, she was capable of forming words in a dysarthric pattern. She was not oriented and poorly cooperative. Gross examination of the cranial nerves revealed no abnormality. Muscle strength was determined as 4/5 in the proximal parts of upper extremities and 3/5 in the distal parts and as 3/5 in the proximal parts of lower extremities and 0/5 in the distal parts. Muscle tone was reduced. Sensory and cerebellar tests could not be performed. Deep tendon reflexes were absent and plantar responses were extensor. Previous routine blood biochemistry and hematological tests were within normal limits. Amino acid levels were found to be within normal limits in an AA analysis using tandem MS (LC-MS-MS) method. C8/C12 ratio was found to be mildly elevated in the acylcarnitine/carnitine analysis; however, the result of the repeat test was normal. Serum levels of vitamin E, AFP, lactate, IgA, IgE, IgG, and IgM were found to be within normal levels. Urine organic acid assessment revealed an excretion of 50 mmol/mol of succinic acid. The excretion of oxalic acid was equal to the internal standard and the excretion of homovanillic acid and vanillylmandelic acid was equal to half of the internal standard along with elevated excretion of pyruvic acid, 3-OH isobutyric acid, ethylmalonic acid, adipic acid, 3-indol acetic acid, and 3-OH propionic acid and trace amount of erythrov 4,5 diOH hexanoate lactone, tiglylglycine, and methyl citrate. The excretion of other organic acids was within normal limits. Increased SCA-specific CAG repeat was not found in any of the SCA 1, 2, 3, 6, and 7 loci. Personal-social development was determined at the level of 18.5 months of age, fine motor skills were found at the level of 14–19 months, language skills were found at the level of 22–30 months of age, and gross motor development was found to be at the level of 12 months in the Denver II developmental screening test. ECG and echocardiography tests were normal. Previous EEGs reported a slow background activity and sharp waves in the right temporooccipital regions and some of them were reported as normal. Motor nerve conduction studies were normal in the lower extremities and no response could be obtained from the sural nerve in the EMG which was interpreted as a technical issue. Cerebellar atrophy was reported in the MRI scan of the brain (Figure 2(d)). The repeat EEG was normal. Sensory nerve action potentials could not be obtained from the sural and superficial peroneal nerves and sensory nerve action potential amplitudes of the median and ulnar nerves were reduced in the repeat EMG study. Motor conduction studies were normal. The patient had scoliosis concave to the left.

5. DNA Analysis

PCR analysis for the GAA repeat in the frataxin gene revealed the homozygous presence of the GAA repeat in all four affected members of generation II. The young Patient III.5 did not have GAA repeat in this locus. The analysis of her parents validated the result, since her mother was a carrier, whereas the father was normal for the GAA repeat.

6. Discussion

In patients with Friedreich ataxia, MRI scans of the spine show thinning of the cervical spinal cord and signal abnormalities in the posterior and lateral columns [7]. Cerebellar atrophy is not a common finding in CT or MRI images; however, the presence of cerebellar atrophy indicates a severe, advanced disease [7, 8]. Brain MRI may be a useful diagnostic procedure, since the absence of cerebellar atrophy may point out other forms of hereditary recessive ataxia rather than Friedreich ataxia [2, 7]. However, as far as we know, no intracranial lesions have been reported in FRDA. Arachnoid cyst was reported in two of our patients and cavum septum pellucidum and cavum vergae variation and nodular signal changes were detected in Patient II.11. Arachnoid cysts and congenital intra-axial midline cysts (cavum septum pellucidum, cavum vergae, and cavum velum interpositum) are nonneoplastic neurological cysts [9]. Arachnoid cysts are fluid-filled duplications or splittings of the arachnoid layer with a content mildly different from the cerebrospinal fluid [10]. They may occur sporadically as isolated variations or may be associated with other malformations or diseases [10]. Usually arachnoid cysts are incidentally detected on imaging studies of the brain [11]. Although most cases are sporadic, intracranial arachnoid cysts in several members of the same family have been reported in a few publications [11]. In one of these reports, arachnoid cysts were accompanied by a deletion in chromosome 16 in the same family [11]. Jadeja and Grewal presented an unusual association of genetic myopathy, oculopharyngeal muscular dystrophy, and arachnoid cysts in the same family [12]. Değerliyurt et al. described two siblings with porencephaly, hemiparesis, epilepsy, and atrophic kidney associated with an arachnoid cyst in one of the siblings and in the asymptomatic mothers. Col4A1 gene mutation screening revealed a novel mutation in mother and both children [13]. Bayrakli et al. presented an intracranial arachnoid cyst family from southern Turkey with six out of seven offspring with intracranial arachnoid cysts in different localizations [14]. Arachnoid cyst was found to be present in two male siblings with FRDA in our study.

When a septum pellucidum has a separation between its two leaflets, it is referred to as cavum septum pellucidum (CSP). This condition takes place when there is separation between the leaflets of the septum pellucidum and posterior extension to the splenium of the corpus callosum. The anterior columns of the fornix separate the anterior cavum septum pellucidum and the posterior cavum vergae (CV). CSP may persist in up to 20% of adults. CV is present in up to 30% of newborns, although it may persist in less than 1% of the adult individuals. CV cysts are usually associated with

CSP [9]. The CSP and CV cyst association was detected also in our patient.

Preadolescent onset is commonly regarded as crucial for the diagnosis of FRDA. Harding revised the diagnostic criteria in order to include patients with late onset up to the age of 25 years [3]. The complaints of Patient II.1 started after the age of 25. Late onset Friedreich ataxia, defined by symptom onset after the age of 25, accounts for 14% of the cases, while very late onset Friedreich ataxia, characterized by disease onset after the age of 40, is very rare [15].

Nerve conduction studies reveal axonal sensory neuropathy along with small or absent sensory action potentials in FRDA patients [2]. Motor conduction velocities are normal or mildly reduced in comparison to the sensory nerve potentials [2]. Nerve conduction studies of Patients II.1 and II.11 shared these characteristics; however, the motor nerve studies of our index case revealed demyelinating characteristics. According to Harding's criteria, a marked reduction of motor nerve conduction velocities is a finding that may exclude the diagnosis of FRDA [3]. However, Panas et al. reported three unrelated families with four affected children who suggested a hereditary motor and sensory neuropathy according to the clinical findings; however, the molecular genetic analysis was consistent with FRDA [16]. They claimed that the mutation identified in all four patients supports that these cases are representatives of a "variant" form of FRDA [16]. Similarly, Benomar et al. also reported that, in four out of seven FRDA patients, electromyography revealed a severe demyelinating neuropathy and severe demyelination and axonal neuropathy in the other three patients [1].

Cardiomyopathy is present in two-thirds of the patients with FRDA which is primarily symmetric concentric hypertrophic cardiomyopathy; in addition, some patients exhibit asymmetric septal hypertrophy [2]. Electrocardiogram reveals widespread T wave inversions and signs of ventricular hypertrophy [2]. The Acadian Type (Louisiana Form), which is observed in a specific population of French origin living in North America, was distinguished from typical FRDA by its milder course and lower incidence of cardiomyopathy [2]. Similarly to the Acadian Type, no significant cardiomyopathy was detected in our cases.

The EMG patterns and ages of onset were heterogeneous in our cases. The interfamilial clinical variability in FRDA patients was explained by mutation heterogeneity before the elucidation of the molecular basis of FRDA. The knowledge that almost all cases of FRDA are caused by the same dynamic mutation provided another way to interpret phenotypic heterogeneity [16]. According to Illarioshkin et al., the cooccurrence of distinct clinical variants of the disorder is associated with different combinations of the mutated alleles inherited from parents [4].

The genetic study of Patient III.5 was negative for FRDA. Bouhlal et al. have described three distinct gene defects leading to an autosomal recessive ataxia in a consanguineous Tunisian family [5]. A study conducted by Zlotogora asserted that a chance phenomenon, the migration of families with

affected patients or a digenic inheritance, might be responsible for the genetic heterogeneity observed in some autosomal recessive disease. However, these explanations are not persuasive in most cases. Although the selection mechanism was demonstrated to explain most of the observations, it is difficult to prove [17]. The hypothesis of a coincidental association seemed to be the most logical explanation; however, it is also difficult to explain it on a statistical basis [5].

Description of FRDA families with different ethnic backgrounds may assist in identifying possible phenotypic and genetic features of the disease. Furthermore, the genetic heterogeneity observed in this family draws attention to the difficulty of genetic counseling in an inbred population and to the need for genotyping all affected members before delivering a comprehensive genetic counseling.

References

[1] A. Benomar, M. Yahyaoui, F. Meggouh et al., "Clinical comparison between AVED patients with 744 del a mutation and Friedreich ataxia with GAA expansion in 15 Moroccan families," *Journal of the Neurological Sciences*, vol. 198, no. 1-2, pp. 25–29, 2002.

[2] G. Alper and V. Narayanan, "Friedreich's ataxia," *Pediatric Neurology*, vol. 28, no. 5, pp. 335–341, 2003.

[3] A. E. Harding, "Friedreich's ataxia: a clinical and genetic study of 90 families with an analysis of early diagnostic criteria and intrafamilial clustering of clinical features," *Brain*, vol. 104, no. 3, pp. 589–620, 1981.

[4] S. N. Illarioshkin, G. K. Bagieva, S. A. Klyushnikov, I. V. Ovchinnikov, E. D. Markova, and I. A. Ivanova-Smolenskaya, "Different phenotypes of Friedreich's ataxia within one 'pseudo-dominant' genealogy: relationships between trinucleotide (GAA) repeat lengths and clinical features," *European Journal of Neurology*, vol. 7, no. 5, pp. 535–540, 2000.

[5] Y. Bouhlal, M. Zouari, M. Kefi, C. Ben Hamida, F. Hentati, and R. Amouri, "Autosomal recessive ataxia caused by three distinct gene defects in a single consanguineous family," *Journal of Neurogenetics*, vol. 22, no. 2, pp. 139–148, 2008.

[6] S. J. Oh, *Clinical Electromyograhy Nerve Conduction Studies*, Lippincott Williams & Wilkins, Philadelphia, Pa, USA, 3rd edition, 2003.

[7] J. B. Schulz, S. Boesch, K. Bürk et al., "Diagnosis and treatment of Friedreich ataxia: a European perspective," *Nature Reviews Neurology*, vol. 5, no. 4, pp. 222–234, 2009.

[8] M. Anheim, C. Tranchant, and M. Koenig, "The autosomal recessive cerebellar ataxias," *The New England Journal of Medicine*, vol. 366, no. 7, pp. 636–646, 2012.

[9] R. S. Tubbs, S. Krishnamurthy, K. Verma et al., "Cavum velum interpositum, cavum septum pellucidum, and cavum vergae: a review," *Child's Nervous System*, vol. 27, no. 11, pp. 1927–1930, 2011.

[10] T. Westermaier, T. Schweitzer, and R.-I. Ernestus, "Arachnoid cysts," *Advances in Experimental Medicine and Biology*, vol. 724, pp. 37–50, 2012.

[11] G. Arriola, P. De Castro, and A. Verdú, "Familial arachnoid cysts," *Pediatric Neurology*, vol. 33, no. 2, pp. 146–148, 2005.

[12] K. J. Jadeja and R. P. Grewal, "Familial arachnoid cysts associated with oculopharyngeal muscular dystrophy," *Journal of Clinical Neuroscience*, vol. 10, no. 1, pp. 125–127, 2003.

[13] A. Değerliyurt, G. Ceylaner, H. Koçak et al., "A new family with autosomal dominant porencephaly with a novel COL4A1 mutation. Are arachnoid cysts related to COL4A1 mutations?" *Genetic Counseling*, vol. 23, no. 2, pp. 185–193, 2012.

[14] F. Bayrakli, A. I. Okten, U. Kartal et al., "Intracranial arachnoid cyst family with autosomal recessive trait mapped to chromosome 6q22.31-23.2," *Acta Neurochirurgica*, vol. 154, no. 7, pp. 1287–1291, 2012.

[15] M. B. Delatycki and L. A. Corben, "Clinical features of Friedreich ataxia," *Journal of Child Neurology*, vol. 27, no. 9, pp. 1133–1137, 2012.

[16] M. Panas, N. Kalfakis, G. Karadima, P. Davaki, and D. Vassilopoulos, "Friedreich's ataxia mimicking hereditary motor and sensory neuropathy," *Journal of Neurology*, vol. 249, no. 11, pp. 1583–1586, 2002.

[17] J. Zlotogora, "Multiple mutations responsible for frequent genetic diseases in isolated populations," *European Journal of Human Genetics*, vol. 15, no. 3, pp. 272–278, 2007.

14

Motor Improvement in Adolescents Affected by Ataxia Secondary to Acquired Brain Injury

Elisabetta Peri, Daniele Panzeri, Elena Beretta, Gianluigi Reni, Sandra Strazzer, and Emilia Biffi ⓘ

Scientific Institute IRCCS Eugenio Medea, Bosisio Parini, Lecco, Italy

Correspondence should be addressed to Emilia Biffi; emilia.biffi@bp.lnf.it

Academic Editor: Mario U. Manto

Aim. To assess changes in locomotion and balance in adolescents affected by ataxia secondary to acquired brain injury after a rehabilitation treatment with physiotherapy and the Gait Real-time Analysis Interactive Lab (GRAIL), an immersive virtual reality platform. *Methods.* 11 ataxic adolescents (16(5) years old, 4.7(6.7) years from injury) underwent 20 45-minute sessions with GRAIL plus 20 45-minute sessions of physiotherapy in one month. Patients were assessed before and after rehabilitation with functional scales and three-dimensional multiple-step gait analysis. *Results.* Results showed significant improvements in ataxia score assessed by the Scale for the Assessment and Rating of Ataxia, in dimension D and E of Gross Motor Function Measure, in walking endurance and in balance abilities. Moreover, the training fostered significant changes at hip, knee, and ankle joints, and the decrease of gait variability, toward healthy references. *Interpretation.* In spite of the pilot nature of the study, data suggest that training with immersive virtual reality and physiotherapy is a promising approach for ataxic gait rehabilitation, even in chronic conditions.

1. Introduction

Ataxia is a neurological sign resulting in cognitive and motor deficits that have a significant impact on quality of daily life. The locomotion ability is impaired by decreased balance due to loss of coordination, dysmetria, tremors, and hypotonia [1]. Cerebellar ataxia is a form of ataxia that originates from a deficit located in the cerebellum [2]. Its etiology is either genetic or it is a consequence of an acquired brain injury (ABI). In the latter case, it can be due to a focal lesion as a result of hemorrhagic events, traumatic brain injury or brain tumor, often located in the posterior cranial fossa. Ataxia in children and adolescents usually entails a relevant social and economic burden, since it involves young subjects that may need assistance and restorative treatments to be paid by the community throughout all life.

Cerebellar ataxic gait shows some common clinical signs: a generalized irregular gait pattern, reduced gait speed and cadence, shorter step and stride length, reduced swing phase, increase of the step width[3], augmented stance phase and double limb support time [4], increased variability in timing [1, 5], knee hyperextension, reduced power at the ankle joint,

loss of smoothness during the gait, and decomposition of multijoint movements into a series of single-joint movements [6]. These signs can increase the exposure to fall risk, reduce the endurance during the walk and, in more severe cases, require the use of orthosis, limiting a complete access to peer activities.

Therefore, the recovery of locomotion is commonly considered one of the primary goals in rehabilitation of ataxic patients.

Previous studies described motor recovery [7] and reported successful outcome in patients with degenerative ataxia [8–11], while only few low-level evidence publications tackle the rehabilitation of patients with ataxia secondary to ABI [7].

Two main rehabilitative approaches are usually considered [12], named as restorative and compensatory strategy. The former aims at restoring the functional ability through the recovery of the neuro-musculoskeletal system, while the latter consists of a series of strategies that the patient has to learn to get access to a determinate function.

The choice is guided by the distance from the injury: a very early intervention exploits the plasticity mechanisms and the subject has a better chance to regain functions working with a restorative approach, trying to re-learn the more correct patterns. In contrast, when the distance from the injury increases and the residual potential relearning declines, the compensatory approach is usually preferred.

In the last years, the advent of advanced technologies in rehabilitation and, specifically, of Virtual Reality (VR)-based devices, has unfolded new possibilities in the world of rehabilitation [13–16]. VR is a promising strategy that incorporates many principles recognized as crucial for motor relearning, such as high intensity, repetitive and goal-oriented tasks, enhanced synchronized sensorial cues and active participation [17–19]. Furthermore, the combination of biofeedback has already shown to be effective [20]. The virtual environment is suitable for a tailor-made work too, as it can be adapted to the individual needs of each patient.

Platforms integrating immersive VR (IVR) with an instrumented treadmill and a motion capture system combine assessment and rehabilitation purposes. Instrumented treadmills are able to acquire gait data recording many consecutive steps, differently to traditional gait analysis devices. This allows to evaluate the step variability, which is particularly relevant in the ataxic population [21], who exhibits an increased variability in terms of step length, excursion, and timing of hip, knee, and ankle joints [5].

VR training with these kinds of platforms has been previously studied on children affected by Cerebral Palsy (CP) [22] and with ABI [23].

Since there are no studies about the rehabilitation of ataxic children and adolescents by means of similar platforms, the aim of this work is to investigate the potential of the use of IVR, biofeedback, and treadmill walking combined with physiotherapy, in this population and to highlight the advantages given by the assessment of the multistep gait analysis in ataxic subjects.

2. Methods

2.1. Participants. Patients affected by ABI who exhibited ataxia secondary to trauma, brain tumor, stroke, encephalitis, anoxia, or arteriovenous malformation were recruited at the Scientific Institute Medea. The inclusion criteria were: signs of ataxia, identified by clinical assessment; age between 7 and 30; mild to moderate gross motor ability–level I–III of Gross Motor Function Classification System (GMFCS) [24, 25]; compliance and ability to understand and execute test instructions. The exclusion criteria were: severe muscle spasticity, a diagnosis of severe learning disability or behavioral problems, and visual difficultiesthat would impact on function and participation.

The protocol was approved by the ethics committee of Scientific Institute Medea and conducted in accordance with the Declaration of Helsinki. Patients or their parents subscribed a written informed consent.

2.2. Gait Real-Time Analysis Interactive Lab. Medea is equipped with an IVR system, the Gait Real-time Analysis Interactive Lab (GRAIL) by Motekforce Link (the Netherlands). This device integrates IVR with an instrumented treadmill and a motion capture system, that can be used for rehabilitation and assessment purposes. It includes a semicircular screen where the virtual reality environment is projected and a dual-belt treadmill, which integrates two force platforms and is synchronized with the projected environment. To assure a safe use, a harness and two lateral handrails are used (Figure 1(a)).

As a rehabilitative tool, the GRAIL provides biofeedback based on kinematic or kinetic gait features, allowing to train left and right body side thanks to the split-belt treadmill, and to coach balance and coordination control.

As assessment tool, the GRAIL is equipped with 10 optoelectronic cameras and three video cameras that, together with the two force platforms, can be used to acquire spatial, temporal, kinematic, and kinetic parameters of many consecutive steps in real time. These data can also be exploited as visual feedback to the operator and patient during the training.

2.3. Study Design and Intervention. Patients underwent 20 45-minute sessions of training with GRAIL plus 20 45-minute sessions of physiotherapy within one month. The therapeutic scheme was customized over the patients' need, tailoring the setting and the difficulty of proposed exergames on patients' skills, and it was oriented to the recovery of balance ability and of a correct locomotion pattern.

The balance training encompassed left-right shifting of body weight, monopodalic support, or balance maintenance while receiving external swinging stimuli (Figure 1(b)).

The gait training included gradually increasing difficulty exercises, from the control of the center of mass during walking without the upper limb support to more challenging tasks, like multitasking activities during walking, external perturbations (i.e., changes of treadmill slope, single belt sliding, mediolateral belt sways) and locomotion with decreased step width (i.e., one belt only activated). The kinetics and kinematics of target districts were projected in real time as feedback and overlaid to healthy reference values (Figure 1(c)).

Concerning physiotherapy, exercises were aimed at reinforcing the activities trained with VR, focusing on monopodalic balance training, walking on narrow path, walking on irregular path, get up and down the stairs, jump and run.

2.4. Outcome Measures. Patients' performance was evaluated before (T0) and after (T1) rehabilitation by means of functional scales and three-dimensional gait analysis.

The Scale for the Assessment and Rating of Ataxia (SARA) is a scale developed to quantify the severity of the ataxia from 0 (no ataxia) to 40 (severe ataxia). It includes motor tasks (that investigate the most common deficits, like imbalance, tremors, dysmetria, and rhythmic movements) and speech [26].

The gross motor ability of patients was assessed by means of Gross Motor Function Measure (GMFM-88): it ranges from 0 (severe deficit) to 100 and is composed of 88 items divided into 5 sections: A–lying and rolling; B–sitting; C–crawling and kneeling; D–standing; E–walking, running, and jumping [27].

The six-minute walking test (6MWT) evaluated walking endurance [28], measuring the distance covered over six minutes of self-paced walking along a standardized path.

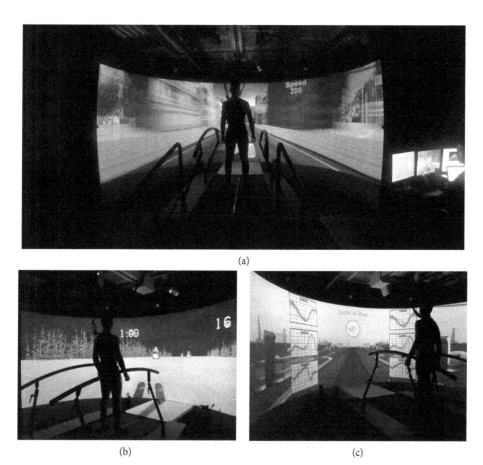

FIGURE 1: (a) The GRAIL system. (b) Example of balance training exercise: the subject performs a slalom on the snow by shifting the body weight left and right. (c) Example of exercise to train locomotion and gait pattern: the kinetics and kinematics of joints during walking are projected in real time as feedback.

The Berg Balance Scale (BBS) assesses patients' fall risk and was used to evaluate patient's balance ability [29]. BBS is composed of 14 items scored with a five-point scale (0–4) according to functional level. The total score ranges from 0 (high fall risks) to 56 (low fall risks).

The 3D gait analysis (GA) was acquired on the GRAIL. Subjects were asked to walk wearing socks for an adaptation period of six minutes on the instrumented treadmill at a fixed velocity, customized over the patient's ability. Then, about 20 steps were acquired. During this assessment no biofeedback was provided with the GRAIL.

At the end of the treatment, qualitative improvements of each patient in terms of activities and participation were collected by patients and their families.

2.5. Data Analysis. Concerning GA data, the Gait Offline Analysis Tool was used to load the .mox file, to filter data (2nd order Butterworth filter, cut off frequency at 6 Hz), to exclude strides with misplaced feet (e.g., foot on both belts or on the opposite belt) and to export the kinematics and kinetics traces in a .csv file. The gait parameters were then computed with an ad-hoc MATLAB (The MathWorks®) software that, for each step, extracted gait features at hip, knee, and ankle levels for left and right side. Since ataxia is not characterized by laterality, the mean value between the right and left parameters was considered.

The gait parameters computed were: the stance period, computed as the percentage ratio between the stance phase (from the initial contact of foot and the toe off of the same limb) and the gait cycle, the step length, the step width, and the gait speed as spatio-temporal parameters; the peak flexion power for the ankle, knee, and hip joints for kinetic evaluations; the peak of flexion and extension for the three joints in the sagittal plane; the range of motion (ROM) of hip abduction/adduction, and the ROM of pelvis in the three planes (tilt, obliquity and rotation).

To evaluate the variability of gait, for each parameter the coefficient of variation (CV) was computed as the percentage ratio between the SD and the mean of the steps of each i-th subject [30], as in Equation (1).

$$CV_i = \frac{SD_i}{mean_i} 100. \qquad (1)$$

The coefficient of variation is not appropriate for negative datasets or with values around zero [31]. For parameters that assumed values ≤ 0, the SD has been reported.

The normality of the data was checked with the Shapiro–Wilk test. Since not all the measures were normal, nonparametric statistical analysis was carried out; medians and interquartile ranges are reported.

A within-group comparison was performed by means of the Wilcoxon test.

To help the interpretation of GA, patients outcomes were compared with those obtained by a healthy control group of 16 subjects (mean (SD) age of 10.0 (1.3) years, 15 males). These data were included in a previous study on autism [32]. The between-group comparison of GA outcomes was performed with Mann–Whitney U-test.

The analysis was carried out with IBM SPSS Statistics v15 and the significance level was set at 5%.

3. Results

According to the inclusion criteria, 11 subjects (age from 9 to 27) were recruited for the study. Demographic characteristics are summarized in Table 1. Accidentally, only patients with GMFCS level of II agreed to participate.

Table 2 shows the results in terms of functional scales.

The signs of ataxia significantly diminished across the training, with a reduction of 20% of the SARA. GMFM-88, and its subscales, 6MWT and balance ability showed significant improvements after the treatment.

Table 3 summarizes results obtained in terms of GA.

A significant variation of step length, gait speed, maximal ankle power, maximal degree of knee flexion, and ROM of hip during abduction was obtained over time. Furthermore, the significant differences observed with respect to the healthy control group in terms of step length, gait speed, maximal ankle power, maximal knee extension and ROM of pelvic rotation disappeared after treatment.

Finally, the CV of step length, gait speed, maximal ankle power, and ROM of pelvic obliquity and rotation significantly reduced after therapy. This was supported by an overall trend of reduction of CV in almost all the parameters.

All the data were collected for the whole group.

Concerning qualitative changes of each patient in terms of activities and participation, improvements for 9 patients out of 11 were observed. Specifically, three patients had significant improvement in terms of safety during activities in standing and walking; three patients, that had reported difficulties in dual task activities such as walking and speaking before the treatment, enhanced their ability to fix a trajectory and keep balance while interacting with other people; one patient was able to go out alone, using public transports after the treatment; two patients showed pain decrease due to the improvement of their gait pattern.

4. Discussion

Children and adolescents with ataxia exhibit coordinative limitations, which often affect their locomotion and balance. In recent years, more and more attention has been devoted to training that exploit the potential of VR in rehabilitative context, but up to now only few studies described improvements on children with ABI treated with VR [23, 33], and, to our knowledge, none specifically on ataxic patients.

This manuscript aims at investigating the feasibility and effectiveness of a rehabilitation program that exploits IVR, biofeedback, and treadmill walking coupled to physiotherapy

TABLE 1: Demographic features of the patients included into the study.

Age (y)	16.0 (5.0)
Gender (M/F)	6/5
Time from injury (y)	4.7 (6.7)
Etiology (tumor/AVM/TBI)	9/1/1
GMFCS (I/II/III)	0/11/0

Data are reported as median (interquartile ranges). M: male; F: female; y: years; AVM: arteriovenous malformation; TBI: traumatic brain injury; GM-FCS: gross motor function classification system.

TABLE 2: Results of functional scales before (T0) and after (T1) training.

	T0	T1	p-value
SARA	10.5 (4.5)	8.5 (2.8)	0.012
GMFM-88	97.0 (4.0)	98.0 (2.5)	0.004
GMFM-D	92.0 (4.0)	97.0 (3.5)	0.008
GMFM-E	90.0 (14.0)	94.0 (7.5)	0.001
6MWT	500 (96)	548 (100)	0.005
BBS	53.0 (3.5)	54.0 (2.0)	0.016

Data are reported as median (interquartile ranges). p-values refer to the non parametric paired Wilcoxon test. SARA: Scale for the assessment and rating of ataxia; GMFM-88: gross motor function measure expressed as percentage, dimension D (standing) and E (walking); 6MWT: six minute walking test; BBS: Berg balance scale.

for the recovery of locomotion and balance in adolescents affected by ataxia secondary to ABI.

The study showed that the training was feasible and well tolerated by patients. No subject withdrew from the study, and patients and their families gave positive feedbacks in terms of engagement and functional recovery.

Our findings support that 20 sessions of treadmill training augmented by IVR together with 20 sessions of physiotherapy are effective for a significant improvement of balance and locomotion functions in ataxic adolescents. The ataxia level was significantly diminished, the gross motor ability was significantly improved in terms of standing and walking, and the balance and the walking endurance improved as well.

In terms of GA, subjects showed at T0 reduced gait speed, shorter step length and swing phase, diminished maximal ankle power, reduced knee flexion, and a generalized increase in step variability, with respect to their healthy pairs. These gait features well match with the typical clinical signs of cerebellar ataxic gait [3–6].

Data obtained after the proposed treatment showed improvements towards the pattern of typically developing subjects in terms of step length, gait speed, kinetic of the movement at ankle, and kinematic of knee, hip and pelvic joints. Evidence of reduction of the variability among steps was also obtained, suggesting the achievement of a more regular gait pattern. Furthermore, a reduction of step width, even if not significant, was observed and the two patients that were affected by knee hyperextension showed improvements after the combination of IVR and physiotherapy treatment.

TABLE 3: Temporal, spatial, kinematics and kinetics characteristics acquired with gait analysis on GRAIL before (T0) and after (T1) training.

	T0	T1	Healthy	p-val T0 vs T1	p-val T0 vs healthy	p-val T1 vs healthy
Stance%	69.4 (1.7)	69.1 (2.1)	67 (2.5)	0.123	*0.001*	*0.008*
CV%	4 (1.6)	3 (1.8)	2.1 (1.3)	0.175	*0.013*	0.094
Step length [cm]	36.6 (2.5)	42.7 (8)	42.1 (10)	*0.001*	*0.019*	0.863
CV%	12 (3.6)	9.4 (3.4)	7.5 (2.3)	*0.001*	*0.004*	0.225
Step width [cm]	18.9 (7)	16.6 (4.1)	15 (5)	0.206	0.190	0.387
CV%	16.9 (6.2)	19.6 (8.9)	14 (5)	0.147	0.226	0.132
Gait speed [cm/s]	66.9 (10.7)	78.1 (12.1)	88.4 (24.9)	*0.001*	*0.000*	0.057
CV%	10.2 (4.8)	8.5 (3.2)	5.4 (1.1)	*0.019*	*0.000*	*0.000*
Max ankle power [W]	0.9 (0.2)	1.3 (0.5)	1.3 (1.3)	*0.020*	*0.008*	0.477
CV%	31.5 (15)	24.1 (8.5)	28.2 (12.4)	*0.002*	0.215	0.692
Max knee power [W]	0.6 (0.3)	0.6 (0.3)	0.9 (0.3)	0.322	*0.003*	*0.014*
CV%	27 (12.9)	26.1 (7.4)	29.8 (13.6)	0.492	0.895	0.732
Max hip power [W]	0.4 (0.2)	0.5 (0.1)	0.9 (0.4)	0.105	*0.001*	*0.016*
CV%	25.3 (8.7)	23.1 (7.6)	20.8 (9.3)	0.193	0.179	0.895
Max ankle flex [°]	11.9 (2.3)	13.9 (3.1)	17.6 (2.7)	0.067	*0.001*	*0.002*
CV%	11.2 (7.5)	12.3 (7)	7.3 (4.3)	0.520	*0.019*	*0.021*
Max ankle ext [°]	6.1 (3.5)	6.7 (4.9)	5.4 (4.7)	0.577	0.711	0.289
SD*	2.2 (1.2)	2.3 (1)	2.9 (2.5)	0.898	0.474	0.474
Max knee flex [°]	57 (6.8)	59 (5.2)	63.2 (5)	*0.032*	*0.001*	*0.005*
CV%	6.2 (2.9)	6.2 (2.2)	3.8 (1.7)	0.240	*0.004*	*0.007*
Max knee ext [°]	−3.1 (3.4)	−3 (4.3)	0.1 (4.4)	0.966	*0.025*	0.051
SD*	2.2 (0.5)	1.9 (0.8)	1.5 (1.1)	0.966	0.160	0.289
Max hip flex [°]	33.3 (7.3)	35.3 (9.4)	32.4 (10.2)	0.278	0.786	0.388
CV%	6 (2.3)	5.8 (1.5)	5.5 (2.3)	0.638	0.245	0.473
Max hip ext [°]	2.2 (7.5)	1.2 (7.8)	3.4 (9.6)	0.413	0.336	0.388
SD*	2.6 (1.1)	2.5 (1.1)	2.1 (0.8)	0.700	0.098	0.160
ROM hip abd [°]	9.2 (4.3)	11.9 (4)	11.7 (4)	*0.001*	0.145	0.863
CV%	16.9 (7.9)	17 (3.9)	15.3 (1.9)	0.365	0.097	0.287
ROM pelvic tilt [°]	4.9 (0.9)	5.2 (1.8)	4.2 (1.2)	0.102	*0.022*	*0.005*
CV%	30.2 (4.5)	28.7 (3.1)	26 (6.2)	0.240	*0.040*	0.174
ROM pelvic ob [°]	5.7 (2.1)	6.4 (1.9)	6.6 (2.4)	0.413	0.604	0.980
CV%	23.7 (4.8)	18.3 (7.2)	17.7 (4.8)	*0.010*	*0.006*	0.415
ROM pelvic rot [°]	10.8 (4.4)	11.5 (4.7)	8.4 (5.1)	0.175	0.120	*0.013*
CV%	28.1 (9.1)	28.5 (6.6)	28.8 (8.9)	*0.042*	0.711	*0.748*

Data are reported as median (interquartile ranges); CV: coefficient of variation; SD: standard deviations; ROM: range of motion; flex: flexion; ext: extension; p-val: p values. P values refer to the nonparametric paired Wilcoxon test in column "T0 vs T1", while they refer to the nonparametric Mann–Whitney U-test in column "T0 vs healthy" and "T1 vs healthy".

Comparison among our results and what was previously reported is limited by the paucity and low-level of evidence reported on ataxia [7]. Previous case-studies have shown some improvements induced by treadmill training or virtual exergames on ataxic adults. Three case reports evaluated five adult ataxic patients (three secondary to traumatic brain injury and two secondary to tumor resection) who underwent trunk exercises and treadmill training with body weight support (15 and 30 sessions). The participants obtained some improvements in terms of BBS and gait [34–36]. Differently, no evidence of improvements induced by a four-week training with VR exergames on five ataxic adults have been reported in terms of balance ability and gait parameters, although SARA highlighted progresses [37].

The effectiveness of IVR treadmill training plus physiotherapy on ataxic adolescents has never been investigated.

However, its performance in young patients with ABI has been previously studied [23], with comparable improvements in terms of gross motor abilities (GMFM-D improved of 6.6% in ABI and of 5.4% in ataxic patients; GMFM-E improved of 11.5% in ABI and of 4.4% in ataxic patients), but smaller ones in terms of 6MWT (improvements of 60.0% in ABI and of 9.6% in ataxic subjects). However the different mean value at baseline (277 m vs 500 m in the current work) may have limited the improvements due to ceiling effect (95% of confidence interval in age-matched healthy population is 651–742 m [38]).

Modifications induced by training based on IVR and physiotherapy look effective in modifying both the locomotion pattern as a whole and the control of the local districts in ataxic patients. Indeed, the present work supports that the treatment induces a modification of the gait kinematics. With respect to other technologically-advanced tools, such as robot-assisted gait training applied in the context of ABI rehabilitation, the effects obtained combining physiotherapy with IVR treadmill training seems to be particularly promising at ankle and knee levels. Indeed, a previous study on 23 children with ABI showed improvements induced by 20 sessions of robot-assisted gait training in terms of gross motor abilities, walking endurance and gait kinematics at hip level, while no changes were observed for more distal districts [39].

One of the strengths of the present work is that we exploited the GRAIL technology to quantitatively analyze the variability of the locomotion, which is a crucial aspect of ataxic patients. Their high gait irregularity prevents from obtaining reliable results by using standard gait analysis, during which the user usually selects one or few steps that should represent the gait pattern of a single patient. Due to the specificity of ataxia, it is mandatory to use a multistep approach to quantify ataxic locomotion. Our results, based on the multistep gait analysis available through GRAIL, give encouraging evidence of reduction of step variability, toward the pattern of healthy individuals.

A limit of this work is that, although GMFCS has been used in the past for the description of patients with ABI [25], we are not aware of any systematic validation in children with this pathology. Furthermore, the increased effectiveness of a combined IVR treadmill training plus physiotherapy with respect to traditional approaches has to be deepened in the future by means of randomized controlled trials. The generalizability of the results of the present work is currently limited by the little sample size, the heterogeneity of patients in terms of age, and the absence of a control group.

However, it is noteworthy that the population analyzed had a median (interquartile) distance from trauma of 4.7 (6.7) years. As studied by Kuper and colleagues, the spontaneous recovery of balance ability in children after cerebellar tumor resection is relevant over the first three months post-surgery and continues over the first year post surgery [40]. The recovery of the remaining motor ability shown in the present work may thus be ascribed to the rehabilitation treatment.

5. Conclusion

To conclude, the present study shows the first evidence of the effectiveness of immersive virtual reality treadmill training together with standard physiotherapy on ataxic adolescents. The intervention proposed was customized on patients' need; it was ecological and highly motivating. Forty sessions of such training produced significant improvements in locomotion pattern, balance, and reduction of gait variability, towards healthy references. Finally, although specific goals in terms of activity and participation were not defined, the proposed protocol improved patients' participation to social life, as reported both by patients and their parents.

What This Paper Adds

(i) Assessment of preliminary effectiveness of IVR devices in the ataxic patient rehabilitation.
(ii) Modifiability of locomotion and balance of ataxic adolescents, even in chronic condition.
(iii) Reliable evaluation of gait pattern and step variability in ataxic population.

Abbreviations

VR:	Virtual reality
GMFCS:	Gross motor function classification system
GRAIL:	Gait real-time analysis interactive lab
SARA:	Scale for the assessment and rating of ataxia
GMFM-88:	Gross motor function measure-88 items
6MWT:	Six minute walking test
BBS:	Berg balance scale
GA:	Gait analysis
ROM:	Range of motion
CV:	Coefficient of variation
AVM:	Arteriovenous malformation
TBI:	Traumatic brain injury
SD:	Standard deviations.

Authors' Contributions

Bi.E., Be.E., G.R., and S.S. substantially contributed to conception and design of the study. P.E. analyzed data. P.E., P.D., and Bi.E interpreted results. P.E., P.D. were the major contributors in writing the manuscript. P.D. was the major responsible of data acquisition. All authors critically read and approved the final manuscript. Elisabetta Peri and Daniele Panzeri equally contributing authors.

Acknowledgments

Authors would like to thank Alessandro Crippa and Silvia Busti for their help in collecting data of the healthy control group. Authors also thank the physiotherapists that performed functional evaluations and patients and their families.

References

[1] W. Ilg, H. Golla, P. Thier, and M. A. Giese, "Specific influences of cerebellar dysfunctions on gait," *Brain*, vol. 130, no. 3, pp. 786–798, 2007.

[2] H.-C. Diener and J. Dichgans, "Pathophysiology of cerebellar ataxia," *Movement Disorders*, vol. 7, no. 2, pp. 95–109, 1992.

[3] W. Hoogkamer, S. M. Bruijn, S. Sunaert, S. P. Swinnen, F. Van Calenbergh, and J. Duysens, "Toward new sensitive measures to evaluate gait stability in focal cerebellar lesion patients," *Gait & Posture*, vol. 41, no. 2, pp. 592–596, 2015.

[4] E. Buckley, C. Mazzà, and A. McNeill, "A systematic review of the gait characteristics associated with cerebellar ataxia," *Gait & Posture*, vol. 60, pp. 154–163, 2018.

[5] Y. Moon, J. Sung, R. An, M. E. Hernandez, and J. J. Sosnoff, "Gait variability in people with neurological disorders: a systematic review and meta-analysis," *Human Movement Science*, vol. 47, pp. 197–208, 2016.

[6] S. M. Morton and A. J. Bastian, "Mechanisms of cerebellar gait ataxia," *The cerebellum*, vol. 6, no. 1, pp. 79–86, 2007.

[7] A. Marquer, G. Barbieri, and D. Pérennou, "The assessment and treatment of postural disorders in cerebellar ataxia: a systematic review," *Annals of Physical and Rehabilitation Medicine*, vol. 57, no. 2, pp. 67–78, 2014.

[8] I. Miyai, M. Ito, N. Hattori et al., "Cerebellar ataxia rehabilitation trial in degenerative Cerebellar diseases," *Neurorehabilitation and Neural Repair*, vol. 26, no. 5, pp. 515–522, 2012.

[9] W. Ilg, M. Synofzik, D. Brötz, S. Burkard, M. A. Giese, and L. Schöls, "Intensive coordinative training improves motor performance in degenerative cerebellar disease," *Neurology*, vol. 73, no. 22, pp. 1823–1830, 2009.

[10] W. Ilg, D. Brötz, S. Burkard, M. A. Giese, L. Schöls, and M. Synofzik, "Long-term effects of coordinative training in degenerative cerebellar disease," *Movement Disorders*, vol. 25, no. 13, pp. 2239–2246, 2010.

[11] K. Armutlu, R. Karabudak, and G. Nurlu, "Physiotherapy approaches in the treatment of ataxic multiple sclerosis: a pilot study," *Neurorehabilitation and Neural Repair*, vol. 15, no. 3, pp. 203–211, 2001.

[12] J. Marsden and C. Harris, "Cerebellar ataxia: pathophysiology and rehabilitation," *Clinical Rehabilitation*, vol. 25, no. 3, pp. 195–216, 2011.

[13] W. Ilg, C. Schatton, J. Schicks, M. A. Giese, L. Schöls, and M. Synofzik, "Video game-based coordinative training improves ataxia in children with degenerative ataxia," *Neurology*, vol. 79, no. 20, pp. 2056–2060, 2012.

[14] M. K. Holden, "Virtual environments for motor rehabilitation: review," *CyberPsychology & Behavior*, vol. 8, no. 3, pp. 187–211, 2005.

[15] C. Cho, W. Hwang, S. Hwang, and Y. Chung, "Treadmill training with virtual reality improves gait, balance, and muscle strength in children with cerebral palsy," *The Tohoku Journal of Experimental Medicine*, vol. 238, no. 3, pp. 213–218, 2016.

[16] N. S. Hamed and M. S. Abd-elwahab, "Pedometer-based gait training in children with spastic hemiparetic cerebral palsy: a randomized controlled study," *Clinical Rehabilitation*, vol. 25, no. 2, pp. 157–165, 2011.

[17] J. W. Krakauer, "Motor learning: its relevance to stroke recovery and neurorehabilitation," *Current Opinion in Neurology*, vol. 19, no. 1, pp. 84–90, 2006.

[18] E. J. Lyons, "Cultivating engagement and enjoyment in exergames using feedback, challenge, and rewards," *Games for Health Journal*, vol. 4, no. 1, pp. 12–18, 2015.

[19] H. Huang, S. L. Wolf, and J. He, "Recent developments in biofeedback for neuromotor rehabilitation," *Journal of Neuroengineering and Rehabilitation*, vol. 3, Article ID 11, 2006.

[20] A. T. C. Booth, A. I. Buizer, J. Harlaar, F. Steenbrink, and M. M. van der Krogt, "Immediate effects of immersive biofeedback on gait in children with cerebral palsy," *Archives of Physical Medicine and Rehabilitation*, vol. 100, no. 4, pp. 598–605, 2019.

[21] W. Ilg and D. Timmann, "Gait ataxia-specific cerebellar influences and their rehabilitation," *Movement Disorders*, vol. 28, no. 11, pp. 1566–1575, 2013.

[22] C. Gagliardi, A. C. Turconi, E. Biffi et al., "Immersive virtual reality to improve walking abilities in cerebral palsy: a pilot study," *Annals of Biomedical Engineering*, vol. 46, no. 9, pp. 1376–1384, 2018.

[23] E. Biffi, E. Beretta, A. Cesareo et al., "An immersive virtual reality platform to enhance walking ability of children with acquired brain injuries," *Methods of Information in Medicine*, vol. 56, no. 02, pp. 119–126, 2017.

[24] R. Palisano, P. Rosenbaum, S. Walter, D. Russell, E. Wood, and B. Galuppi, "Development and reliability of a system to classify gross motor function in children with cerebral palsy," *Developmental Medicine & Child Neurology*, vol. 39, no. 4, pp. 214–223, 1997.

[25] M. Jackman, I. Novak, and N. Lannin, "Effectiveness of functional hand splinting and the cognitive orientation to occupational performance (CO-OP) approach in children with cerebral palsy and brain injury: two randomized controlled trial protocols," *BMC Neurology*, vol. 14, no. 1, p. 144, 2014.

[26] H. Hartley, B. Pizer, S. Lane et al., "Inter-rater reliability and validity of two ataxia rating scales in children with brain tumours," *Child's Nervous System*, vol. 31, no. 5, pp. 693–697, 2015.

[27] M. Linder-Lucht, V. Othmer, M. Walther et al., "Gross motor function measure-traumatic brain injury study group. validation of the gross motor function measure for use in children and adolescents with traumatic brain injuries," *Pediatrics*, vol. 120, no. 4, pp. e880–e886, 2007.

[28] C. Andersson, L. Asztalos, and E. Mattsson, "Six-minute walk test in adults with cerebral palsy. A study of reliability," *Clinical Rehabilitation*, vol. 20, no. 6, pp. 488–495, 2006.

[29] S.-M. Gan, L.-C. Tung, Y.-H. Tang, and C.-H. Wang, "Psychometric properties of functional balance assessment in children with cerebral palsy," *Neurorehabilitation and Neural Repair*, vol. 22, no. 6, pp. 745–753, 2008.

[30] C. E. Brown, "Coefficient of variation," *in: Applied Multivariate Statistics in Geohydrology and Related Sciences*, Springer, Berlin Heidelberg, Berlin, Heidelbergpp. 155–157, 1998.

[31] L. Sachs, *Applied Statistics : A Handbook of Techniques*, Springer, New York, 1984.

[32] E. Biffi, C. Costantini, S. B. Ceccarelli et al., "Gait pattern and motor performance during discrete gait perturbation in children

with autism spectrum disorders," *Frontiers in Psychology*, vol. 9, 2018.

[33] E. Biffi, E. Beretta, E. Diella et al., "Gait rehabilitation with a high tech platform based on virtual reality conveys improvements in walking ability of children suffering from acquired brain injury," in *37th Annual International Conference of the IEEE Engineering in Medicine and Biology Society (EMBC)*, IEEE, pp. 7406–7409, Milan, Italy, 2015.

[34] J. E. Freund and D. M. Stetts, "Use of trunk stabilization and locomotor training in an adult with cerebellar ataxia: a single system design," *Physiotherapy Theory and Practice*, vol. 26, no. 7, pp. 447–458, 2010.

[35] K. M. Gill-Body, R. A. Popat, S. W. Parker, and D. E. Krebs, "Rehabilitation of balance in two patients with cerebellar dysfunction," *Physical Therapy*, vol. 77, no. 5, pp. 534–552, 1997.

[36] R. Teixeira, V. R. Cavalcanti Furtado, S. R. de Mello, and E. Figueiredo, "Treadmill training for ataxic patients: a single-subject experimental design," *Clinical Rehabilitation*, vol. 22, no. 3, pp. 234–241, 2008.

[37] R.-Y. Wang, F.-Y. Huang, B.-W. Soong, S.-F. Huang, and Y.-R. Yang, "A randomized controlled pilot trial of game-based training in individuals with spinocerebellar ataxia type 3," *Scientific Reports*, vol. 8, no. 1, p. 7816, 2018.

[38] R. Geiger, A. Strasak, B. Treml et al., "Six-minute walk test in children and adolescents," *The Journal of Pediatrics*, vol. 150, no. 4, pp. 395–399.e2, 2007.

[39] E. Beretta, M. Romei, E. Molteni, P. Avantaggiato, and S. Strazzer, "Combined robotic-aided gait training and physical therapy improve functional abilities and hip kinematics during gait in children and adolescents with acquired brain injury," *Brain Injury*, vol. 29, no. 7-8, pp. 955–962, 2015.

[40] M. Küper, K. Döring, C. Spangenberg et al., "Location and restoration of function after cerebellar tumor removal—a longitudinal study of children and adolescents," *The Cerebellum*, vol. 12, no. 1, pp. 48–58, 2013.

15

A Novel CACNA1A Nonsense Variant [c.4054C>T (p.Arg1352*)] Causing Episodic Ataxia Type 2

Sean Lance ⓘ, Stuart Mossman, and Gemma Poke

Wellington Hospital, Wellington, New Zealand

Correspondence should be addressed to Sean Lance; sean.lance@huttvalleydhb.org.nz

Academic Editor: Majaz Moonis

Episodic ataxia is a heterogenous group of uncommon neurological disorders characterised by recurrent episodes of vertigo, dysarthria, and ataxia for which a variety of different genetic variations have been implicated. Episodic ataxia type two (EA2) is the most common and also has the largest number of identified causative genetic variants. Treatment with acetazolamide is effective in improving symptoms, so accurate diagnosis is essential. However, a large proportion of patients with EA2 have negative genetic testing. We present a patient with a typical history of EA2 who had a novel variant in the CACNA1A gene not previously described. Report of such variations is important in learning more about the disease and improving diagnostic yield for the patient.

1. Case Report

We describe the case of a 47-year-old male who presented to neurology clinic with recurrent episodes of acute vertigo and unsteadiness, associated with severe nausea and vomiting. The symptoms of vertigo and ataxia typically lasted 1–3 hours, with persistent nausea often for the following 24 hours. He was having several episodes per week, with the observation by himself that they were more likely to occur in warmer weather and on exertion, with an improvement in symptoms when attempting to cool himself.

These episodes had been recurrent since approximately age 10 and were previously labelled as seizures. However, there was no reported loss of consciousness or observed seizure-like activity. Additionally, treatment with an unknown anticonvulsant (presumed to be phenytoin given his age) in his teenage years had actually exacerbated the symptoms.

Other relevant history includes intermittent migraines without any other associated neurological symptoms. He had a mild intellectual disability recognised since childhood which was unquantified. The patient was unaware of any family members being affected by similar problems and specifically no reports of suffering from ataxia, seizures, or migraine. No further history was obtainable directly from his family members.

On examination there was mild dysarthria. Eye movements revealed slightly jerky pursuit with a small target which was normal with a larger target; saccades were normal and there was no nystagmus. Head impulse test was normal. He had mild intention tremor on finger nose testing and gait assessment revealed a broad based ataxic gait with an inability to tandem walk with an otherwise normal neurological examination.

MRI brain was unremarkable. Previous EEG from 1991 was normal.

Given his history of recurrent attacks of vertigo and ataxia, he was started on acetazolamide with a significant reduction in symptoms, in both severity and frequency, to once per month, compared to several times per week.

Genetic testing showed a novel heterozygous variant in exon 25 of the *CACNA1A* gene, c.4054C>T (p.Arg1352*). Nonsense mutations are an established cause of episodic ataxia type 2, and the variant did not appear in the GnomAD population database. This variant was therefore predicted to be pathogenic. This finding confirmed the diagnosis of episodic ataxia type 2 and represents another newly identified variant which can now be searched for in other patients.

Referral to the genetic service was made, with his family members declining screening.

2. Discussion

Episodic ataxia (EA) is rare, with incidence thought to be less than 1 per 100,000 [1]. Several different types of episodic ataxia have been described, with types one and two making up the majority of cases. EA type two (EA2) is the most common type and characterised by recurrent episodes of vertigo, ataxia, and dysarthria which typically last for a period of hours (as compared to EA type one (EA1) where symptoms last only minutes) [1, 2]. Additionally, findings of ataxia, dysarthria, and nystagmus may persist in between attacks in EA2 but are not classically a persistent feature of EA1. Attacks may be precipitated by various environmental factors including heat and exertion, as well as drugs such as caffeine and phenytoin [1, 2].

The underlying pathological mechanism for the episodic ataxias likely relates to abnormal neurotransmission, explained by the seven described subtypes of EA having underlying variants in genes coding for various channelopathies, pumps, and transporters [1].

In EA2, the genetic abnormality involves the *CACNA1A* gene located on chromosome 19p13. This gene encodes the alpha-1A subunit of the P/Q-type voltage-gated calcium channel. This is found throughout the nervous system but in higher density in the cerebellum, accounting for the prominent cerebellar symptoms and signs [3].

There have been over 50 different mutations described with the majority being nonsense mutations leading to loss of function of this channel [1–4]. These lead to reduced calcium currents and alteration in calcium dependent neurotransmitter release and subsequently the typical phenotypic presentation as described.

In addition to EA2, the *CACNA1A* gene is implicated in at least two other autosomal dominant neurological disorders: familial hemiplegic migraine type 1 (FHM1) and spinocerebellar ataxia type 6 (SCA6). In general, missense mutations are associated with FHM1 and trinucleotide (CAG) expansions associated with SCA6. However, a number of reports more recently have identified a significant lack of genotype-phenotype correlation, for example, missense mutations causing EA2 [5–7]. Also reported is the significant variability of clinical phenotype within families who have the same underlying mutation [8], a complex feature of the *CACNA1A* gene which is not yet fully understood.

Additionally, *CACNA1A* gene mutations are known to be associated with epilepsy and biallelic mutations have been reported with an epileptic encephalopathy associated with progressive neurological decline, adding further to the complexity of this gene and the wide phenotypic variability [9].

Despite multiple mutations being described, 30–50% of patients with the classic clinical presentation of EA2 have negative genetic testing [1–3]. This observation, as well as the lack of genotype-phenotype correlation, makes diagnosis and subsequent familial screening difficult.

Our patient had a typical clinical presentation with typical associated features such as migraine and interictal dysarthria and ataxia. Initially thought to represent seizures, the description of his events fit well with a diagnosis of EA2 and also worsening of symptoms in EA2 is seen with phenytoin (which

we suspect he was treated with when he was younger, although we were not able to confirm). Additionally, intellectual disability and psychological symptoms are often seen in EA. These factors and the predicted response to acetazolamide make the diagnosis of EA2 reasonably secure. The nonsense variant in *CACNA1A*, whilst previously undescribed, is considered to be pathogenic.

With a large number of patients with EA2 not having an identifiable genetic abnormality a number of whole-genome sequencing studies are attempting to identify novel mutations in such patients. Maksemous et al. identified nine novel variants in 31 patients with EA2, of which six were missense changes [10]. Although it is unclear whether all of these new variants were likely to be pathogenic, these results do highlight the high proportion of patients *without* a known genetic mutation (52%) and also that variants in genes other than *CACNA1A* may well contribute to the EA2 phenotype [10].

3. Conclusion

The identification of a *CACNA1A* variant such as ours is important in the further characterisation of this disorder and can offer another target for testing in similar patients and those in whom the genetic abnormality remains unknown. This can assist with their ongoing management and with genetic counselling. Reporting of such variants and further research into whole-genome sequencing will help to expand our knowledge of EA2 and assist with genetic diagnosis and subsequent management.

References

[1] S. Kipfer and M. Strupp, "The Clinical Spectrum of Autosomal-Dominant Episodic Ataxias," *Movement Disorders Clinical Practice*, vol. 1, no. 4, pp. 285–290, 2014.

[2] J. Jen, G. W. Kim, and R. W. Baloh, "Clinical spectrum of episodic ataxia type 2," *Neurology*, vol. 62, no. 1, pp. 17–22, 2004.

[3] J. C. Jen, T. D. Graves, E. J. Hess, M. G. Hanna, R. C. Griggs, and R. W. Baloh, "Primary episodic ataxias: diagnosis, pathogenesis and treatment," *Brain*, vol. 130, no. 10, pp. 2484–2493, 2007.

[4] I. F. A. C. Fokkema, P. E. M. Taschner, G. C. P. Schaafsma, J. Celli, J. F. J. Laros, and J. T. den Dunnen, "LOVD v.2.0: the next generation in gene variant databases," *Human Mutation*, vol. 32, no. 5, pp. 557–563, 2011.

[5] K. Bürk, F. J. Kaiser, S. Tennstedt et al., "A novel missense mutation in *CACNA1A* evaluated by *in silico* protein modeling is associated with non-episodic spinocerebellar ataxia with slow progression," *European Journal of Medical Genetics*, vol. 57, no. 5, pp. 207–211, 2014.

[6] Š. Sivák, E. Kurča, A. Krajčiová et al., "Novel missense variant of CACNA1A gene: A case report of a family with episodic ataxia type 2," *Journal of the Neurological Sciences*, vol. 376, pp. 119-120, 2017.

[7] A. Petrovicova, M. Brozman, E. Kurca et al., "Novel missense variant of CACNA1A gene in a Slovak family with episodic ataxia type 2," *Biomedical Papers*, vol. 161, no. 1, pp. 107–110, 2017.

[8] L. Pradotto, M. Mencarelli, M. Bigoni, A. Milesi, A. Di Blasio, and A. Mauro, "Episodic ataxia and SCA6 within the same family due to the D302N CACNA1A gene mutation," *Journal of the Neurological Sciences*, vol. 371, pp. 81–84, 2016.

[9] K. Reinson, E. Õiglane-Shlik, I. Talvik et al., "Biallelic CACNA1A mutations cause early onset epileptic encephalopathy with progressive cerebral, cerebellar, and optic nerve atrophy," *American Journal of Medical Genetics Part A*, vol. 170, no. 8, pp. 2173–2176, 2016.

[10] N. Maksemous, B. Roy, R. A. Smith, and L. R. Griffiths, "Next-generation sequencing identifies novel *CACNA1A* gene mutations in episodic ataxia type 2," *Molecular Genetics & Genomic Medicine*, vol. 4, no. 2, pp. 211–222, 2016.

16

Novel Mutation in *CACNA1A* Associated with Activity-Induced Dystonia, Cervical Dystonia and Mild Ataxia

Benjamin Stampfl and **Dominic Fee**

Department of Neurology, Medical College of Wisconsin, Milwaukee, WI, USA

Correspondence should be addressed to Dominic Fee; nickkarin2@gmail.com

Academic Editor: Roberto Massa

CACNA1A encodes the pore-forming α1 subunit of the neuronal voltage-gated Cav2.1 (P/Q-type) channels, which are predominantly localized at the presynaptic terminals of the brain and cerebellar neurons and play an important role in controlling neurotransmitter release. Mutations in *CACNA1A* have been associated with several autosomal dominant neurologic disorders, including familial hemiplegic migraine type 1, episodic ataxia type 2 (EA2), and spinocerebellar ataxia type 6. A 37-year-old woman presented with a history of slowly progressive, activity-induced stiffness, and pain in her right leg since age 15 and cervical dystonia since age 20. She denied any right leg stiffness or pain at rest, but when she began to walk, her right foot turned in and her right leg stiffened up. She also had neck pain, stiffness, and spams. There was no family history of similar symptoms. On physical exam, her strength, tone, and reflexes were normal in all extremities at rest. There was mild head titubation and very mild past pointing on finger-to-nose testing. MRI of the brain and spinal cord was unremarkable. This patient's clinical picture was felt to be most consistent with paroxysmal kinesigenic dyskinesia, as she has attacks of dystonia that are triggered by voluntary movement, last from a few seconds to a minute, and are relieved with rest. She was trialed on carbidopa/levodopa without improvement. A dystonia panel showed two potentially pathologic mutations, one in *CACNA1A* and the other in *PNKP*, along with a variant of unknown significance in *ATP7B*. The mutation in *CACNA1A* is C2324 G < A. It is heterozygous, autosomal dominant, and computer modeling suggests pathogenicity. This mutation has not been reported previously and is likely the cause of her paroxysmal dystonia; dystonia is sometimes seen during episodes of ataxia in EA2, and *CACNA1A* knockout mice exhibit dystonia and cerebellar atrophy. After receiving her genetic diagnosis, the patient was trialed on acetazolamide without improvement in her dystonia symptoms. This is the second case report of a patient with cervical dystonia and cerebellar ataxia associated with a mutation in *CACNA1A*.

1. Introduction

CACNA1A encodes the pore-forming α1 subunit of the neuronal voltage-gated Cav2.1 (P/Q-type) channels, which are predominantly localized at the presynaptic terminals of the brain and cerebellar neurons and play an important role in controlling neurotransmitter release [1]. Additionally, it has been shown that *CACNA1A* contains an internal ribosome entry site that initiates the translation of a second protein called α1ACT, which is a transcription factor that is important in cerebellar development [2].

Mutations in *CACNA1A* have been associated with several autosomal dominant neurologic disorders, including familial hemiplegic migraine type 1 (FHM1), episodic ataxia type 2 (EA2), and spinocerebellar ataxia type 6 (SCA6) [3]. Familial hemiplegic migraine is characterized by severe headache preceded by an aura with unilateral weakness; the weakness is sometimes accompanied by other neurologic symptoms such as numbness, tingling, hemianopia, ataxia, and aphasia [4]. Patients usually recover fully between episodes, but some develop permanent ataxia. More than 25 pathologic variants in *CACNA1A* have been associated with FHM1, the majority of which are missense, gain-of-function mutations that result in increased calcium influx, and excessive neurotransmission [1]. EA2 is characterized by spells of ataxia lasting hours to days that can be accompanied by vertigo, diplopia, dysarthria, dystonia, and generalized weakness. Between spells, patients often demonstrate persistent nystagmus. In some cases, secondarily progressive ataxia can develop [5]. Unlike FHM1, EA2 is typically caused by loss-of-function mutations that lead to decreased calcium influx. More than 80 pathologic variants in *CACNA1A* have been associated with EA2 [1]. SCA6 is characterized by progressively worsening gait ataxia, dysarthria, dysphasia, diplopia, and mild cognitive impairment. It is caused by 20–33 CAG (polyglutamine) repeats near the C-terminus of the *CACNA1A* gene, which is important for channel function. These repeats may lead to abnormal aggregations of proteins and impaired channel function, contributing to cell dysfunction and death. While SCA6 was previously thought to cause only cerebellar damage, it is now known to cause degeneration of the cortex, thalamus, midbrain, pons, and medulla as well [6]. Dystonia occurs in up to 25% of patients with SCA6. Acetazolamide has been shown to reduce the number of ataxia episodes [7]. There is clinical overlap between FHM1, EA2, and SCA6; about 50% of patients with EA2 also have migraines, and episodic headaches and nausea are also common in SCA6 [1].

2. Case

We report the case of a 37-year-old woman with a history of slowly progressive, activity-induced stiffness and pain in her right leg since age 15. Her birth and early childhood history were unremarkable. The patient's symptoms began as a limp in her right leg around age 15; she denied any illnesses, exposures, or trauma around this time. Additionally, at age 20, the patient began having neck pain and stiffness, with occasional neck spasms associated with decreased range of motion.

When evaluated in clinic, she denied any right leg stiffness or pain at rest, but when she began to walk, her right foot turned in and her right leg, knee, proximal thigh, and hip stiffened up. She denied any numbness, tingling, or burning. She denied significant right arm, left arm, or left leg symptoms. The patient denied any gait instability or feeling of imbalance. The patient was using a cane and wearing left and right leg braces, which helped with her walking. She endorsed great difficulty with stairs and with walking long distances. There was no family history of similar symptoms. On physical exam, her strength, tone, and reflexes were normal in all extremities at rest. She also has mild retrocolis, right laterocolis, and right torticolis at rest. There was mild head titubation and very mild past pointing on finger-to-nose testing. There were no other signs of dysmetria or ataxia on exam. MRI of the brain and spinal cord was unremarkable. EMG/NCS of the left arm was unremarkable; lower extremity study was deferred because of recently receiving botulinum toxin injections to the right leg. In light of her history, symptoms, and physical exam, a tentative diagnosis of activity-induced dystonia was made. Given the possibility of it being dopamine-responsive dystonia, the patient was trialed on carbidopa/levodopa without improvement. She also was receiving regular botulinum toxin injections for her cervical dystonia and right leg stiffness,

with some improvement in her symptoms. The patient was prescribed cyclobenzaprine as well, with some improvement in her right foot pain and neck spasms. For a table summarizing the patient's clinical characteristics and genetic testing results, please see Figure 1.

A dystonia panel was sent, and it showed two potentially pathologic mutations, one in *CACNA1A* and the other in *PNKP*, along with a variant of unknown significance in *ATP7B*. The mutation in *CACNA1A* is C2324 G < A, protein W775X. It is heterozygous, autosomal dominant, and computer modeling suggests pathogenicity. This mutation has not been reported previously. She also has a heterozygous pathological mutation in *PNKP*, C1029 + 2 T < C, though this is autosomal recessive. The variant of unknown significance in *ATP7B* is C2544, C < T, protein G848G, and is also autosomal recessive. After receiving her genetic diagnosis, the patient was trialed on acetazolamide without improvement in her dystonia symptoms.

3. Discussion

This patient's clinical picture is most consistent with paroxysmal kinesigenic dyskinesia, as she has attacks of dystonia that are triggered by voluntary movement, last from a few seconds to a minute, and are relieved with rest [8]. Her paroxysmal dystonia is likely due to her mutation in *CACNA1A*, as it is sometimes seen during episodes of ataxia in EA2 [9], there are other case reports of *CACNA1A* mutations being associated with dystonia, and *CACNA1A* knockout mice (Ca$_V$2.1$^{-/-}$) exhibit dystonia and cerebellar atrophy [3]. Dystonia, usually cervical, can occur in EA2 during paroxysmal episodes of ataxia and can become chronic if secondarily progressive ataxia develops. There have also been case reports of patients with EA2 who went on to develop interictal dystonia later in their disease course [9].

Interestingly, there is a 2020 case report of a 62-year-old man with long-standing cerebellar ataxia and cervical dystonia who was found to have a novel mutation in *CACNA1A*. He had a 40-year history of slowly progressive gait instability and a 15-year history of cervical dystonia; he had begun requiring unilateral support 5 years prior to presentation. On exam, he had clear rightward deviation of the head, shoulder flexion, and dysmetria of both the lower limbs and right arm. The patient had an ataxic gait with increased base of support, inability to walk in tandem, and a mild positive Romberg sign. Brain MRI was significant for cerebellar atrophy predominantly affecting the vermis. The novel mutation was a one-nucleotide insertion (c.4056_4057insG), which causes a reading frame shift resulting in a premature stop codon three amino acids after the insertion. This was predicted to cause a truncated and nonfunctional protein [10]. Our patient also had cerebellar ataxia and cervical dystonia, in addition to the paroxysmal dystonia in her right leg. Unlike the other patient, her paroxysmal dystonia appeared first, followed by cervical dystonia, followed by her cerebellar ataxia, which is very mild and associated with subtle findings on neurological exam. However, it is possible that her ataxia could slowly progress over time, as it did in

Sex	Female
Age of onset	15
Initial symptom	Stiffness and pain in her right leg with activity (started age 15)
Other symptoms	Neck pain and stiffness, with occasional neck spasms (started age 20)
Functional impact	Difficulty with stairs and with walking long distances
Personal medical history	Unremarkable birth and early childhood history
Family history	No family history of similar symptoms
Exam findings	Normal strength, tone, and reflexes in all extremities at rest Mild retrocolis, right laterocolis, and right torticolis at rest Mild head titubation and very mild past pointing on finger-to-nose testing
Imaging	Unremarkable MRI of the brain and spinal cord
Other diagnostic studies	EMG/NCS of the left arm was unremarkable
Attempted treatments	Carbidopa/levodopa: no improvement Botulinum toxin injections: symptomatic relief of cervical dystonia Cyclobenzaprine: symptomatic relief Acetazolamide: no improvement
Genetic testing	*CACNA1A*, C2324 G < A: novel mutation, heterozygous, autosomal dominant, computer modeling suggests pathogenicity *PNKP*, C1029 + 2 T < C: heterozygous, autosomal recessive, known pathological mutation *ATP7B*, C2544 C < T: autosomal recessive, variant of unknown significance

FIGURE 1: Clinical characteristics and genetic testing.

the other patient. Additionally, although her most recent brain MRI at age 37 was normal, she could go on to develop cerebellar atrophy like the other patient. The report of another patient with cervical dystonia and a mutation in *CACNA1A* supports the idea that our patient's cervical dystonia is due to her mutation in *CACNA1A*.

Mice designed to have a homozygous null mutation in *CACNA1A* develop severe ataxia, dystonia, and cerebellar degeneration, supporting the notion that mutations in *CACNA1A* can cause dystonia in humans [3]. This is consistent with the discovery that *CACNA1A* encodes α1ACT, a transcription factor that is important for cerebellar development; this transcription factor may also be important for the survival of cerebellar neurons [2]. Additionally, three homogeneous, loss-of-function *CACNA1A* mouse models, *tottering*, *rocker*, and *tottering-4j*, exhibit stress-induced attacks of dystonia, which is thought to be due to cerebellar dysfunction. This provides further evidence in support of our patient's novel *CACNA1A* mutation being the cause of her paroxysmal dystonia. An important limitation to *CACNA1A* mouse models is that a single defective *CACNA1A* allele is sufficient to cause disease in humans, while heterozygous mice are minimally symptomatic (though some aged mice have clear motor deficits) [3].

In our patient, it makes sense that her mutation in *CACNA1A* would be associated with ataxia, given the importance of *CACNA1A* channels to normal cerebellar function; it is less intuitive that such a mutation would led to dystonia. Dystonia has classically been associated with the basal ganglia, especially the striatum. However, more recent research has shown that dystonia is better explained as a network disorder involving the basal ganglia, cortex, thalamus, and cerebellum. In particular, some monogenic animal models of dystonia show changes in cerebellar output that may be associated with basal ganglia dysfunction [11].

Thus, our patient's dystonia may be due in part to cerebellar dysfunction related to her *CACNA1A* mutation.

In summary, we report a novel *CACNA1A* variant associated with activity-induced dystonia of the right leg, cervical dystonia, and mild ataxia.

Authors' Contributions

Benjamin Stampfl wrote the manuscript, with concept guidance from Dominic Fee.

References

[1] H. G. Sutherland, C. L. Albury, and L. R. Griffiths, "Advances in genetics of migraine," *The Journal of Headache and Pain*, vol. 20, no. 1, p. 72, 2019.

[2] X. Du, J. Wang, H. Zhu et al., "Second cistron in CACNA1A gene encodes a transcription factor mediating cerebellar development and SCA6," *Cell*, vol. 154, no. 1, pp. 118–133, 2013.

[3] D. Pietrobon, "CaV2.1 channelopathies," *Pflügers Archiv - European Journal of Physiology*, vol. 460, no. 2, pp. 375–393, 2010.

[4] V. Di Stefano, M. G. Rispoli, N. Pellegrino et al., "Diagnostic and therapeutic aspects of hemiplegic migraine," *Journal of Neurology, Neurosurgery & Psychiatry*, vol. 91, no. 7, pp. 764–771, 2020.

[5] E. L. Guterman, B. Yurgionas, and A. B. Nelson, "Pearls & oysters: episodic ataxia type 2," *Neurology*, vol. 86, no. 23, pp. e239–e241, 2016.

[6] Z. Rentiya, R. Hutnik, Y. Q. Mekkam, and J. Bae, "The pathophysiology and clinical manifestations of spinocerebellar ataxia type 6," *The Cerebellum*, vol. 19, no. 3, pp. 459–464, 2020.

[7] H. L. Casey and C. M. Gomez, *Spinocerebellar Ataxia Type 6*, M. P. Adam, H. H. Ardinger, and R. A. Pagon, Eds., GeneReviews®. Seattle (WA): University of Washington, Seattle, WA, USA, 2019.

[8] A. Méneret and E. Roze, "Paroxysmal movement disorders: an update," *Revue neurologique*, vol. 172, no. 8-9, pp. 433–445, 2016.

[9] E. Indelicato and S. Boesch, "From genotype to phenotype: expanding the clinical spectrum of CACNA1A variants in the era of next generation sequencing," *Frontiers in Neurology*, vol. 12, p. 639994, 2021.

[10] A. Fuerte-Hortigón, R. Pérez-Noguera, J. Dotor García-Soto, I. Royo Boronat, S. Álvarez de Andrés, and J. M. García-Moreno, "Novel CACNA1A variant may cause cervical dystonia and cerebellar ataxia syndrome," *Journal of the Neurological Sciences*, vol. 415, p. 116909, 2020.

[11] T. Schirinzi, G. Sciamanna, N. B. Mercuri, and A. Pisani, "Dystonia as a network disorder: a concept in evolution," *Current Opinion in Neurology*, vol. 31, no. 4, pp. 498–503, 2018.

Six Novel ATM Gene Variants in Sri Lankan Patients with Ataxia Telangiectasia

D. Hettiarachchi (ID),[1] Hetalkumar Panchal (ID),[2] B. A. P. S. Pathirana,[1] P. D. Rathnayaka,[3] A. Padeniya,[3] P. S. Lai (ID),[4] and V. H. W. Dissanayake (ID)[1]

[1]*Human Genetics Unit, Faculty of Medicine, University of Colombo, Colombo, Sri Lanka*
[2]*Post Graduate Department of Bioscience, Sardar Patel University, Vallabh Vidyanagar, Gujarat, India*
[3]*Lady Ridgway Hospital for Children, Colombo, Sri Lanka*
[4]*Department of Paediatrics, Yong Loo Lin School of Medicine, National University of Singapore, Singapore*

Correspondence should be addressed to D. Hettiarachchi; dinebine@gmail.com

Academic Editor: Balraj Mittal

Introduction. Ataxia telangiectasia is a rare genetic condition with an estimated prevalence of 1 in 40,000–100,000 live births. This condition predominantly affects the nervous and immune systems. It is characterized by progressive ataxia beginning from early childhood. The neurological deficit associated with this condition affects one's balance, coordination, walking, and speech and can be accompanied by chorea, myoclonus, and neuropathy. They may also have ocular telangiectasias and high levels of blood alpha-fetoprotein (AFP). The ataxia telangiectasia mutated gene (ATM) is associated with this condition and codes for the ATM protein which is a phosphatidylinositol 3-kinase. This gene occupies 150 kb on chromosome 11q22–23 and contains 66 exons encoding a 13 kb transcript. ATM is a relatively large protein with a molecular weight of 350 kDa and 3,056 amino acids. *Methods.* Four patients of Sri Lankan origin presenting with features suggestive of ataxia telangiectasia were referred to our genetics center for specialized genetic counseling and testing. Whole-exome sequencing followed by Sanger sequencing was used to confirm the candidate variants. Protein modeling and genotype to phenotype correlation was performed in the identified variants. *Results.* We observed 6 novel ATM gene variants in four patients with ataxia telangiectasia. The identified variants are as follows: homozygous c.7397C > A (p.Ala2466Glu) and c.510_511delGT (p.Tyr171fs) and compound heterozygous c.5347_5350delGAAA (p.Glu1783fs), c.8137A > T (p.Arg2713*) and c.1163A > C (p.Lys388Thr), and c.5227A > C (p.Thr1743Pro). Variant analysis was followed by modeling of the native and altered protein structures. *Conclusion.* We report novel *ATM* gene variants that have implications on the molecular diagnosis of ataxia telangiectasia.

1. Introduction

The ataxia telangiectasia mutated gene (ATM) codes for the ATM protein which is a phosphatidylinositol 3-kinase that responds to DNA damage. It is a key substrate in DNA repair and cell cycle control [1, 2]. ATM gene occupies a 150 kb space on chromosome 11q22–23 which contains 66 exons encoding a transcript of 13 kb. ATM is a relatively large protein with a molecular weight of 350 kDa containing 3,056 amino acids. Many ATM transcripts have been identified which share almost the same open reading frames of 9.2 kb

and exhibit numerous 5′-untranslated regions (5′-UTRs) which are formed by complex alternative splicing and several alternative 3′-UTRs [3, 4]. Ataxia telangiectasia (A-T; MIM# 208900) is an autosomal recessive genetic disorder caused by biallelic inactivation of the ATM gene [5]. This condition is primarily characterized by cerebellar degeneration dominated by gradual cerebellar cortical atrophy which results in progressive ataxia beginning from early childhood. Neurological deficit affects one's balance, coordination, walking, and speech and can be accompanied by chorea, myoclonus, and neuropathy as well as telangiectasias in the eyes and sometimes on the facial skin. Thymic degeneration, immunodeficiency, recurrent sino-pulmonary infections, retarded somatic growth, premature aging, gonadal dysgenesis, predisposition to lymphoreticular malignancies, and acute sensitivity to ionizing radiation are some of the other associated features. It is reported that AT carriers are suspected to be cancer-prone which is often due to genomic instability or DNA damage response syndrome. The worldwide prevalence of AT is estimated to range from 1 in 40,000 and 1 in 100,000 live births [6, 7]. In this study, we describe 6 novel ATM gene variants in 4 patients with clinical features of ataxia telangiectasia using next generation sequencing.

2. Methods

2.1. Selection of Patients. Four patients who were clinically diagnosed with AT were referred for genetic testing and counseling to the Human Genetics Unit, Faculty of Medicine, the University of Colombo. Written informed consent was obtained from the patient's parents following a protocol approved by the Ethics Review Committee, Faculty of Medicine, University of Colombo, Sri Lanka.

2.2. Sample Collection and DNA Extraction. Venous blood samples in EDTA tubes were obtained from the patients and extraction of genomic DNA from peripheral blood leukocytes was performed using a QIAamp DNA Mini Kit according to the manufacturer's protocol [8].

2.3. Next Generation Sequencing. The patients underwent whole-exome sequencing on an Illumina HiSeq platform followed by library preparation using the Agilent SureSelect Human All Exon + UTR Kit according to the manufacturer's protocol [9]. Genetic analysis of the paired-end sequencing data was performed using an in-house bioinformatics pipeline. FASTQ files were mapped with the (GRCh37/hg19) human reference sequence using the BWA-mem algorithm and Genome Analysis Tool Kit (GATK). The annotation of the VCF file was performed using SNP-eff with Refseq, clinical databases, and population frequency databases available online [10–12]. All sequence variants were confirmed by visual inspection of alignments, followed by Sanger sequencing.

Genes that matched the AT phenotype (ATM, MRE11A, and NBS1) and other genes associated with cerebellar ataxia (RAD50, RNF168, APTX, SETX, TWNK, POLG, and ABCB7) were analyzed in all four probands. They were classified according to standard ACMG guidelines (https://www.acgs.uk.com/media/11631/uk-practice-guidelines-for-variant-classification-v4-01-2020.pdf). *In-silico* functional prediction tools were employed to study the pathogenicity of the identified variants.

2.4. Protein Modeling. Modeling of the native and truncated structure of the ATM protein was performed for each identified variant using the SWISS-MODEL server (http://swissmodel.expasy.org). The mRNA sequence of serine-protein kinase/ataxia telangiectasia mutated ATM protein was retrieved in FASTA format from GenBank with GenBank ID: U33841.1.

3. Results

3.1. Case Presentation. Case 1 was a 6-year-old girl representing one of the two affected siblings of a non-consanguineous marriage (Figure 1(a)). She was born at term without complications following a normal pregnancy. She developed cerebellar ataxia with asynergy (lack of co-ordination between muscles) and spasticity (increase in tendon reflexes) around 3 years of age. Her brain MRI showed no abnormalities. Her alpha-fetoprotein (AFP) level was 172.2 µg/ml (elevated). However, other blood investigations were within the normal range. She was clinically diagnosed with AT. She did not have any ocular telangiectasias or immunological features. Her brother also showed similar signs of cerebellar ataxia during his early years. Both parents were unaffected. However, with age, their symptoms gradually reduced. Currently, the proband suffers from minimal writing and walking difficulty and her brother is almost asymptomatic.

Case 2 was a 9-year-old girl born to consanguineous parents (Figure 1(b)). She was born without complications at term following a normal pregnancy. Her sister and parents are unaffected. She was diagnosed with epilepsy at 2 years of age and developed difficulty in walking and other cerebellar signs around 7 years of age. Currently, she is experiencing frequent syncopal attacks. She also has dysarthric speech, dystonia, tremors, ocular telangiectasias and suffers from recurrent respiratory tract infections. Her AFP levels are between 200–300 µg/ml. Her other blood parameters are within normal range and there are no abnormalities in her brain MRI scan. However, the severity of her condition has progressed over the years.

Case 3 was a 7-year-old boy born at term to non-consanguineous parents following a normal uneventful pregnancy (Figure 1(c)). He showed signs of cerebellar ataxia and difficulty in walking during early childhood. At the age of 2 years, he was clinically diagnosed with AT. His blood AFP level was elevated at 320.1 µg/ml. His other blood parameters and MRI of the brain were normal. Currently, he suffers from dysarthria, dystonia, ocular telangiectasias, and recurrent respiratory tract infections. His parents and sibling (sister) are asymptomatic and healthy.

Case 4 was a 24-year-old male born to non-consanguineous parents following an uneventful pregnancy. He presented with late-onset ataxia, dysarthria, dystonia, and difficulty in walking. He has no ocular telangiectasias or immunological features. He also shows signs of dystonia. His symptoms have not shown any progression or improvement for the past 2 years. His blood AFP level is only mildly elevated 49 µg/ml with other blood parameters within the normal range. His MRI brain is normal and his parents and sibling (sister) are unaffected (Figure 1(d)).

Genotype to phenotype characteristics along with alpha-fetoprotein (AFP) levels, family history of neurological,

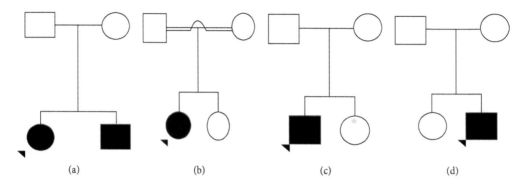

FIGURE 1: Pedigrees of the patients diagnosed with AT following whole-exome sequencing.

immunological disorders, and cancers are described in Table 1.

3.2. Variant Identification. We observed 6 novel ATM gene variants in four patients with AT. The variants were as follows: homozygous c.7397C > A (p.Ala2466Glu) and c.510_511delGT (p.Tyr171fs) and compound heterozygous c.5347_5350delGAAA (p.Glu1783fs), c.8137A > T (p.Arg2713*) and c.1163A > C (p.Lys388Thr), and c.5227A > C (p.Thr1743Pro). These variants were confirmed using Sanger sequencing.

3.3. Comparison of Variants with AT Phenotype. We compared the phenotypic severity with the functional predictions observed for each variant (Table 1). *In-silico* tools were employed to derive the altered protein structure.

3.4. Pathogenicity of the Variants. The variants observed in this study were predicted to be damaging when analyzed using functional prediction software tools such as Mutation Taster, disease mutation; Provean, deleterious; Polyphen2, damaging; SIFT damaging. Variants predicted as damaging are likely to be pathogenic.

4. Discussion and Conclusion

Ataxia telangiectasia is a clinically heterogeneous neurological condition resulting from the loss of ATM protein which is a relatively large protein (350 kDa). It comprises of 3056 amino acids (Figure 2(a)) and belongs to the family of phosphatidylinositol 3-kinase-like protein kinases [13]. It was observed that severe forms were associated with a total loss of ATM protein while milder, slow-progressing, or late-onset forms of AT were caused by nontruncating variants such as missense or splice site variants which rendered some residual ATM kinase activities within the cells [14]. To date, over 1700 variants in the ATM gene have been reported, and among them, over 800 variants have shown to be associated with the AT phenotype (http://www.hgmd.cf.ac.uk/ac/gene.php?gene=ATM). The majority of the pathogenic variants resulting in the total loss of the ATM protein account for about 75% of the AT phenotype [15, 16]. Molecular cloning studies targeted at the cDNA spanning the complete open reading frame of the ATM gene and the ATM protein shows

significant sequence similarities to several large proteins across species, e.g., *Drosophila*, yeast, and mammals, as they all share a similar PI 3-kinase domain. Mutations in their genes confer a variety of phenotypes with features similar to those observed in human cells affected with AT [13]. Hence, those missense variants residing over highly conserved domains across species are more likely to be pathogenic.

In our study, we have observed a similar correlation between the type of variants and phenotypic severity. Thus, in Case 1, homozygous missense variant (c.7397C > A) was located in exon 48. This region has 11 overlapping transcripts; studies have shown the 48th exon, which spans 114 bp, affects the mitochondrial function related to ataxia telangiectasia [17, 18]. It was observed that at 2466th position the mutated protein had a substitution in one amino acid (i.e., Ala to Glu), while the rest of the amino acids remained unchanged (Figure 2(b)). It was also observed that the change in a single amino acid did not affect the secondary and tertiary structures of the protein. However, this change was situated in a highly conserved protein domain across species (Table 2).

In Case 2, homozygous frameshift variant (c.510_511delGT) was located on exon 3 which spans 113 bps. We observed the amino acids coded by mutated mRNA remained unchanged up to the 510th position. However, the deletion of G and T nucleotides at the 510th and 511th positions respectively results in a frameshift in the remaining mRNA sequence. This change caused the formation of a premature stop codon immediately after the 511th position, thus resulting in the synthesis of a truncated protein with only 2708 amino acids compared to the 3056 amino acids in the wild type protein (Figure 2(c)). The frequent occurrence of truncated mutations in AT patients suggests that the PI 3-kinase domain at the 3′ end of the gene is indispensable, therefore resulting in a more severe phenotype. Several studies have shown that truncating variants lead to a more severe early-onset AT [19].

In Case 3, a compound heterozygous variant was observed. One was a frameshift (c.5347_5350delGAAA) and the other was a missense variant (c.8137 A > T). c.5347_5350delGAAA resides on exon 33 which spans 96 bps. Deleted GAAA nucleotides from 5347–5350 positions in mRNA sequence resulted in the formation of a stop codon immediately after the 5370th position and a truncated protein of 1790 amino acids was synthesized (Figure 2(d)).

TABLE 1: Comparison of mutation positions of the cases and its effect on protein sequence and phenotypic severity.

Case	Novel variants	Current evidence on the effect of the variant	Effect on ATM	Protein structure	AFP level (<10 μg/ml)	Phenotypic severity
1	c.7397C > A homozygous, missense	This variant is located in exon 48 of the ATM gene. Variants in this region overlaps 11 transcripts which code for mitochondrial fission factor interactor, a protein required for mitochondrial function.	p.Ala2466Glu	This single amino acid change did not affect the secondary and tertiary structures.	172.2	Mild ataxia; no family history of neurological, immunological disorders, or cancers
2	c.510_511delGT, homozygous, frameshift	This variant is located in exon 3 and has 14 overlapping transcripts. Frameshift variants lead to truncation of the ATM protein. This type of variants is associated with a more severe phenotype.	p.Tyr171fs	A partial protein was synthesized with only 2708 amino acids (wild type protein had 3056 amino acids)	200–300	Severe phenotype with multisystem involvement and recurrent infections; no family history of neurological, immunological disorders, or cancers
3	c.5347_5350delGAAA and c.8137A > T compound heterozygous	A deletion in the exon 33 of the ATM gene was observed. There are 8 overlapping transcripts in this region. The first variant leads to the formation of a truncated ATM protein and the second missense variant leads to a premature stop codon	p.Glu1783fs p.Arg2713*	The synthesized protein had only 1790 amino acids.	320.1	Severe early-onset ataxia, dysarthria, dystonia, and recurrent respiratory tract infections; no family history of neurological, immunological disorders, or cancers
4	c.1163A > C and c.5227A > C compound heterozygous	The first missense variant resides on exon 8; the second variant resides on exon 32 which is also a missense variant; missense variants were observed to result in a milder phenotype	p.Lys388Thr p.Thr1743Pro	The secondary and the tertiary structures of the protein remained unchanged	49	Mild late-onset AT phenotype; no family history of neurological, immunological disorders, or cancers

The second variant in this patient c.8137 A > T resides in exon 52 spanning 159 bps and has 12 overlapping transcripts. This variant leads to a premature stop codon at p.Arg2713* position further leading to the truncation of the ATM protein. In previous studies, similar compound, heterozygous variants have shown phenotypic heterogeneity and late-onset AT [20]. However, this was mainly observed when variants reside outside the PI 3-kinase domain (aa 2857–2915). This suggests that missense mutations outside the catalytic domain may result in residual ATM activity. However, we observed that this hypothesis was subjective as frameshift variants residing outside this domain also resulted in a severe early onset form of AT.

In Case 4, there was a compound heterozygous missense variant denoted as c.1163A > C and c.5227A > C residing on exon 3 and 32, respectively. As per our findings, we changed the nucleotides at 1163A > C and 5227A > C manually in the mRNA sequence. In the translated protein sequence, it was found that there is a substitution of Lys > Thr at the 388th

position and Thr > Pro at the 1743rd position but the remaining amino acids were unchanged. These compound heterozygous variants do not appear to have a marked impact on the 3D structure of the protein. However, the second amino acid change (p.Thr1743Pro) appears to occur in a domain that is highly conserved across species (Table 2). This patient had a late-onset milder form. In addition to variants exhibiting milder forms of AT, other clinical features such as dystonia have also been described along with the late presentation [19].

Variant detection in the ATM gene has advanced since the advent of next generation sequencing as it is a relatively large gene with 63 exons and no documented hotspot regions [21]. Current studies are predominantly based on Caucasian populations [22, 23]. There are not many studies conducted in southeast Asian patients and none describing the genotype of Sri Lankan AT patients. Identifying new disease-causing variants is becoming increasingly important for genetic testing and it is leading to a significant change in

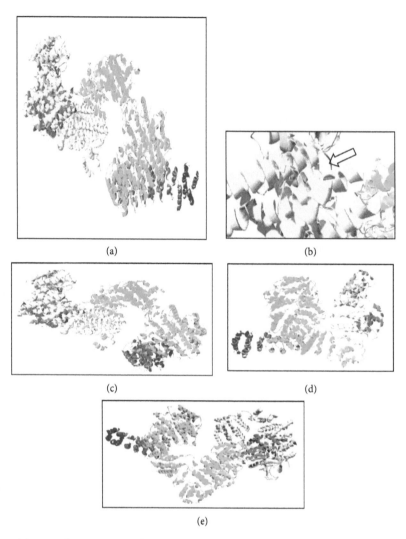

FIGURE 2: Protein modeling. (a) Normal ATM protein, (b) ATM protein structure with Glu at 2466 in helix, (c) structure of the protein with a missing helix, (d) structure of the ATM protein synthesized after deletion of GAAA from normal ATM mRNA at 5347_5350, and (e) 3D structure unaltered.

TABLE 2: Conservation of the mutated domain across species in comparison to Cases 1 and 4.

Proband in Case 1	QRELELDEL *E* LRALKEDRKRF	Proband in Case 4	NTLVEDCVKVRSAAV *P* CL
Homo sapiens Human	QRELELDEL *A* LRALKEDRKRF	*Homo sapiens* Human	NTLVEDCVKVRSAAV *T* CL
Mus musculus House mouse	QRELELDEC *A* LRALREDRKRF	*Mus musculus* House mouse	NTLVEDSVKIRSAAA *T* CL
Rattus norvegicus Norway rat	QRELELDEC *A* LRALKEDRKRF	*Rattus norvegicus* Norway rat	NTLVEDSVKIRSAAA *T* CL
Sus scrofa Pig	QRELELDEG *A* LRALKKDRKR	*Sus scrofa* Pig	STLVEDCVKVRSAAV. *T* CL
Canis lupus familiaris Dog	QRELELDEC *A* LRALKEDRKRF	*Canis lupus familiaris* Dog	NTLVEDCVKVRSAAV. *T* CL
Macaca mulatta Rhesus monkey	QRELELDEL *A* LHALKEDRKRF	*Macaca mulatta* Rhesus monkey	NTLVEDCVKVRAAAV *T* CL
Xenopus tropicalis Tropical clawed frog	QRELELDEC *A* ILALREDRKRF	*Xenopus tropicalis* Tropical clawed frog	NTLVEDCVKVRSAAV. *T* CL
Pan troglodytes Chimpanzee	QRELELDEL *A* LRALKEDRKRF	*Pan troglodytes* Chimpanzee	NALTDHCIQVRSAAA. *T* CL

the scale and sensitivity of molecular genetic analysis in AT. The hope of a new therapy to reverse the effects of the absence of a functional ATM kinase is on the horizon [24]. In keeping with already published literature, the results from our study showed that truncating variants resulted in an earlier onset disease with increased severity and vice versa for missense variants where some residual activities of the ATM kinase would be present. In conclusion, we have demonstrated the 6 novel ATM gene variants resulting in AT in Sri Lankan patients.

4.1. Limitations. The main limitation of this study is the sample size. We would like to expand WES to other patients who are clinically diagnosed with AT. Furthermore, for missense variants, functional studies can complement *in silico* analysis to further decipher the exact effect on ATM kinase.

4.2. Future Work. It should be possible to detect AT shortly after birth and early referral for genetic studies for confirmation should take precedence, as it will enable individualized patient interventions and genetic counseling for the family members, especially those who are carriers for ATM gene variants. They can also be followed up for neurological, immunological disorders and cancers, as they will have a higher risk of developing malignancies.

Abbreviations

ATM: Ataxia telangiectasia mutated
AT: Ataxia telangiectasia
WES: Whole-exome sequencing
cDNA: Complementary DNA
SPDBV: Swiss-PdbViewer.

Acknowledgments

The authors wish to acknowledge their collaborators and the laboratory staff for their contribution.

References

[1] K. Savitsky, A. Bar-Shira, S. Gilad et al., "A single ataxia telangiectasia gene with a product similar to PI-3 kinase," *Science*, vol. 268, no. 5218, pp. 1749–1753, 1995.

[2] P. J. McKinnon, "ATM and ataxia telangiectasia," *EMBO Reports*, vol. 5, no. 8, pp. 772–776, 2004.

[3] K. Savitsky, T. Uziel, S. Gilad et al., "Ataxia-telangiectasia: structural diversity of untranslated sequences suggests complex post-transcriptional regulation of ATM gene expression," *Nucleic Acids Research*, vol. 25, no. 9, pp. 1678–1684, 1997.

[4] G. Rotman and S. Yosef, "ATM: from gene to function," *Human Molecular Genetics*, vol. 7, no. 10, pp. 1555–1563, 1998.

[5] A. FiévetD. Bellanger et al., "Functional classification of ATM variants in ataxia-telangiectasia patients," *Human Mutation*, vol. 40, no. 10, pp. 1713–1730, 2019.

[6] C. Rothblum-Oviatt, J. Wright, M. A. Lefton-Greif, S. A. McGrath-Morrow, T. O Crawford, and H. M. Lederman, "Ataxia telangiectasia: a review," *Orphanet Journal of Rare Diseases*, vol. 11, no. 1, 159 pages, 2016.

[7] M. F. Lavin and Y. Shiloh, "The genetic defect in ataxia-telangiectasia," *Annual Review of Immunology*, vol. 15, no. 1, pp. 177–202, 1997.

[8] Qiagen.Com, 2020, https://www.qiagen.com/ch/resources/download.aspx?id=62a200d6-faf4-469b-b50f-2b59cf738962&lang=en.

[9] Agilent.Com, 2020, https://www.agilent.com/cs/library/datasheets/public/SureSelect%20V6%20DataSheet%205991-5572EN.pdf.

[10] Index of/pub/Clinvar/Vcf_Grch37". Ftp.Ncbi.Nlm.Nih.Gov, 2020, https://ftp.ncbi.nlm.nih.gov/pub/clinvar/vcf_GRCh37/.

[11] The Genome aggregation database (gnomad) | gnomad blog". Gnomad.Broadinstitute.Org, 2020, https://gnomad.broadinstitute.org/blog/2017-02-the-genome-aggregation-database/.

[12] Exac allele frequency of pathogenic clinvar variants - dave tang's blog". Dave Tang's Blog, 2020, https://davetang.org/muse/2017/01/30/exac-allele-frequency-pathogenic-clinvar-variants/.

[13] N. J. H. Van Os, A. F. M. Jansen, M. Van Deuren et al., "Ataxia-telangiectasia: immunodeficiency and survival," *Clinical Immunology*, vol. 178, pp. 45–55, 2017.

[14] M. M. M. Verhagen, J. I. Last, F. B. L. Hogervorst et al., "Presence of ATM protein and residual kinase activity correlates with the phenotype in ataxia-telangiectasia: a genotype-phenotype study," *Human Mutation*, vol. 33, no. 3, pp. 561–571, 2012.

[15] V. Jacquemin, G. Rieunier, S. Jacob et al., "Underexpression and abnormal localization of ATM products in ataxia telangiectasia patients bearing ATM missense mutations," *European Journal of Human Genetics*, vol. 20, no. 3, pp. 305–312, 2012.

[16] A. Pourahmadiyan, P. Alipour, N. Golchin, and M. A. Tabatabaiefar, "Next generation sequencing reveals a novel pathogenic variant in the ATM gene," *International Journal of Neuroscience*, pp. 1–8, 2020.

[17] F. V. Pallardó, A. Lloret, M. Lebel et al., "Mitochondrial dysfunction in some oxidative stress-related genetic diseases: ataxia-telangiectasia, down syndrome, fanconi anaemia and werner syndrome," *Biogerontology*, vol. 11, no. 4, pp. 401–419, 2010.

[18] K. Nakamura, L. Du, R. Tunuguntla et al., "Functional characterization and targeted correction of ATM mutations identified in Japanese patients with ataxia-telangiectasia," *Human Mutation*, vol. 33, no. 1, pp. 198–208, 2012.

[19] S. Gilad, L. Chessa, R. Khosravi et al., "Genotype-phenotype relationships in ataxia-telangiectasia and variants," *The American Journal of Human Genetics*, vol. 62, no. 3, pp. 551–561, 1998.

[20] S. SaviozziA. Saluto et al., "A late onset variant of ataxia-telangiectasia with a compound heterozygous genotype, A8030G/7481insA," *Journal of Medical Genetics*, vol. 39, no. 1, pp. 57–61, 2002.

[21] S. Martin-Rodriguez, A. Calvo-Ferrer, N. Ortega-Unanue, L. Samaniego-Jimenez, M. P. Sanz-Izquierdo, and I. Bernardo-Gonzalez, "Two novel variants in the ATM gene causing ataxia-telangiectasia, including a duplication of 90 kb:

utility of targeted next-generation sequencing in detection of copy number variation," *Annals of Human Genetics*, vol. 83, pp. 266–273, 2019.

[22] Y. Shiloh and Y. Ziv, "The ATM protein kinase: regulating the cellular response to genotoxic stress, and more," *Nature Reviews Molecular Cell Biology*, vol. 14, no. 4, pp. 197–210, 2013.

[23] E. Suspitsin, A. Sokolenko, I. Bizin et al., "ATM mutation spectrum in Russian children with ataxia-telangiectasia," *European Journal of Medical Genetics*, vol. 63, no. 1, Article ID 103630, 2020.

[24] D. A. Ovchinnikov, S. L. Withey, H. C. Leeson et al., "Correction of ATM mutations in iPS cells from two ataxia-telangiectasia patients restores DNA damage and oxidative stress responses," *Human Molecular Genetics*, vol. 29, no. 6, pp. 990–1001, 2020.

18

A Case of Ataxia with Isolated Vitamin E Deficiency Initially Diagnosed as Friedreich's Ataxia

Michael Bonello and Partha Ray

The Walton Centre NHS Foundation Trust, Lower Lane, Liverpool L9 7LJ, UK

Correspondence should be addressed to Michael Bonello; michaelbonello@gmail.com

Academic Editor: Dominic B. Fee

Ataxia with isolated vitamin E deficiency (AVED) is a rare autosomal recessive condition that is caused by a mutation in the alpha tocopherol transfer protein gene. It is almost indistinguishable clinically from Friedreich's ataxia but with appropriate treatment its devastating neurological features can be prevented. Patients can present with a progressive cerebellar ataxia, pyramidal spasticity, and evidence of a neuropathy with absent deep tendon reflexes. It is important to screen for this condition on initial evaluation of a young patient presenting with progressive ataxia and it should be considered in patients with a long standing ataxia without any diagnosis in view of the potential therapeutics and genetic counselling. In this case report we present a patient who was initially diagnosed with Friedreich's ataxia but was later found to have AVED.

1. Introduction

Ataxia with isolated vitamin E deficiency (AVED) is a rare autosomal recessive condition that is characterised by progressive cerebellar ataxia, dorsal column signs, and pyramidal deficits on examination. It is caused by a mutation in the alpha tocopherol transfer protein gene on chromosome 8 and was first described by Burck et al. in 1981 in a paediatric patient [1]. Clinically it is almost indistinguishable from Friedreich's ataxia but with appropriate treatment most of its devastating neurological features can be prevented. Below we discuss a patient who had a diagnosis of Friedreich's ataxia but was later found to have AVED.

2. Case Presentation

A 28-year-old Iranian male was referred to the regional neurology centre for assessment of his progressive ataxia and dysarthria. He was an asylum seeker that arrived in the UK from Tehran 3 months prior to being seen in clinic. His first symptoms started when he was 15 years old with progressive gait difficulties. He was noted to have wasting of his muscles and paraesthesia of his legs. He developed cerebellar dysarthria 5 years later. He managed to do his first

year as a medical student in Iran, but unfortunately due to illness he was unable to complete his studies. He recently became wheelchair bound. Two of his cousins have speech difficulties but no further family history was obtainable. There was no parent consanguinity or gastrointestinal symptoms. Neurological examination confirmed a broad based gait which was clearly ataxic. Bedside examination of the cranial nerves revealed dysarthria, nystagmus, and normal fundoscopy. Upper and lower limb examination confirmed cerebellar ataxia with intention tremor and absent deep tendon reflexes. Plantar responses were extensor on the left and absent on the right. There was absent vibration sense and joint position sense bilaterally. Genetic analysis of the frataxin gene confirmed two alleles in the normal size range and no evidence of an expansion. Further investigation confirmed evidence of vitamin E deficiency. The concentration of alpha tocopherol was measured at <1.0 μmol/L (normal range: 9.5–41.5 μmol/L). The vitamin E/cholesterol ratio was 0.3 μmol/mmol suggesting pure vitamin E deficiency. Other laboratory investigations confirmed a normal full blood count, glucose, liver, kidney function, coeliac antibodies, fasting lipids, thyroid function tests, copper, and ceruloplasmin. Magnetic Resonance Imaging (MRI) of the brain confirmed normal intracranial appearances including no cerebellar atrophy. The diagnosis of AVED was confirmed by mutations in the TTPA gene. There was a homozygous pathogenic frame shift mutation in the TTPA gene *c.706del (p.(His236fs))* which results in loss of activity of the α-TTP. The patient started treatment with high dose vitamin E in the form of D-alpha tocopherol supplementation at 800 mg/day. Serum vitamin E concentration improved at 1-year follow-up. His ataxia and dysarthria had stabilised although he was still significantly disabled requiring support in his ADLs.

3. Discussion

The role of vitamin E deficiency and neurological disease was first described in 1981 in a 12-year-old with progressive cerebellar ataxia and low serum vitamin E [1]. Further reports followed in the literature until a case series was presented in 1993 of eight patients with Friedreich's ataxia phenotype but low vitamin E [2]. Genetic locus was mapped to chromosome 8q in the same year [3]. In 1995 mutations in the gene encoding hepatic α-tocopherol transfer protein (α-TTP) were identified in this condition and since then have been termed ataxia with vitamin E deficiency (AVED) [4]. The majority of patients reported in the literature are from Mediterranean countries, particularly North African countries and Japan, although it has been reported in other countries including the United Kingdom [5]. Pathological studies from post-mortem examinations of two patients confirmed atrophy of the brainstem, spinal cord, cerebral hemispheres, and cerebellum. There was cell loss in the third cortical layer, giant cells of the striatum, the dentate nucleus, anterior horn cells, neurons of the twelfth and ambiguous nuclei, and the inferior olive. There was Purkinje cell loss in the cerebellum as well as degeneration of the posterior columns and moderate degeneration of the lateral corticospinal tracts [6, 7]. Nerve biopsy shows mild to moderate axonal neuropathy associated with regeneration as opposed to Friedreich's ataxia where the peripheral neuropathy is mainly sensory and severe from the early stages of the disease [8].

α-TTP is a liver transfer protein that acts as a carrier molecule for RRR-α-tocopherol and binds it preferentially to very low density lipoproteins (VLDL). Thus it acts as an important step in the circulation of RRR-α-tocopherol to the nervous system [9]. Vitamin E is an antioxidant and is thought to play a crucial role in neurological function although the specific role is still uncertain. It is thought that oxidative stress in the lack of vitamin E results in damage to the various parts of the nervous system resulting in the clinical signs [10].

The age of onset of clinical signs varies from early childhood to very late adult life [11]. Patients develop a progressive cerebellar ataxia that can lead to severe gait disturbances and disability if not treated early. The type of mutation seems to determine the age of needing a wheelchair, the age of onset, and the progression of the disease [12, 13]. Posterior column involvement is evident in most patients. Romberg's sign is found in most patients and joint position sense is usually impaired. Lateral corticospinal tracts are usually affected late [12]. Pyramidal spasticity is usually evident. Tendon reflexes are normally absent similar to Friedreich's ataxia phenotype.

Gaze paralysis and nystagmus often happen. Distal amyotrophy is also noticed in such patients [11]. Other features reported include myoclonus, focal dystonia, deafness, and urinary symptoms [11]. Retinitis pigmentosa is more frequent in Japanese patients and seems to be more prominent with an *H101Q* mutation [14]. Other features include pes cavus and kyphoscoliosis. Cardiac involvement is seen in up to 31% of patients [15].

High dose vitamin E supplementation in patients with AVED results in stabilisation of the neurological features and in some cases can result in improvement [12]. This is an important point which signifies that if treatment is started early, most of the disability could potentially be prevented. This confirms the importance of genetic counselling in patients with AVED.

We advocate that vitamin E levels should form part of the initial screen for a patient with young onset progressive ataxia. In the literature there are a number of cases of patients who have been clinically diagnosed prior to genetic testing being widely available. We do recommend that such patients have their frataxin gene checked and if negative have a vitamin E blood level tested as adequate treatment with high dose vitamin E can halt progression of the condition and can be invaluable in genetic counselling.

References

[1] U. Burck, H. H. Goebel, H. D. Kuhlendahl, C. Meier, and K. M. Goebel, "Neuromyopathy and vitamin E deficiency in man," *Neuropediatrics*, vol. 12, no. 3, pp. 267–278, 1981.

[2] M. Ben Hamida, S. Belal, G. Sirugo et al., "Friedreich's ataxia phenotype not linked to chromosome 9 and associated with selective autosomal recessive vitamin E deficiency in two inbred Tunisian families," *Neurology*, vol. 43, no. 11, pp. 2179–2183, 1993.

[3] C. Ben Hamida, N. Doerflinger, S. Belal et al., "Localization of Friedreich ataxia phenotype with selective vitamin E deficiency to chromosome 8q by homozygosity mapping," *Nature Genetics*, vol. 5, no. 2, pp. 195–200, 1993.

[4] K. Ouahchi, M. Arita, H. Kayden et al., "Ataxia with isolated vitamin E deficiency is caused by mutations in the α-tocopherol transfer protein," *Nature Genetics*, vol. 9, no. 2, pp. 141–145, 1995.

[5] S. R. Hammans and C. R. Kennedy, "Ataxia with isolated vitamin E deficiency presenting as mutation negative Friedreich's ataxia," *Journal of Neurology, Neurosurgery & Psychiatry*, vol. 64, no. 3, pp. 368–370, 1998.

[6] A. Larnaout, S. Belal, M. Zouari et al., "Friedreich's ataxia with isolated vitamin E deficiency: a neuropathological study of a Tunisian patient," *Acta Neuropathologica*, vol. 93, no. 6, pp. 633–637, 1997.

[7] T. Yokota, T. Uchihara, J. Kumagai et al., "Postmortem study of ataxia with retinitis pigmentosa by mutation of the α-tocopherol transfer protein gene," *Journal of Neurology, Neurosurgery & Psychiatry*, vol. 68, no. 4, pp. 521–525, 2000.

[8] M. Zouari, M. Feki, C. Ben Hamida et al., "Electrophysiology and nerve biopsy: comparative study in Friedreich's ataxia

and Friedreich's ataxia phenotype with vitamin E deficiency," *Neuromuscular Disorders*, vol. 8, no. 6, pp. 416–425, 1998.

[9] M. G. Traber, R. J. Sokol, G. W. Burton et al., "Impaired ability of patients with familial isolated vitamin E deficiency to incorporate α-tocopherol into lipoproteins secreted by the liver," *The Journal of Clinical Investigation*, vol. 85, no. 2, pp. 397–407, 1990.

[10] R. Meier, T. Tomizaki, C. Schulze-Briese, U. Baumann, and A. Stocker, "The molecular basis of vitamin E retention: structure of human alpha-tocopherol transfer protein," *Journal of Molecular Biology*, vol. 331, no. 3, pp. 725–734, 2003.

[11] F. Hentati, G. El-euch, Y. Bouhlal, and R. Amouri, "Ataxia with vitamin E deficiency and abetalipoproteinemia," *Handbook of Clinical Neurology*, vol. 103, pp. 295–305, 2012.

[12] S. Gabsi, N. Gouider-Khouja, S. Belal et al., "Effect of vitamin E supplementation in patients with ataxia with vitamin E deficiency," *European Journal of Neurology*, vol. 8, no. 5, pp. 477–481, 2001.

[13] R. J. Sokol, J. M. McKim Jr., M. C. Goff et al., "Vitamin E reduces oxidant injury to mitochondria and the hepatotoxicity of taurochenodeoxycholic acid in the rat," *Gastroenterology*, vol. 114, no. 1, pp. 164–174, 1998.

[14] M. Hoshino, N. Masuda, Y. Ito et al., "Ataxia with isolated vitamin E deficiency: a Japanese family carrying a novel mutation in the alpha-tocopherol transfer protein gene," *Annals of Neurology*, vol. 45, no. 6, pp. 809–812, 1999.

[15] N. Marzouki, A. Benomar, M. Yahyaoui et al., "Vitamin E deficiency ataxia with (744 del A) mutation on α-TTP gene: genetic and clinical peculiarities in Moroccan patients," *European Journal of Medical Genetics*, vol. 48, no. 1, pp. 21–28, 2005.

19

Autophagy Promoted the Degradation of Mutant ATXN3 in Neurally Differentiated Spinocerebellar Ataxia-3 Human Induced Pluripotent Stem Cells

Zhanhui Ou, Min Luo, Xiaohua Niu, Yuchang Chen, Yingjun Xie, Wenyin He, Bing Song, Yexing Xian, Di Fan, Shuming OuYang, and Xiaofang Sun

Key Laboratory for Major Obstetric Diseases of Guangdong Province, Key Laboratory of Reproduction and Genetics of Guangdong Higher Education Institutes, The Third Affiliated Hospital of Guangzhou Medical University, Guangzhou 510150, China

Correspondence should be addressed to Xiaofang Sun; xiaofangsun@gzhmu.edu.cn

Academic Editor: Wiep Scheper

Spinocerebellar ataxia-3 (SCA3) is the most common dominant inherited ataxia worldwide and is caused by an unstable CAG trinucleotide expansion mutation within the *ATXN3* gene, resulting in an expanded polyglutamine tract within the ATXN3 protein. Many *in vitro* studies have examined the role of autophagy in neurodegenerative disorders, including SCA3, using transfection models with expression of pathogenic proteins in normal cells. In the current study, we aimed to develop an improved model for studying SCA3 *in vitro* using patient-derived cells. The patient-derived iPS cells presented a phenotype similar to that of human embryonic stem cells and could be differentiated into neurons. Additionally, these cells expressed abnormal ATXN3 protein without changes in the CAG repeat length during culture for at least 35 passages as iPS cells, up to 3 passages as neural stem cells, and after 4 weeks of neural differentiation. Furthermore, we demonstrated that neural differentiation in these iPS cells was accompanied by autophagy and that rapamycin promoted autophagy through degradation of mutant ATXN3 proteins in neurally differentiated spinocerebellar ataxia-3 human induced pluripotent stem cells ($p < 0.05$). In conclusion, patient-derived iPS cells are a good model for studying the mechanisms of SCA3 and may provide a tool for drug discovery *in vitro*.

1. Introduction

Spinocerebellar ataxia-3 (SCA3) is one of nine polyglutamine (polyQ) disorders caused by a CAG expansion mutation within the *ATXN3* gene, which encodes the ATXN3 protein [1]. Expansion of the polyQ tract results in neuronal cytotoxicity, with calpain-dependent proteolysis of the mutant ATXN3, thereby generating expanded polyQ fragments and insoluble aggregates and leading to the formation of inclusions in the nucleus and cytoplasm of neurons, including axonal tracts [2, 3]. The onset of SCA3 occurs during adulthood and is associated with gait and stance abnormalities, limb ataxia, dysarthria, dysphagia, oculomotor dysfunction, pyramidal and extrapyramidal signs, peripheral neuropathy, and aspiration pneumonia resulting from dysphagia [4]. The pathogenic mechanisms of SCA3 and other polyQ disorders

are not well understood, and there are currently no effective cures for these disorders.

Cells continuously turn over proteins through cycles of synthesis and degradation to maintain cellular homeostasis. The ubiquitin-proteasome system is a process for selective degradation of proteins, and recent studies have highlighted the role of lysosomes in this selective degradation process via autophagy [5]. Autophagy is a highly conserved biological process involving bulk degradation of proteins and organelles, during which portions of the cytoplasm are sequestered into double-membrane vesicles known as autophagosomes. These autophagosomes then fuse with lysosomes to form single-membrane autolysosomes; ultimately, the contents of autolysosomes are degraded by lysosomal hydrolases and recycled for energy utilization. This process helps to maintain cellular homeostasis and protects organisms from damage and diseases [6]. Dysregulation of autophagy is involved in many human diseases, including cancer, infection, immunity, heart disease, liver disease, aging, myopathies, and neurodegeneration [7]. Alzheimer's disease (AD), Parkinson's disease (PD), Huntington's disease (HD), and dominant spinocerebellar ataxia (SCA) are the most common neurodegenerative diseases exhibiting accumulation of abnormal protein aggregates. Several studies have demonstrated that inhibition of mammalian target of rapamycin (mTOR) complex 1 (mTORC1) by rapamycin promotes the degradation of mutant proteins *in vitro* and reduces the severity of neurodegeneration in animal models [8–10].

Induced pluripotent stem (iPS) cells, which are generated by transduction with a set of transcript factors in human somatic cells, offer an alternative cellular model for mechanistic studies [11]. Patient-derived iPS cells can preserve the genetic mutations carried by the patient in a functional human genomic background. Furthermore, these cells can be differentiated into human cells of neural lineage, which could be advantageous for investigating the pathogenic mechanisms of a disease and identifying potential therapies.

In this study, we used an episomal reprogramming assay to produce SCA3-iPS cells from skin fibroblasts of a woman with SCA3. We then examined the effects of autophagy during the neural differentiation of SCA3-iPS cells. Our results suggested that patient-specific iPS cells may represent an effective model system for analysis of potential therapies in a variety of diseases, including SCA3.

2. Materials and Methods

2.1. Cell Culture. The study was performed in accordance with the Declaration of Helsinki and has been approved by the ethical committee of The Third Affiliated Hospital of Guangzhou Medical University. Informed consent was obtained from all patients. hESC line 10 (hES-10), which was used as a positive control, was established in our hospital [12]. SCA3-iPS cells were generated using episomal reprogramming assays (Invitrogen, Carlsbad, CA, USA) from a woman (skin fibroblasts) with SCA3 who suffered from gait and stance abnormalities, limb ataxia, dysarthria, dysphagia, and oculomotor dysfunctions and had 81 CAG repeats in the *ATXN3* gene, as determined using polymerase chain reaction (PCR), fragment analysis, and sequencing. Two clones from the patient (SCA3-iPS-1 and SCA3-iPS-2) were used for the experiments. Cell lines were cultured using Essential 8 Medium (Gibco, USA)/Geltrex LDEV-Free hESC-qualified Reduced Growth Factor Basement Membrane Matrix (Invitrogen) in a feeder-independent culture system, as previously described [13].

2.2. CAG Repeats Length Analysis. The primers used for detection of the CAG repeat in the *ATXN3* gene by PCR and fragment analysis were as follows: Fam-CAGTGACTACTT-TGATTCG and TGGCCTTTCACATGGATGTGAA. The primers for sequencing were described previously [3].

2.3. Stem Cell and Pluripotency Analysis. Reverse-transcription PCR (RT-PCR) was performed to detect the expression of endogenous pluripotency genes according to the manufacturer's instructions (TaKaRa, Japan). The primers were as follows: *Oct4*, 5′-GACAGGGGGAGGGGAGGAGCT-AGG-3′ and 5′-CTTCCCTCCAACCAGTTGCCCCAAAC-3′; Nanog, 5′-CAGCCCCGATTCTTCCACCAGTCC-3′ and 5′-CGGAAGATTCCCAGTCGGGTTCACC-3′. AP staining and immunofluorescence analysis were performed as previously described [14]. The primary antibodies used were as follows: anti-SSEA-3 (1:100; Sigma, USA), anti-TRA1-60 (1:200; Sigma), anti-TRA1-81 (1:500; Sigma), anti-alpha-fetoprotein (AFP; 1:500; Sigma), anti-Nestin (1:100; Abcam, England), anti-PAX6 (1:200; Sigma), anti-NeuN (1:100; Abcam), beta-tubulin III (1:100; Abcam), and anti-smooth muscle actin (SMA; 1:500; Sigma).

2.4. In Vivo and In Vitro Differentiation. The colonies were harvested and subcutaneously injected into the inguinal grooves of 6-week-old male mice with severe combined immunodeficiency (SCID) as previously described [15]. Embryoid body (EB) formations were performed as previously described [16].

2.5. Karyotype Analysis. After Giemsa staining, at least 20 cells were examined in each group for chromosome analysis as previously described [14].

2.6. Neural Stem Cells (NSCs) and Neural Differentiation. NSCs were cultured using Gibco PSC neural induction medium and StemPro NSC SFM (Life Technologies, USA), and neural differentiation was performed according to the manufacturer's instructions. Briefly, about 24 h after hESCs and iPS cells were split into six-well plates, the culture medium was switched to Gibco PSC neural induction medium containing neurobasal medium and Gibco PSC neural induction supplement. The neural induction medium was changed every other day from the beginning of neural induction. The neural induction medium was changed every day after 4 days of neural induction. At day 7, primitive NSCs were dissociated using Accutase (Life Technologies) and plated on Geltrex-coated dishes in an NSC expansion medium containing 50% neurobasal medium, 50% Advanced DMEM/F12, and neural induction supplement. The NSC expansion medium was changed every other day until NSCs reached confluence at day 5 after plating of primitive NSCs [17]. For neural differentiation, NSCs were plated onto laminin (10 μg/mL; Life Technologies) coated six-well chamber slides at a density of 5×10^4 cells/cm^2 in a neuronal differentiation medium consisting of neurobasal medium, B-27, and GlutaMAX (Life Technologies). The culture medium was changed every 2-3 days, according to the manufacturer's instructions (Life Technologies).

2.7. Western Blot Analysis. The protein content was determined using a BCA protein assay kit (Thermo Fisher) according to the manufacturer's instructions. Equivalent amounts of protein were separated on 10–15% sodium dodecyl sulfate-

(SDS-) polyacrylamide gels and blotted onto nitrocellulose membranes. After being blocked at room temperature for 2 h with 5% nonfat milk in TBS with 0.1% Tween-20, the membranes were probed with anti-LC3B (1:1000; Cell Signaling Technology, USA), anti-p62 (1:1000; Abcam), anti-GAPDH (1:5000; Cell Signaling Technology), anti-ATXN3 (1:1000; Abcam), and horseradish peroxidase- (HRP-) conjugated IgG antibodies (1:10000; Cell Signaling Technology). The volumes of the bands were determined by standard scanning densitometry with normalization of densitometry measures to the expression of GAPDH.

2.8. Flow Cytometry Assay. Single cells derived from NSCs were fixed and permeabilized following the manufacturer's instructions (BD Pharmingen, USA). Cells were then stained with the following monoclonal fluorochrome-conjugated antibodies: Alexa Fluor® 647 mouse anti-NESTIN (BD Biosciences, USA) and Alexa Fluor® 488 mouse anti-human PAX6 (BD Biosciences, USA). Flow cytometry was performed using FACSAria™III flow cytometer (BD Biosciences, USA).

2.9. Chromosomal Microarray Analysis–Single Nucleotide Polymorphism Array Analysis. Chromosomal microarray analysis–single nucleotide polymorphism array analysis was performed for a higher resolution. DNA was prepared and hybridized to the CytoScan HD array (Affymetrix) platform according to the manufacturer's protocol [18].

2.10. Statistical Analysis. Data are expressed as the mean ± standard error of the mean (SEM) and were compared by one-way analysis of variance (ANOVA). When ANOVA results were significant, differences between groups were assessed by *post hoc* testing using LSD tests (SPSS version 17.0 for Windows). Differences with $p < 0.05$ were considered statistically significant.

3. Results

3.1. Characterization of SCA3-iPS Cells. RT-PCR analysis showed that the cells were positive for endogenous expression of *Oct4* and *Nanog* (Figure 1(a)). Immunofluorescence analysis of stem cell markers in SCA3 and control iPS colonies indicated positive staining for AP, SSEA-3, TRA-1-60, and TRA-1-81 (Figure 1(b)). Karyotyping analysis showed a normal female karyotype (Figure 1(c)).

3.2. Differentiation In Vitro and In Vivo. EBs were used to determine the differentiation ability of SCA3-iPS cells *in vitro*. Immunofluorescence results showed that the differentiated cells were positive for AFP (endoderm), SMA (mesoderm), and Nestin (ectoderm; Figure 1(d)). To demonstrate the pluripotency of SCA3-iPS cells *in vivo*, SCA3-iPS cells were subcutaneously injected into SCID mice. Eight weeks after injection, we observed teratoma formation. Histological examinations showed that the teratomas contained various tissues comprising all three germ layers (Figure 1(e)).

3.3. SCA3-iPS Cells Could Differentiate into NSCs and Neurons. Both SCA3-iPS cells (15–20 passages) and normal control iPS cells (15–20 passages) could be differentiated into NSCs and neurons. Approximately 24 h after passaging, the culture medium was switched to Gibco PSC neural induction medium containing neurobasal medium and Gibco PSC neural induction supplement. At day 7 of induction, primitive NSCs were formed, and immunofluorescence results showed that cells were positive for Pax6 and Nestin, which are NSC markers (Figure 2(a)). And the flow cytometry result showed no difference in these markers (Figure 2(b)). After NSCs expansion for several passages, neural induction medium was added for neural differentiation. Around day 21, immunofluorescence for NeuN and tubulin confirmed their neural lineage (Figure 2(c)).

3.4. CAG Repeats and ATXN3 Protein Remained Stable during Reprogramming and Neural Differentiation. Expansion of the CAG repeats in the *ATXN3* gene was verified by PCR and fragment analysis in fibroblasts (passage 3), SCA3-iPS cells (passages 15 and 30), NSCs (passage 3), and neurons (28 days). All cells showed stable CAG repeats (15 and 81; Figure 3(a)). Western blots were performed to detect the protein expression of ATXN3 in iPS cells, NSCs, and neurons derived from the patient with SCA3. Specific bands around 42 kDa (ATXN3) and 60 kDa (mutant ATXN3) were detected in all cell lines derived from the patient with SCA3, while control iPS cells and hES-10 had only the normal band of nonexpanded ATXN3 at around 42 kDa (Figure 3(b)).

3.5. No Obvious De Novo Mutations in Genome during Reprogram and Differentiation. To detect deletions or duplication across the whole genome, a chromosomal microarray analysis–single nucleotide polymorphism analysis was performed in the fibroblasts, iPS cells, and the neurons. In accordance with the karyotyping results, neither *de novo* deletions nor duplications were found in these cells.

3.6. Involvement of Autophagy during Neural Differentiation. Anti-LC3B antibodies were used to detect the level of autophagy in iPS cells and NSCs (day 3) and during neural differentiation (days 3 and 14) of control iPS cells and SCA3-iPS cells. The results showed that autophagy was increased during neural differentiation ($p < 0.05$). And the levels of LC3-II were increased during the SCA3 neural differentiation compared with the control iPS neural differentiation, but the increase levels were not of significant difference ($p > 0.05$). However, the levels of p62 were increased during the SCA3 neural differentiation compared with the control iPS neural differentiation ($p < 0.05$); these results may indicate impairment in the trafficking to lysosomes and protein degradation (Figure 4(a)).

3.7. Autophagy Promoted the Degradation of Mutant ATXN3 in Neurally Differentiated Spinocerebellar Ataxia-3 Human iPS Cells. Beginning on the first day of neural differentiation, we added 100 nM rapamycin (an autophagy inducer; Sigma) to the neural differentiation medium. The culture medium (with

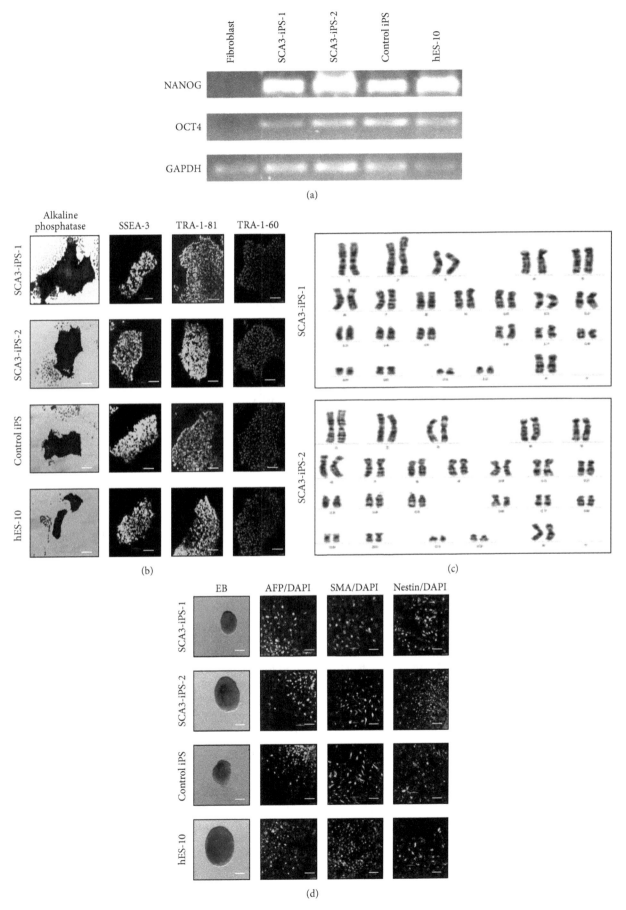

(a)

(b)

(c)

(d)

Figure 1: Continued.

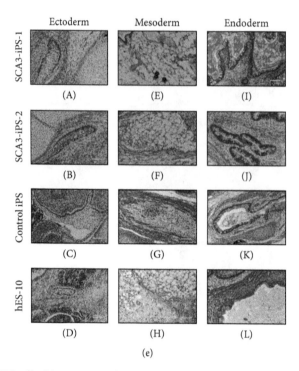

FIGURE 1: Characterization of SCA3-iPS cells. (a) RT-PCR analysis of the expression of undifferentiated hES cell marker genes in SCA3-iPS cells. (b) Immunostaining of iPS cells for cell surface markers, including alkaline phosphatase, SSEA-3, TRA-1-60, and TRA-1-81. Scale bars, 100 μm. (c) Karyotype of SCA3-iPS cells. (d) Immunofluorescence results showed differentiated SCA3-iPS cells expressing AFP (endoderm marker), SMA (mesoderm marker), and Nestin (ectoderm marker). Scale bars, 100 μm. (e) Teratomas contained tissues from all three types of germ layers, including ectoderm, that is, sebaceous glands (A, B, and C) and neural canal (D); mesoderm, that is, adipose tissue (E, F, and H) and smooth muscle (G); and endoderm, that is, glandular tissue (I, J, K, and L). Cell nuclei were stained with DAPI (blue). Scale bars, 20 μm.

20 nM rapamycin) was changed every 2-3 days. Cells were harvested, and western blot analysis was performed on days 0, 7, 14, and 21. Levels of LC3-II protein were increased following rapamycin treatment compared with that in untreated cells ($p < 0.05$), and levels of p62 protein were decreased ($p < 0.05$), indicating upregulation of autophagy. Moreover, the levels of the expanded polyQ ATXN3 protein (60 kDa) were significantly reduced ($p < 0.05$); however, there were no obvious changes in the levels of the wild-type ATXN3 protein (42 kDa; $p > 0.05$). These results suggested that the mutant protein was more efficiently degraded by autophagy than the wild-type protein (Figure 4(b)).

4. Discussion

SCA3 is characterized by the formation of intraneuronal inclusions, particularly in brain regions such as the cerebellum, substantia nigra, and pontine nuclei [19]. However, the mechanism underlying the formation of these inclusions is still poorly understood because of the lack of an appropriate model [10, 20]. Recent studies reported a novel mouse model of SCA3 that could be used to study the pathogenesis and treatment of SCA3. However, there are many differences between mice and humans, and a mouse model may not be completely applicable to humans. Patient-derived iPS cells preserve the genetic mutation carried by the patient on a functional human genomic background and can be differentiated into human cells of a neural lineage. Thus, this feature may be advantageous for investigating the pathogenic mechanisms of SCA3 and for the development of appropriate therapies to treat the disease. SCA3-iPS cell line could differentiate into human cells of neural lineage. Additionally, CAG repeats remained stable during reprogramming and neural differentiation, and the abnormal ATXN3 protein was expressed in SCA3-iPS cells and neurons. Furthermore, the chromosomal microarray analysis–single nucleotide polymorphism analysis showed no obvious *de novo* mutations in whole genome during reprogram and differentiation.

In humans with polyQ expansion disorders, expanded alleles are prone to changes in repeat length. These changes are related to both meiosis and mitosis in male gametes [21]. In our SCA3 iPS cells, both the expanded allele and normal allele remained stable with regard to repeat length during reprogramming, proliferation, and differentiation from iPS cells to neurons, consistent with a previous study by Koch and Xia [3, 22]. We assumed that the stable CAG repeats observed in our cell line may be explained by genomic stability during reprogramming, proliferation, and differentiation.

Autophagy is a bulk lysosomal degradation pathway involved in recycling of long-lived proteins and cytoplasmic organelles for cell survival [23, 24]. On induction of autophagy, the conversion of LC3-I into LC3-II is indicative

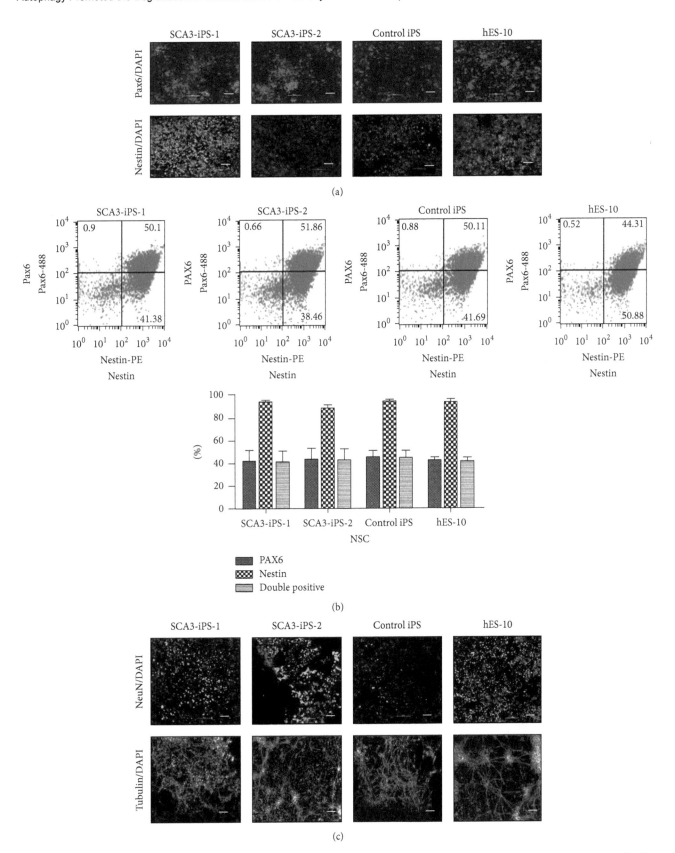

FIGURE 2: SCA3-iPS cells could differentiate into NSCs and neurons. (a) Immunofluorescence results for Pax6 and Nestin. (b) The flow cytometry analysis below showed that no significant difference was observed in the percentage of Pax6 or Nestin positive cells or Pax6 and Nestin-double positive cells ($n = 3$). (c) Immunofluorescence results for NeuN and beta-tubulin III. Cell nuclei were stained with DAPI (blue). Scale bars, 20 μm.

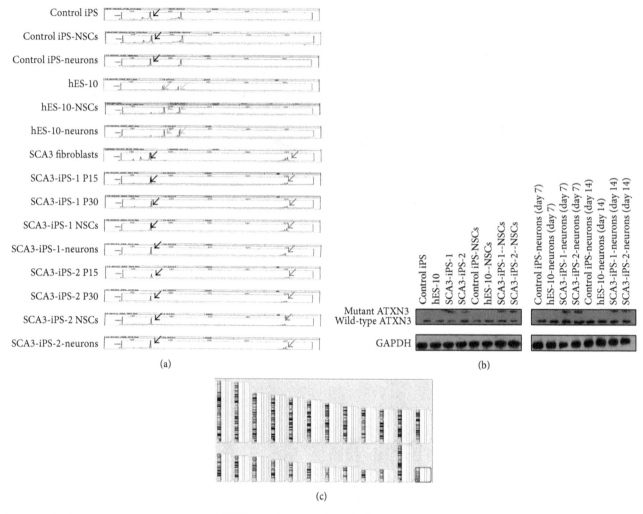

FIGURE 3: CAG repeats, genome, and mutant ATXN3 protein remained stable during reprogramming and neural differentiation. (a) Repeat sizes were confirmed by PCR with fluorescently labeled primers and capillary electrophoresis. The expanded alleles showed no detectable differences (15 (black arrows) and 81 (red arrows)) in fibroblasts (P3), SCA3 iPS cells (P15 and P30), NSCs (P3), and neurons (day 28) (yellow arrows: 30 repeats; green arrows: 23 repeats; blue arrows: 29 repeats). (b) Western blot bands from SCA3-iPS cells, NSCs, neurons, and control cells. P = passage. (c) No obvious *de novo* mutations in the fibroblasts (green), iPS cells (yellow), and the neurons (pink).

of autophagosome formation and is therefore widely used as a marker for autophagosome formation. In many types of tissues, basal autophagy is induced by starvation; in neurons, autophagy is also constitutively active at a low level [25]. Moreover, autophagy is critical for stem cell reprogramming, renewal, proliferation, and differentiation [26–29]. In our results, we also found that basal autophagy was present in control iPS neuronal differentiation. Interestingly, autophagy is typically upregulated in various HD mouse models and in neuronal and nonneuronal cells from patients with HD [30, 31]. Besides, another study reported that accumulation of p62 and light chain 3-positive autophagosomes has been associated with impairment in the trafficking to lysosomes and protein degradation in the putamen of the SCA3 patient [32]. These results were consistent with our *in vitro* neuronal differentiation of SCA3-iPS cells. Growing evidence has revealed that regulation of autophagy is involved in many

human diseases, including neurodegeneration [8, 20]. Aggregation of the mutated form of the disease protein ATXN3 into neuronal nuclear inclusions has been studied extensively in SCA3. The misfolded proteins in cells could be initially cleared by the molecular chaperone and the ubiquitin-proteasome system [33]. When these systems malfunction, the misfolded proteins accumulate and form oligomers and then small aggregates, which are potentially cytotoxic [34]. Several studies have demonstrated that the inhibition of mTORC1 by rapamycin promotes the degradation of mutant proteins *in vitro* and results in a reduction in the severity of neurodegeneration in several models *in vivo* [10, 20, 35]. Studies have also shown that rapamycin plays a role in neuroprotection in a Parkinson's disease murine model by blocking mTORC1-dependent translation of the pro-cell death protein RTP801 [36]. However, many *in vitro* studies investigating the function of autophagy in neurodegenerative disorders have

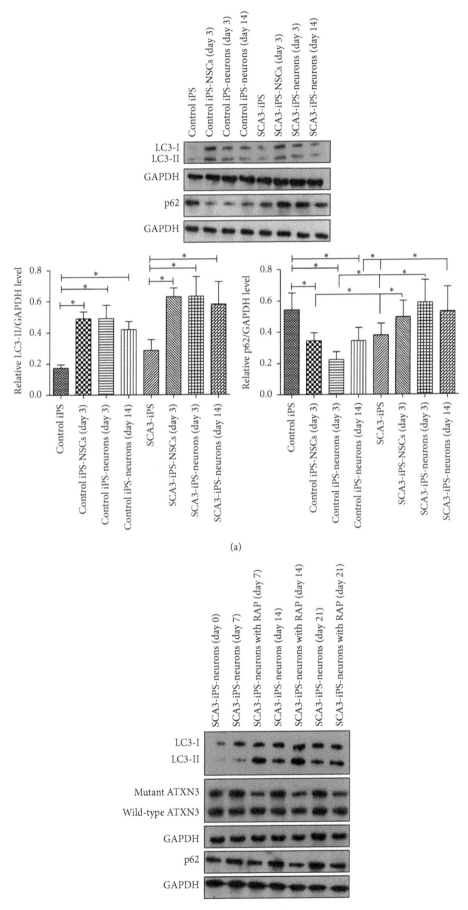

(a)

FIGURE 4: Continued.

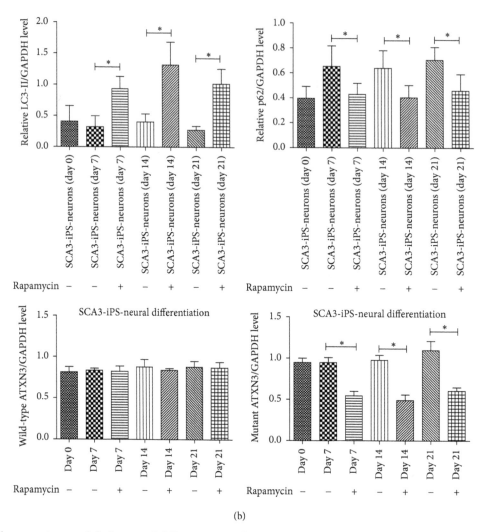

(b)

FIGURE 4: Autophagy was increased during neural differentiation and autophagy promoted the degradation of mutant ATXN3 in neurally differentiated spinocerebellar ataxia-3 human iPS cells. (a) Western blot was used to determine the levels of LC3-II and P62 in various cell types on days 3 and 14. Quantification of the band intensity is shown in the lower panel. (b) Western blot analysis was performed on days 0, 7, 14, and 21. Quantification of the band intensity is shown in the lower panel. $^*p < 0.05$ ($n = 3$).

been based on transfection with genes encoding pathogenic proteins in normal cells [8]. iPS cells generated from SCA3-patient and retaining the disease-causing ATXN3 mutation have been reported by Koch and Hansen, but they did not study the relation between ATXN3 proteins and autophagy [3, 37]. In the present study, we used iPS cells induced from somatic cells of a patient with SCA3. Rapamycin was also added to the neural differentiation medium to promote autophagy to degrade mutant proteins in neurally differentiated spinocerebellar ataxia-3 human iPS cells. The results showed that the amount of mutant ATXN3 protein (about 60 kDa) of rapamycin-treated neuronal differentiation was lower than that without rapamycin treatment, demonstrating that rapamycin-dependent autophagy could reduce the levels of mutant proteins. However, there were no significant effects on wild-type ATXN3. These results were consistent with previous studies suggesting that mutant proteins depend more on autophagy for clearance [38]. Notably, we treated the cells with rapamycin early for the following reasons. First, neurons

are more prone to accumulate cytotoxic proteins than other cell types because they cannot dilute toxic substances by means of cell division [39]. Moreover, mutant proteins need to be packaged into autophagic vacuoles in dendrites and axons and then be retrogradely transported to the cell body for degradation [40]. Additionally, young neurons can clear cytotoxic proteins; however, this process becomes increasingly difficult as neurons age because of the downregulation of chaperone-mediated autophagy and macroautophagy at the transcriptional, translational, and posttranslational levels [25, 41]. Lastly, rapamycin may not be effective during the late stage of these diseases. Therefore, early upregulation of autophagy may have therapeutic potential in treating SCA3. However, autophagy can only eliminate cytoplasmic mutant proteins; hence, the cellular localization of mutant proteins is a key factor when targeting upregulation of autophagy as a therapeutic strategy for their elimination. Different neurodegenerative diseases show different distributions of these aggregates. For example, in spinal and bulbar muscular atrophy SCA1, SCA7, and SCA17, proteins accumulate in the nucleus, whereas, in SCA2 and SCA6, proteins accumulate in the cytoplasm, and, in SCA3 and HD, proteins accumulate in both the nucleus and cytoplasm [42].

5. Conclusion

In summary, we found that SCA3-iPS cells could be differentiated into neurons to maintain patient-specific genome information. We also demonstrated that neural differentiation was accompanied by autophagy and that rapamycin promoted autophagy, which resulted in degradation of mutant ATXN3 in neurally differentiated spinocerebellar ataxia-3 human iPS cells. Thus, patient-derived iPS cells are a good model for studying the mechanisms of SCA3 and may provide a powerful tool for drug discovery.

Acknowledgments

This work was supported by the National Natural Science Foundation of China [31171229 and U1132005]; the Natural Science Foundation of Guangdong Province [2014A030312012]; the International Cooperation Project of Science and Technology Planning Project of Guangdong Province [2013B51000087]; the Science and Information Technology of Guangzhou Key Project [201508020258, 201400000003-4, and 201400000004-4]; and the National Natural Science Foundation of China [81301184].

References

[1] Y. Kawaguchi, T. Okamoto, M. Taniwaki et al., "CAG expansions in a novel gene for Machado-Joseph disease at chromosome 14q32.1," *Nature Genetics*, vol. 8, no. 3, pp. 221–228, 1994.

[2] K. Seidel, W. F. A. den Dunnen, C. Schultz et al., "Axonal inclusions in spinocerebellar ataxia type 3," *Acta Neuropathologica* vol. 120, no. 4, pp. 449–460, 2010.

[3] P. Koch, P. Breuer, M. Peitz et al., "Excitation-induced ataxin-3 aggregation in neurons from patients with Machado-Joseph disease," *Nature*, vol. 480, no. 7378, pp. 543–546, 2011.

[4] P. Coutinho and C. Andrade, "Autosomal dominant system degeneration in Portuguese families of the Azores Islands. A new genetic disorder involving cerebellar, pyramidal, extrapyramidal and spinal cord motor functions," *Neurology*, vol. 28, no. 7, pp. 703–709, 1978.

[5] A. Ciechanover and P. Brundin, "The ubiquitin proteasome system in neurodegenerative diseases: sometimes the chicken, sometimes the egg," *Neuron*, vol. 40, no. 2, pp. 427–446, 2003.

[6] X. Yang, X. Zhong, J. L. Tanyi et al., "mir-30d regulates multiple genes in the autophagy pathway and impairs autophagy process in human cancer cells," *Biochemical and Biophysical Research Communications*, vol. 431, no. 3, pp. 617–622, 2013.

[7] N. Mizushima, B. Levine, A. M. Cuervo, and D. J. Klionsky, "Autophagy fights disease through cellular self-digestion," *Nature*, vol. 451, no. 7182, pp. 1069–1075, 2008.

[8] B. Ravikumar, C. Vacher, Z. Berger et al., "Inhibition of mTOR induces autophagy and reduces toxicity of polyglutamine expansions in fly and mouse models of Huntington disease," *Nature Genetics*, vol. 36, no. 6, pp. 585–595, 2004.

[9] B. Dehay, J. Bové, N. Rodríguez-Muela et al., "Pathogenic lysosomal depletion in Parkinson's disease," *Journal of Neuroscience*, vol. 30, no. 37, pp. 12535–12544, 2010.

[10] F. M. Menzies, J. Huebener, M. Renna, M. Bonin, O. Riess, and D. C. Rubinsztein, "Autophagy induction reduces mutant ataxin-3 levels and toxicity in a mouse model of spinocerebellar ataxia type 3," *Brain*, vol. 133, no. 1, pp. 93–104, 2010.

[11] K. Takahashi, K. Tanabe, M. Ohnuki et al., "Induction of pluripotent stem cells from adult human fibroblasts by defined factors," *Cell*, vol. 131, no. 5, pp. 861–872, 2007.

[12] Y. Fan, Y. Luo, X. Chen, and X. Sun, "A modified culture medium increases blastocyst formation and the efficiency of human embryonic stem cell derivation from poor-quality embryos," *Journal of Reproduction and Development*, vol. 56, no. 5, pp. 533–539, 2010.

[13] B. Song, Y. Fan, W. He et al., "Improved hematopoietic differentiation efficiency of gene-corrected beta-thalassemia induced pluripotent stem cells by CRISPR/Cas9 system," *Stem Cells and Development*, vol. 24, no. 9, pp. 1053–1065, 2015.

[14] W. Liu, Y. Yin, X. Long et al., "Derivation and characterization of human embryonic stem cell lines from poor quality embryos," *Journal of Genetics and Genomics*, vol. 36, no. 4, pp. 229–239, 2009.

[15] X. Sun, X. Long, Y. Yin et al., "Similar biological characteristics of human embryonic stem cell lines with normal and abnormal karyotypes," *Human Reproduction*, vol. 23, no. 10, pp. 2185–2193, 2008.

[16] Y. Luo, Y. Fan, B. Zhou, Z. Xu, Y. Chen, and X. Sun, "Generation of induced pluripotent stem cells from skin fibroblasts of a patient with olivopontocerebellar atrophy," *The Tohoku Journal of Experimental Medicine*, vol. 226, no. 2, pp. 151–159, 2012.

[17] Y. Yan, S. Shin, S. J. Balendu et al., "Efficient and rapid derivation of primitive neural stem cells and generation of brain subtype neurons from human pluripotent stem cells," *Stem Cells Translational Medicine*, vol. 2, no. 11, pp. 862–870, 2013.

[18] X. Yingjun, Z. Yi, W. Jianzhu et al., "Prader-willi syndrome with a long-contiguous stretch of homozygosity not covering the critical region," *Journal of Child Neurology*, vol. 30, no. 3, pp. 371–377, 2015.

[19] K. Nishiyama, S. Murayama, J. Goto et al., "Regional and cellular expression of the Machado-Joseph disease gene in brains of normal and affected individuals," *Annals of Neurology*, vol. 40, no. 5, pp. 776–781, 1996.

[20] A. Silva-Fernandes, S. Duarte-Silva, A. Neves-Carvalho et al., "Chronic treatment with 17-DMAG improves balance and coordination in a new mouse model of machado-joseph disease," *Neurotherapeutics*, vol. 11, no. 2, pp. 433–449, 2014.

[21] S. S. Chong, A. E. McCall, J. Cota et al., "Gametic and somatic tissue-specific heterogeneity of the expanded SCA1 CAG repeat in spinocerebellar ataxia type 1," *Nature Genetics*, vol. 10, no. 3, pp. 344–350, 1995.

[22] G. Xia, K. Santostefano, T. Hamazaki et al., "Generation of human-induced pluripotent stem cells to model spinocerebellar ataxia type 2 in vitro," *Journal of Molecular Neuroscience*, vol. 51, no. 2, pp. 237–248, 2013.

[23] D. J. Klionsky and S. D. Emr, "Autophagy as a regulated pathway of cellular degradation," *Science*, vol. 290, no. 5497, pp. 1717–1721, 2000.

[24] N. Mizushima and M. Komatsu, "Autophagy: renovation of cells and tissues," *Cell*, vol. 147, no. 4, pp. 728–741, 2011.

[25] T. Hara, K. Nakamura, M. Matsui et al., "Suppression of basal autophagy in neural cells causes neurodegenerative disease in mice," *Nature*, vol. 441, no. 7095, pp. 885–889, 2006.

[26] Y. Wu, Y. Li, H. Zhang et al., "Autophagy and mTORC1 regulate the stochastic phase of somatic cell reprogramming," *Nature Cell Biology*, vol. 17, no. 6, pp. 715–725, 2015.

[27] A. L. Morgado, J. M. Xavier, P. A. Dionísio et al., "MicroRNA-34a modulates neural stem cell differentiation by regulating expression of synaptic and autophagic proteins," *Molecular Neurobiology*, vol. 51, no. 3, pp. 1168–1183, 2015.

[28] Y.-H. Cho, K.-M. Han, D. Kim et al., "Autophagy regulates homeostasis of pluripotency-associated proteins in hESCs," *Stem Cells*, vol. 32, no. 2, pp. 424–435, 2014.

[29] M. Zeng and J.-N. Zhou, "Roles of autophagy and mTOR signaling in neuronal differentiation of mouse neuroblastoma cells," *Cellular Signalling*, vol. 20, no. 4, pp. 659–665, 2008.

[30] M. Martinez-Vicente, Z. Talloczy, E. Wong et al., "Cargo recognition failure is responsible for inefficient autophagy in Huntington's disease," *Nature Neuroscience*, vol. 13, no. 5, pp. 567–576, 2010.

[31] E. Wong and A. M. Cuervo, "Autophagy gone awry in neurodegenerative diseases," *Nature Neuroscience*, vol. 13, no. 7, pp. 805–811, 2010.

[32] I. Nascimento-Ferreira, T. Santos-Ferreira, L. Sousa-Ferreira et al., "Overexpression of the autophagic beclin-1 protein clears mutant ataxin-3 and alleviates Machado-Joseph disease," *Brain*, vol. 134, no. 5, pp. 1400–1415, 2011.

[33] P. J. Muchowski and J. L. Wacker, "Modulation of neurodegeneration by molecular chaperones," *Nature Reviews Neuroscience*, vol. 6, no. 1, pp. 11–22, 2005.

[34] C. A. Ross and M. A. Poirier, "What is the role of protein aggregation in neurodegeneration?" *Nature Reviews Molecular Cell Biology*, vol. 6, no. 11, pp. 891–898, 2005.

[35] Z. Z. Chong, Y. C. Shang, S. Wang, and K. Maiese, "Shedding new light on neurodegenerative diseases through the mammalian target of rapamycin," *Progress in Neurobiology*, vol. 99, no. 2, pp. 128–148, 2012.

[36] C. Malagelada, Z. H. Jin, V. Jackson-Lewis, S. Przedborski, and L. A. Greene, "Rapamycin protects against neuron death in in vitro and in vivo models of Parkinson's disease," *Journal of Neuroscience*, vol. 30, no. 3, pp. 1166–1175, 2010.

[37] S. K. Hansen, H. Borland, L. F. Hasholt et al., "Generation of spinocerebellar ataxia type 3 patient-derived induced pluripotent stem cell line SCA3.B11," *Stem Cell Research*, vol. 16, no. 3, pp. 589–592, 2016.

[38] Z. Berger, B. Ravikumar, F. M. Menzies et al., "Rapamycin alleviates toxicity of different aggregate-prone proteins," *Human Molecular Genetics*, vol. 15, no. 3, pp. 433–442, 2006.

[39] S. Lee, Y. Sato, and R. A. Nixon, "Lysosomal proteolysis inhibition selectively disrupts axonal transport of degradative organelles and causes an Alzheimer's-like axonal dystrophy," *Journal of Neuroscience*, vol. 31, no. 21, pp. 7817–7830, 2011.

[40] K. E. Larsen and D. Sulzer, "Autophagy in neurons: a review," *Histology and Histopathology*, vol. 17, no. 3, pp. 897–908, 2002.

[41] N. Mizushima, "The role of the Atg1/ULK1 complex in autophagy regulation," *Current Opinion in Cell Biology*, vol. 22, no. 2, pp. 132–139, 2010.

[42] X. Li, H. Liu, P. L. Fischhaber, and T.-S. Tang, "Toward therapeutic targets for SCA3: insight into the role of Machado-Joseph disease protein ataxin-3 in misfolded proteins clearance," *Progress in Neurobiology*, vol. 132, pp. 34–58, 2015.

Permissions

List of Contributors

Almaguer-Gotay Dennis, Luis E. Almaguer-Mederos, Rodríguez-Aguilera Raúl, Cuello-Almarales Dany and González-Zaldívar Yanetza
Center for the Investigation and Rehabilitation of Hereditary Ataxias (CIRAH), Holguín, Cuba
University of Medical Sciences of Holguín, Cuba

Vázquez-Mojena Yaimeé, Estupiñán-Domínguez Annelié, Rodríguez-Labrada Roberto, Peña-Acosta Arnoy and Torres-Vega Reydenis
Center for the Investigation and Rehabilitation of Hereditary Ataxias (CIRAH), Holguín, Cuba

Velázquez-Pérez Luis
Center for the Investigation and Rehabilitation of Hereditary Ataxias (CIRAH), Holguín, Cuba
Cuban Academy of Sciences, Cuba

Barbara Pietrucha, Edyta Heropolitanska-Pliszka, Malgorzata Pac, Beata Wolska-Kusnierz and Ewa Bernatowska
Clinical Immunology, The Children's Memorial Health Institute, Av. Dzieci Polskich 20, 04-730 Warsaw, Poland

Mateusz Maciejczyk and Halina Car
Department of Experimental Pharmacology, Medical University of Bialystok, Szpitalna 37 Str., 15-295 Bialystok, Poland

Jolanta Sawicka-Powierza
Department of Family Medicine, Medical University of Bialystok, Bialystok, Poland

Radosław Motkowski and Bozena Mikoluc
Department of Pediatrics Rheumatology, Immunology and Metabolic Bone Diseases, Medical University of Bialystok, Waszyngtona 17 Str., 15-274 Bialystok, Poland

Joanna Karpinska and Marta Hryniewicka
Institute of Chemistry, University of Bialystok, Bialystok, Poland

Anna Zalewska
Department of Conservative Dentistry, Medical University of Bialystok, Bialystok, Poland

Vamshi K. Rao
Division of Neurology, Ann & Robert H. Lurie Children's Hospital of Chicago, Chicago, IL 60611, USA

Department of Pediatrics, Feinberg School of Medicine, Northwestern University, Chicago, IL 60611, USA

Christine J. DiDonato
Department of Pediatrics, Feinberg School of Medicine, Northwestern University, Chicago, IL 60611, USA
Human Molecular Genetics Program, Ann & Robert H. Lurie Children's Hospital, Stanley Manne Research Institute, Chicago, IL 60611, USA

Paul D. Larsen
Division of Neurology, Department of Pediatrics, University of Nebraska Medical Center and Children's Hospital and Medical Center, Omaha, NE, USA

Alessandra Bolotta, Provvidenza Maria Abruzzo and Marina Marini
Department of Experimental, Diagnostic and Specialty Medicine, Bologna University, 40126 Bologna, Italy
IRCCS Fondazione Don Carlo Gnocchi, 20148 Milan, Italy

Alessandro Ghezzo and Cinzia Zucchini
Department of Experimental, Diagnostic and Specialty Medicine, Bologna University, 40126 Bologna, Italy

Vito Antonio Baldassarro
Interdepartmental Centre for Industrial Research in Health Sciences and Technologies (ICIR-HST), University of Bologna, 40064 Ozzano, Bologna, Italy

Katia Scotlandi
CRS Development of Biomolecular Therapies, Experimental Oncology Laboratory, Orthopedic Rizzoli Institute, 40136 Bologna, Italy

Xiaoping Chen, Lihui Zheng and Jianqi Yao
Department of Statistics, College of Mathematics and Informatics & FJKLMAA, Fujian Normal University, Fuzhou 350000, China

Teresa Anglada, Mariona Terradas, Laia Hernández, Anna Genescà and Marta Martín
Departament de Biologia Cellular, Fisiologia i Immunologia, Universitat Autònoma de Barcelona, Edifici C, Bellaterra, 08193 Cerdanyola del Vallès, Spain

Camilla Polonini Martins, Carlos Henrique Ramos Horsczaruk, Débora Cristina Lima da Silva and Agnaldo José Lopes
Post-Graduation Program in Rehabilitation Sciences, Augusto Motta University Center (UNISUAM), Rio de Janeiro, RJ, Brazil

Laura Alice Santos de Oliveira
Post-Graduation Program in Rehabilitation Sciences, Augusto Motta University Center (UNISUAM), Rio de Janeiro, RJ, Brazil
School of Physiotherapy, Federal Institute of Rio de Janeiro, Rio de Janeiro, RJ, Brazil

Luiz Felipe Vasconcellos
Institute of Neurology Deolindo Couto, Federal University of Rio de Janeiro (UFRJ), Rio de Janeiro, RJ, Brazil

Míriam Raquel Meira Mainenti
Physical Education College of the Brazilian Army (EsEFEx), Rio de Janeiro, RJ, Brazil

Erika de Carvalho Rodrigues
Post-Graduation Program in Rehabilitation Sciences, Augusto Motta University Center (UNISUAM), Rio de Janeiro, RJ, Brazil
D'Or Institute for Research and Education (IDOR), Rio de Janeiro, RJ, Brazil

Marguerite Blignaut, Sarah Harries, Amanda Lochner and Barbara Huisamen
Centre for Cardio-Metabolic Research in Africa (CARMA), Division of Medical Physiology, Department of Biomedical Sciences, Faculty of Medicine and Health Sciences, Stellenbosch University, South Africa

Amer Awad
Baton Rouge Neurology Associates, Baton Rouge General Medical Center, Baton Rouge, LA, USA

Olaf Stüve
Department of Neurology, The University of Texas Southwestern Medical Center, Dallas, TX, USA
Neurology Section, VA North Texas Health Care Systems, Dallas, TX, USA

Marlyn Mayo
Department of Internal Medicine-Digestive and Liver Diseases, The University of Texas Southwestern Medical Center, Dallas, TX, USA

Rafeed Alkawadri
Neurological Institute, Cleveland Clinic Foundation, Cleveland, OH, USA

Bachir Estephan
Department of Neurology, University of Kansas Medical Center, Kansas, KS, USA

Marcia Belas dos Santos, Arly dos Santos and Ricardo Mario Arida
Physiology Department, Universidade Federal de São Paulo (UNIFESP), São Paulo, SP, Brazil

Viviana Dylewski and Clarissa Barros de Oliveira
Physiotherapy Department, Associação de Assistência a Criança Deficiente (AACD), São Paulo, SP, Brazil

Cristhiane Garabello Pires
Faculty of Medicine, University of Sao Paulo (USP), São Paulo, SP, Brazil

Eric Black
Assistant Professor of Psychiatry, Southern Illinois University, USA

P. Calap-Quintana, M. J. Martínez-Sebastián and J. V. Llorens
Department of Genetics, University of Valencia, Campus of Burjassot, Valencia, Spain

J. A. Navarro
Institute of Zoology, University of Regensburg, Regensburg, Germany

J. González-Fernández
Department of Genetics, University of Valencia, Campus of Burjassot, Valencia, Spain
Biomedical Research Institute INCLIVA, Valencia, Spain

M. D. Moltó
Department of Genetics, University of Valencia, Campus of Burjassot, Valencia, Spain
Biomedical Research Institute INCLIVA, Valencia, Spain
Centro de Investigación Biomédica en Red de Salud Mental (CIBERSAM), Madrid, Spain

Semiha Kurt, Betul Cevik and Durdane Aksoy
Department of Neurology, Gaziosmanpasa University Faculty of Medicine, 60100 Tokat, Turkey

E. Irmak Sahbaz, Aslı Gundogdu Eken and A. Nazli Basak
Suna and Inan Kıraç Foundation Neurodegeneration Research Laboratory, Molecular Biology and Genetics Department, Bogazici University, 34342 Istanbul, Turkey

Elisabetta Peri, Daniele Panzeri, Elena Beretta, Gianluigi Reni, Sandra Strazzer and Emilia Biffi
Scientifc Institute IRCCS Eugenio Medea, Bosisio Parini, Lecco, Italy

Sean Lance, Stuart Mossman and Gemma Poke
Wellington Hospital, Wellington, New Zealand

Benjamin Stampfl and Dominic Fee
Department of Neurology, Medical College of Wisconsin, Milwaukee, WI, USA

D. Hettiarachchi, B. A. P. S. Pathirana and V. H. W. Dissanayake
Human Genetics Unit, Faculty of Medicine, University of Colombo, Colombo, Sri Lanka

Hetalkumar Panchal
Post Graduate Department of Bioscience, Sardar Patel University, Vallabh Vidyanagar, Gujarat, India

P. D. Rathnayaka and A. Padeniya
Lady Ridgway Hospital for Children, Colombo, Sri Lanka

P. S. Lai
Department of Paediatrics, Yong Loo Lin School of Medicine, National University of Singapore, Singapore

Michael Bonello and Partha Ray
The Walton Centre NHS Foundation Trust, Lower Lane, Liverpool L9 7LJ, UK

Zhanhui Ou, Min Luo, Xiaohua Niu, Yuchang Chen, Yingjun Xie, Wenyin He, Bing Song, Yexing Xian, Di Fan, Shuming OuYang and Xiaofang Sun
Key Laboratory for Major Obstetric Diseases of Guangdong Province, Key Laboratory of Reproduction and Genetics of Guangdong Higher Education Institutes, The Third Affiliated Hospital of Guangzhou Medical University, Guangzhou 510150, China

Index

Printed in the USA
CPSIA information can be obtained
at www.ICGtesting.com
JSHW051446221024
72173JS00006B/1596

9 781639 275717